Metabolic Activities of the Lung

Ciba Foundation Symposia are published in collaboration with Excerpta Medica in Amsterdam.

Excerpta Medica, P.O. Box 211, Amsterdam

Metabolic Activities of the Lung

Ciba Foundation Symposium 78 (new series)

1980

Excerpta Medica
Amsterdam · Oxford · New York

ISBN Excerpta Medica 90 219 4084 1
ISBN Elsevier/North-Holland 0 444 90159 0

Published in October 1980 by Excerpta Medica, P.O. Box 211, Amsterdam
and Elsevier/North-Holland, Inc., 52 Vanderbilt Avenue, New York, N.Y. 10017.

Suggested series entry for library catalogues: Ciba Foundation Symposia.
Suggested publisher's entry for library catalogues: Excerpta Medica.

Ciba Foundation Symposium 78 (new series)

401 pages, 80 figures, 38 tables.

Library of Congress Cataloging in Publication Data

Symposium on Metabolic Functions of the Lung, London,
1980.
Metabolic activities of the lung.

(Ciba Foundation symposium; 78 (new ser.))
Bibliography: p.
Includes indexes.
1. Lungs–Congresses. 2. Metabolism–Congresses.
I. Title. II. Series: Ciba Foundation. Symposium;
new ser., 78. [DNLM: 1. Lung–Metabolism–Congresses.
W3 C161F v. 78 1980 / WF600 S9875m 1980]
QP121.S96 1980 599.01'21 80-20318
ISBN 0-444-90159-0 (Elsevier/North-Holland)

Printed in The Netherlands by Casparie, Amsterdam

Contents

Participants

Symposium on Metabolic Functions of the Lung, held at the Ciba Foundation, London, 12th–14th February 1980

The topic of this symposium was suggested by Dr Y.S. Bakhle and Professor M.B.H. Youdim

J. R. VANE *(Chairman)* The Wellcome Research Laboratories, Langley Court, Beckenham, Kent, BR3 3BS, UK

J. W. AIKEN Department of Experimental Biology, Upjohn Co., Kalamazoo, Michigan 49001, USA

K. G. M. M. ALBERTI Department of Clinical Biochemistry, University of Newcastle upon Tyne, The Royal Victoria Infirmary, Newcastle upon Tyne, NE1 4LP, UK

M.S. AYUSO-PARRILLA Instituto G. Marañon, Higher Council of Research, Velazquez 144, Madrid-6, Spain

Y. S. BAKHLE Department of Pharmacology, Institute of Basic Medical Sciences, Royal College of Surgeons of England, 35–43 Lincoln's Inn Fields, London WC2A 3PN, UK

P. L. BALLARD Department of Pediatrics, University of California, School of Medicine, San Francisco, California 94143, USA

P. H. BURRI Anatomisches Institut, Universität Bern, Bühlstrasse 26, Postfach 139, 3000 Bern 9, Switzerland

H. O. J. COLLIER Miles Laboratories Ltd, Stoke Poges, PO Box 37, Slough, SL2 4LY, UK

H. DATTA Department of Clinical Biochemistry, University of Newcastle upon Tyne, The Royal Victoria Infirmary, Newcastle upon Tyne, NE1 4LP, UK

S. H. FERREIRA Departamento de Farmacologia, Faculdade de Medicina de Ribeirão Preto, Caixa Postal 301, 14,100 Ribeirão Preto, Est. São Paulo, Brazil

R. J. FLOWER Department of Prostaglandin Research, The Wellcome Research Laboratories, Langley Court, Beckenham, Kent, BR3 3BS, UK

R. J. GRYGLEWSKI Department of Pharmacology, Copernicus Medical Academy, Grzegórzecka 16, 31-531 Cracow, Poland

K. HERBACZYŃSKA-CEDRO Research Centre of Experimental Medicine, Polish Academy of Sciences, Dworkowa 3, 00784 Warsawa, Poland

A. F. JUNOD Division de Pneumologie, Département de Médecine, Hôpital Cantonal Universitaire, CH-1211 Genève 4, Switzerland

R. B. MELLINS Department of Pediatrics, Pediatric Pulmonary Division, College of Physicians and Surgeons of Columbia University, 630 West 168th Street, New York, NY 10032, USA

B. MEYRICK Department of Pathology, Harvard Medical School, The Children's Hospital Medical Center, 300 Longwood Avenue, Boston, Massachusetts 02115, USA

S. MONCADA Department of Prostaglandin Research, The Wellcome Research Laboratories, Langley Court, Beckenham, Kent, BR3 3BS, UK

W. K. MORISHIGE Department of Physiology, School of Medicine, University of Hawaii at Manoa, Biomedical Sciences Building, T-608, 1960 East-West Road, Honolulu, Hawaii 96822, US

R. PARRILLA Department of Biochemistry (Biophysics), School of Medicine, Universidad Autónoma, Madrid-34, Spain

P. J. PIPER Department of Pharmacology, Institute of Basic Medical Sciences, Royal College of Surgeons of England, 35-43 Lincoln's Inn Fields, London WC2A 3PN, UK

L. M. REID Department of Pathology, Harvard Medical School, The Children's Hospital Medical Center, 300 Longwood Avenue, Boston, Massachusetts 02115, USA

S. I. SAID Department of Internal Medicine, The University of Texas Health Science Center at Dallas, Southwestern Medical School, 5323 Harry Hines Boulevard, Dallas, Texas 75235, USA

M. SIMIONESCU The Institute of Cellular Biology and Pathology, 8 Hasdeu Street, Bucharest 70646, Romania

T. F. SLATER Department of Biochemistry, School of Biological Sciences, Brunel University, Kingston Lane, Uxbridge, Middlesex UB8 3PH, UK

R. L. SOFFER Department of Biochemistry, Cornell University Medical College, 1300 York Avenue, New York, NY 10021, USA

S. A. STALCUP Department of Pediatrics, Pediatric Pulmonary Division, College of Physicians and Surgeons of Columbia University, 630 West 168th Street, New York, NY 10032, USA

W. A. STUBBS Department of Medicine, St Bartholomew's Hospital, West Smithfield, London EC1A 7BE, UK

H. F. WOODS Departments of Clinical Pharmacology and Therapeutics, Royal Hallamshire Hospital, University of Sheffield, Glossop Road, Sheffield, S10 2JF, UK

M. B. H. YOUDIM* Department of Pharmacology, Faculty of Medicine, Israel Institute of Technology, 12 Haalyah Street, Bat-Galim, PO Box 9649, Haifa, Israel

Editors: RUTH PORTER *(Organizer)* and JULIE WHELAN

---

* *In absentia.*

Introduction

J.R. VANE

Wellcome Research Laboratories, Langley Court, Beckenham, Kent, BR3 3BS, UK

It is now well established that the pulmonary circulation has another function apart from that associated with the exchange of gases. This is a pharmacokinetic function, in which enzyme systems in the cells of the pulmonary vascular bed change the biological activity of a variety of substances presented to them in the passing blood. In this symposium we shall also hear about the metabolic utilization of substrates.

Our own contribution to the field started some 15 years ago with a study of the metabolic fate of several vasoactive amines, peptides and prostaglandins. The initiation of the study probably coincided with the arrival of Sergio Ferreira in our laboratories at the Royal College of Surgeons in 1965. Since then there has been a continuing growth of knowledge, so much so that the Ciba Foundation now feels that a three-day symposium is justified. For more detailed and fully referenced reviews the reader is referred to Bakhle & Vane (1974) and Bakhle & Vane (1977). First let us consider the inactivation of amines.

5-HYDROXYTRYPTAMINE

Almost sixty years ago Starling & Verney (1925) found that they could not maintain adequate circulation through an isolated perfused kidney with a simple perfusion circuit. A substance was present in defibrinated blood which caused intense vasoconstriction in the kidneys. They removed this substance by perfusing the kidney from a heart–lung preparation and concluded that the blood was 'detoxicated' in the lungs. The isolation of the serum vasoconstrictor substance and its identification as 5-hydroxytryptamine (5-HT) started a whole field of new research; it was some years later that Gaddum et al (1953) showed that the perfused lung of the cat removed the pharmacological activity

Metabolic activities of the lung
(Ciba Foundation symposium 78) p 1-10

of 5-HT from the blood. The pulmonary circulation of dogs *in vivo* removed up to 98% of intravenous infusions of 5-HT (Thomas & Vane 1967).

In experiments with isolated lungs, the involvement of monoamine oxidase in this removal process is clearly shown in several species. Alabaster & Bakhle (1970) perfused rat isolated lungs with Krebs' solution and found a 92% removal of the biological activity of 5-HT. When labelled 5-HT was infused for 4 min, 10% of the radioactivity appeared in the lung effluent as 5-HT within the first 5 min and the rest of the radioactivity could be recovered as a metabolite, probably 5-HIAA, over the next 50 min. Monoamine oxidase inhibitors inhibited the initial removal only slightly; their main effect was to preserve the 5-HT taken up and this slowly reappeared in the effluent from the lungs. Inhibitors of 5-HT uptake in platelets, such as amitriptyline and desmethylimipramine, substantially prevented the removal of 5-HT by the lungs. The removal process involves uptake followed by metabolism rather than uptake followed by storage. Junod (1972b) showed that the removal process for 5-HT in rat isolated lungs was saturable, with transport of 5-HT into the cell as the rate-limiting step.

The liver, which receives only a portion of the cardiac output, inactivates 5-HT to rather less an extent than do the lungs, and circulating platelets can only remove 5-HT from the blood by a relatively slow process (Vane 1964). It must be concluded, therefore, that the major site of inactivation of 5-HT in the body is the lungs and not the liver or platelets. Predominantly right-sided heart lesions associated with carcinoid tumour may be linked with the pulmonary removal of 5-HT and there is evidence that the removal mechanism in man may sometimes fail.

Cross et al (1974) studied the disposition of labelled 5-HT in rat lung by autoradiography and suggested that endothelial cells of pulmonary arterioles and the cells in the alveolar region are the sites of uptake and metabolism. Strum & Junod (1972) established by autoradiography at the electron microscope level that the uptake of radioactivity after infusions of [^{3}H]5-HT was concentrated in the endothelial cells of arterioles and capillaries of isolated rat lungs. Both studies agree that mast cells and smooth muscle cells are not labelled.

CATECHOLAMINES

Adrenaline and noradrenaline have a half-life in the circulation of the cat of less than 20 s (Ferreira & Vane 1967) so they must be substantially removed from the blood in one circulation. In 1905, Elliot showed that adrenaline did not disappear in the lungs but did so in other vascular beds. Experiments *in vivo* have confirmed that there is no significant removal of adrenaline in the pulmonary circulation of dogs, cats, rats and man. Two other catecholamines, dopamine and isoprenaline, also survive passage through the lung.

However, noradrenaline is subject to inactivation by the pulmonary circulation *in vivo* and in isolated lungs. In several animal species there was 20–35% inactivation of histamine. The pulmonary removal in man has been estimated at 17% and 23% by two different methods. Gillis et al (1972), using patients undergoing total cardiopulmonary bypass, found that the removal of noradrenaline after bypass (50%) was more than double that immediately before bypass.

In isolated lungs, perfused with blood or Krebs' solution, the removal is also about 30%. In rat isolated lungs radioactivity derived from infusions of [^{3}H]noradrenaline is concentrated by lung tissue through a saturable uptake mechanism. However, only 20% of the retained radioactivity is noradrenaline, the remainder being methylated and deaminated metabolites. The endothelial cells of capillaries were the major sites of accumulation of radioactivity.

Thus, noradrenaline shares with 5-HT a removal process comprising uptake followed by metabolism. These mechanisms will be discussed in detail later (Youdim et al, p 105–128). The endothelial cells of the capillaries seem to be important sites of uptake for both amines. The pulmonary uptake of these two amines may therefore be illustrative of properties unique to endothelial cells of the pulmonary circulation.

ACETYLCHOLINE AND HISTAMINE

The actions of acetylcholine are usually terminated by acetylcholinesterase close to the site of its release from nerve endings. Cholinesterases in the blood are also highly active and can reduce the concentration of acetylcholine in blood to less than half in two seconds (Vane 1969). In addition to these inactivating mechanisms, dog isolated lungs perfused with a dextran–saline solution rapidly inactivate large amounts of acetylcholine. Thus rapid metabolism shields the arterial circulation from acetylcholine.

Histamine is not removed by the pulmonary circulation of rats and dogs *in vivo,* nor is it inactivated in heart–lung or perfused lung preparations from dogs. This lack of pulmonary metabolism of histamine must reflect the lack of a carrier mechanism into the cell, for lung slices or homogenates from man, cat, guinea-pig and rat all inactivate histamine readily.

BRADYKININ

Bradykinin is fairly rapidly destroyed in blood with a half-life in rats, cats and dogs of about 17 s. Thus, bradykinin formed in, or injected into, venous blood is likely to reach the pulmonary circulation. The lungs avidly remove bradykinin, about 80% disappearing in one passage through cat lungs. Pulmonary inactivation of bradykinin has since been confirmed in several species, including rat, guinea-pig, dog and sheep.

Ryan et al (1970) showed that bradykinin was inactivated in the pulmonary circulation of rats by enzymic hydrolysis of peptide bonds. The circulation time was identical with that of blue dextran (mol. wt. 2 000 000), indicating that, in the lung, bradykinin does not leave the vascular space. They concluded that the enzymes responsible for degradation of bradykinin in the lung are bound on or near the vascular endothelial cells.

CONVERTING ENZYME AND BRADYKININASE

In 1968 Ng & Vane suggested that the pulmonary conversion of angiotensin I (AI) and inactivation of bradykinin might be catalysed by the same peptidase. In subsequent years this idea has been tested by many experiments and much discussion. Converting enzyme purified to homogeneity also inactivates bradykinin. In the lung, there are several peptidases capable of hydrolysing the angiotensins. However, angiotensin II is unaffected by passage through the pulmonary circulation, *in vivo* or in isolated lungs, of all species so far studied including rats, dogs, guinea-pigs, cats and man.

OTHER PEPTIDES

The selectivity of the pulmonary inactivation mechanism is strikingly demonstrated by the way in which the lungs inactivate bradykinin but allow three other vasodepressor peptides – eledoisin, substance P and physalaemin – to pass through without change. Similarly, vasopressin survives passage through the pulmonary circulation of rats, rabbits, cats, dogs and man, as does oxytocin.

Little is known of the way in which the lung treats fibrinopeptides although Bayley et al (1967) suggested that the lung may be an active site for fibrinopeptide metabolism. Similarly, it is not known whether the lungs have any effects on the activity of cholecystokinin, pancreozymin, glucagon and other peptide hormones of gastrointestinal origin.

PROSTAGLANDINS

The metabolism of prostaglandins (PGs) in the pulmonary circulation *in vivo* was first studied by Ferreira & Vane (1967) who showed that more than 90% of PGE_1, PGE_2 or $PGF_{2\alpha}$ was removed in one passage through the lung. In the ewe, as well as in dogs, cats and rabbits, the hypotensive effects of PGs of the E and F series are greater with intra-aortic than with intravenous injections. Their removal in the pulmonary circulation, therefore, takes place in all species so far studied. McGiff et al (1969) confirmed that PGE_1 and PGE_2 were removed by dog lung *in vivo* and further showed that PGA_1 and PGA_2 survived the passage through the lungs without change. More interestingly, Dusting et al (1978) showed that prostacyclin passes through the pulmonary circulation unchanged. Thus, within this very closely related group of substances, the inactivation process can distinguish between the individual members. Again, as with the amines, the selectivity depends upon whether the particular PG is a substrate for a carrier mechanism (Bito et al 1977), for the inactivating enzyme is present in lung tissues as an intracellular enzyme.

The location of PG-inactivating enzymes is of particular interest as the lung is also capable of PG synthesis and of PG release. Does synthesis of PGs from blood-borne precursors occur 'upstream' or 'downstream' of the inactivating enzymes? Are the PGs that are released (following, say, an infusion of bradykinin) the severely attenuated remainder of a much larger release in the lung, or does release take place 'downstream'?

The lung is also capable of accumulating, without metabolism, non-biogenic amines. Many basic drugs are known to be concentrated in the lung after administration to the whole animal, for example tripelennamine, diphenhydramine and mepacrine. Junod (1972a) has investigated the accumulation of imipramine in rat isolated lungs. [^{14}C]imipramine infused through the pulmonary circulation was concentrated by the tissue giving tissue/fluid ratios of 17 and 2.9 over a range of imipramine concentrations (0.5 μM to 2 μM). The amine was not metabolized and the concentration process was unaffected by cold, cocaine or 5-HT. However, chlorpromazine or, equally effectively, non-radioactive imipramine could displace the radioactive, previously accumulated imipramine. These results imply that there is in the lung a saturable binding site of limited specificity (perhaps on cell membranes) for some types of basic drugs. Basic metabolites of cyproheptadine are concentrated particularly in the lungs of rats and mice. All these experiments suggest the possibility of competition for these binding sites between different basic drugs and metabolites and the consequent possibility of drug interactions *in vivo* analogous to those due to competition between drugs for binding sites on plasma proteins.

ENDOCRINE FUNCTION OF THE LUNG

As well as inactivating circulating vasoactive hormones, the lung is also capable of adding to the blood biologically active substances which may then act throughout the systemic circulation.

HYDROLYSIS OF ANGIOTENSIN I TO ANGIOTENSIN II

This hydrolysis results in an increase in biological activity, for angiotensin II (AII) is much more potent than AI in raising the systemic arterial blood pressure and in causing contraction of smooth muscle. Indeed, the intrinsic myotropic activity of AI is very low (2% of AII) and most of its apparent activity *in vitro* arises from formation of AII in the tissue being used to measure the activity (Aiken & Vane 1970).

The hydrolysis is catalysed by converting enzyme (CE), first described by Skeggs et al (1954) and partially purified by these authors from horse plasma (Skeggs et al 1956). Considerably later, much more converting enzyme activity was discovered in the pulmonary circulation of dogs *in vivo* (Ng & Vane 1967). The assay, preparation and properties of CE *in vivo* and *in vitro* have been extensively reviewed (see Bakhle & Vane 1977).

The discovery by Ng & Vane (1967) of the importance of the pulmonary conversion of AI to AII *in vivo* has been confirmed in guinea-pig, rat, cat, dog and man. Isolated lungs perfused with physiological salt solutions will also convert AI to AII and with such preparations the problem of recirculation does not arise. Furthermore, estimates of conversion may be made without allowing for blood angiotensinase activity as AII is not inactivated on passage through the pulmonary circulation, at least until the preparation shows signs of oedema. Aiken & Vane (1970) first suggested that CE activity was associated with the surface of the endothelial cells and this has been elegantly demonstrated by the Ryans (see Bakhle & Vane 1977).

RELEASE OF ACTIVE SUBSTANCES

During anaphylaxis, histamine and SRS-A are released from the lungs of man and guinea-pig, and kallikrein, which then generates kinins from plasma precursors, is released from guinea-pig lungs. The release of dopamine and 5-HT from lung has been suggested during anaphylaxis in cattle.

RELEASE BY CHEMICAL STIMULI

Spasmogens other than histamine, notably PGs and a potent rabbit aorta contracting substance (RCS), have been detected in the effluent from guinea-pig isolated lungs during anaphylaxis (Piper & Vane 1969a, b). RCS is now known to be thromboxane A_2 (TXA_2). The PGs were identified on the basis of chromatographic mobilities and biological activity as mainly PGE_2 and $PGF_{2\alpha}$. More recent evidence (see Gryglewski, p 147–164, Moncada & Vane, p 165–183) now suggests that prostacyclin is the main PG released by the lungs and that the release (probably from the endothelial cells) occurs also in man.

RELEASE BY PHYSICAL STIMULI

Biologically active lipids are also liberated from lung by physical means, ranging from over-ventilation of lungs *in vivo* to the stirring of chopped lungs. Here again, E-type PGs, prostacyclin and TXA_2 are most frequently identified. The release of 'spasmogens' from embolized lungs was first studied by Lindsey & Wyllie (1970). Infusions of a variety of suspensions into guinea-pig and rat isolated lungs caused spasmogen release and sometimes an increase in perfusion pressure. They identified PGE_2 as one component of the spasmogen activity and subsequently Palmer et al (1973) were able to identify RCS as another component released from embolized lungs. However, the latter authors routinely used lungs from sensitized guinea-pigs, noting that spasmogen release from lungs of unsensitized animals was much less. The reason for this difference is unknown. In both sets of experiments, histamine (from guinea-pig lungs) and 5-HT (from rat lungs) were released but in amounts small compared with those present during anaphylaxis.

Handling of lungs or of lung tissue is another potent stimulus for release. The handling can be 'gentle squeezing' or as vigorous as stirring chopped lung tissue. Human, passively sensitized, chopped lung released histamine and SRS-A-like activity along with PGs, RCS and histamine, but no SRS-like spasmogen was detected (Palmer et al 1973).

Hyperventilation, another stimulus for PG release *in vitro,* may also release PGs from lungs *in vivo*. A fall in blood pressure of anaesthetized dogs produced by hyperventilation was partially prevented by giving indomethacin (Kitamura et al 1973). E-type PGs are released from hyperventilated isolated lungs (Said et al 1972).

CONCLUSIONS

Because the lung processes the entire blood volume every 20 seconds or so in man, and because it has a relatively large capillary surface area, it has a unique opportunity to exert a control function over the contents of arterial blood.

The control by the lungs of pharmacological agents in blood is achieved by a variety of methods: uptake and enzymic inactivation, enzymic inactivation without uptake, formation of active materials from cell constituents or from blood-borne substrates. The control acts on a variety of hormones and drugs, biogenic amines, peptides, and fatty acid derivatives, but at the same time acts selectively within each group, removing 5-HT but not histamine, hydrolysing bradykinin but not oxytocin, inactivating PGE but not prostacyclin. The control mechanisms may be inhibited or stimulated by exogenous agents.

Although only the pharmacokinetic properties of the lung have been discussed, it is worth pointing out analogies between these and the other better-known properties of the lung. Thus, just as the lungs remove carbon dioxide, emboli, leucocytes and cellular debris from the blood by the physical processes of diffusion and filtration, so they remove 5-HT, bradykinin and PGs from blood by biochemical processes. On the other hand, the respiratory function of lung adds oxygen to blood and platelets are released from megakaryocytes in the lung to maintain blood platelet levels. In an analogous manner, the pharmacokinetic systems of the lung maintain angiotensin II levels by converting angiotensin I and, when stimulated, add histamine, prostacyclin or other substances to the blood entering the systemic arterial circulation.

Some of the questions that I hope we shall address in this symposium are as follows. Is the metabolic function of the lung mainly related to the endothelial cells? If so, is this simply a reflection of the large mass of endothelial cells contained in the lungs (some 50% of the totality in the body), and do the other endothelial cells of the body have a similar metabolic property; or is there something special about the pulmonary endothelial cell? When we come to consider converting enzyme and the metabolism of bradykinin, is this the only enzyme responsible for activating angiotensin I and for metabolizing bradykinin, or does the lung contain other enzymes which affect these substances?

When we come to the liberation of active substances from the lungs into the arterial blood, is this really an endocrine or secretory activity, and, if so, does this happen all the time or only in special circumstances such as during stress, or is it simply a coincidental overspill of substances into the arterial blood, arising because of the large endothelial cell mass in the lungs?

Other questions which need answering are: how does the respiratory function interlink with the metabolic one; what happens when the lungs are overstretched? We know that prostaglandins are released when tissue is stretched; is their release from the lungs simply due to the fact that the lungs are moving all the time and the cells are being distorted? What can we consider to be the normal pathway of arachidonic acid metabolism in the lungs, and can this normal pathway, if there is one, be diverted or altered by pathological states? Is slowly reacting substance in anaphylaxis (SRS-A) a normal or abnormal metabolite? If it turns out to be a metabolite that is expressed only during anaphylaxis, what is it that specifically diverts arachidonic acid metabolism away from the other products and towards SRS-A?

Does prostacyclin, formed by the lung endothelial cells, help to break up circulating platelet aggregates which get trapped in the lung capillaries? Is this a function of prostacyclin formation? Does it also break up megakaryocytes that are trapped in the lungs? Do the cells of various kinds that are known to be trapped in the lungs contribute to the release of active substances such as thromboxane A_2, which has been shown to be released from lung tissue?

Is there some relationship between the lungs and the kidneys, thinking of the renin–angiotensin and bradykinin systems? And, finally, we shall probably be considering the antihypertensive activity of converting enzyme inhibitors; is this simply a reduction in the formation of angiotensin II or is something else also involved, such as an increase in bradykinin formation? I look forward to discussing some of these questions during this symposium.

References

Aiken JW, Vane JR 1970 The renin-angiotensin system; inhibition of converting enzyme in isolated tissues. Nature (Lond) 228:30-34

Alabaster VA, Bakhle YS 1970 Removal of 5-hydroxytryptamine in the pulmonary circulation of rat isolated lungs. Br J Pharmacol 40:468-482

Bakhle YS, Vane JR 1974 The pharmacokinetic function of the pulmonary circulation. Physiol Rev 54:1007-1045

Bakhle YS, Vane JR 1977 (eds) Metabolic functions of the lung (Lung biology in health and disease, vol 4) Dekker, New York

Bayley T, Clements JA, Osbahr AJ 1967 Pulmonary and circulatory effects of fibrinopeptides. Circ Res 21:469-485

Bito LZ, Baroody RA, Reitz ME 1977 Dependence of pulmonary prostaglandin metabolism on carrier-mediated transport processes. Am J Physiol 232(4):E382-E387

Cross SAM, Alabaster VA, Bakhle YS, Vane JR 1974 Sites of uptake of ^{3}H-5-hydroxytryptamine in rat isolated lung. Histochemie 39:83-91

Dusting GJ, Moncada S, Vane JR 1978 Recirculation of prostacyclin (PGI_2) in the dog. Br J Pharmacol 64:315-320

Elliot TR 1905 The action of adrenaline. J Physiol (Lond) 32:401-467

Ferreira SH, Vane JR 1967 Prostaglandins. Their disappearance from and release into the circulation. Nature (Lond) 216:868-873

Gaddum JH, Hebb CO, Silver A, Swan AAB (1953) 5-Hydroxytryptamine. Pharmacological action and destruction in perfused lungs. Q J Exp Physiol Cogn Med Sci 38:255-262

Gillis CN, Green NM, Cronau LH, Hammond GL 1972 Pulmonary extraction of 5-hydroxytryptamine and norepinephrine before and after cardiopulmonary bypass in man. Circ Res 30:666-674

Junod AF 1972a Accumulation of ^{14}C-imipramine in isolated perfused rat lungs. J Pharmacol Exp Ther 183:182-187

Junod AF 1972b Uptake, metabolism and efflux of ^{14}C-imipramine in isolated perfused rat lungs. J Pharmacol Exp Ther 183:341-355

Kitamura S, Preskitt J, Yoshida T, Said SI 1973 Prostaglandin release, respiratory alkalosis and systemic hypotension during mechanical ventilation. Fed Proc 32:341

Lindsey HE, Wyllie JH 1970 Release of prostaglandins from embolized lungs. Br J Surg 57:738-741

McGiff JC, Terragno NA, Strand JC, Lee JB, Lonigro AJ, Ng KKF 1969 Selective passage of prostaglandins across the lung. Nature (Lond) 223:742-745

Ng KKF, Vane JR 1967 The conversion of angiotensin I to angiotensin II. Nature (Lond) 216:762-766

Ng KKF, Vane JR 1968 Fate of angiotensin I in the circulation. Nature (Lond) 218:144-150

Palmer MA, Piper PJ, Vane JR 1973 Release of rabbit aorta contracting substance (RCS) and prostaglandins induced by chemical or mechanical stimulation of guinea-pig lungs. Br J Pharmacol 49:226-242

Piper PJ, Vane JR 1969a Release of additional factors in anaphylaxis and its antagonism by anti-inflammatory drugs. Nature (Lond) 223:29-35

Piper PJ, Vane JR 1969b The release of prostaglandins during anaphylaxis in guinea-pig isolated lungs. In: Mantegazza P, Horton EW (eds) Prostaglandins, peptides and amines. Academic Press, London, p 15-19

Ryan JW, Roblero J, Stewart JM 1970 Inactivation of bradykinin in rat lung. Adv Exp Med Biol 8:263-271

Said SI, Kitamura S, Vreim C 1972 Prostaglandins; release from the lungs during mechanical ventilation at large tidal volumes. J Clin Invest 51:83a-84a

Skeggs LT, Marsh WH, Kahn JR, Shumway NP 1954 The existence of two forms of hypertensin. J Exp Med 99:275-282

Skeggs LT, Kahn JR, Shumway NP 1956 Preparation and function of the hypertensin converting enzyme. J Exp Med 103:295-299

Starling EH, Verney EB 1925 The secretion of urine as studied on the isolated kidney. Proc R Soc Lond B Biol Sci 97:321-363

Strum JM, Junod AF 1972 Radioautographic demonstration of 5-hydroxytryptamine-^{3}H uptake by pulmonary epithelial cells. J Cell Biol 54:456-467

Thomas DP, Vane JR 1967 5-Hydroxytryptamine in the circulation of the dog. Nature (Lond) 216:335-338

Vane JR 1964 The use of isolated organs for detecting active substances in the circulating blood. Br J Pharmacol Chemother 23:360-373

Vane JR 1969 The release and fate of vasoactive hormones in the circulation. Br J Pharmacol 35:209-242

Ultrastructural organization of the alveolar-capillary unit

MAYA SIMIONESCU

Institute of Cellular Biology and Pathology, 8 Hasdeu Street, Bucharest 70646, Romania

Abstract As a result of its special position in the circulatory system the lung can screen and monitor the composition of the blood which comes from and is returned to all the tissues. This function, together with the exchange of gases, takes place at the level of the alveolar-capillary unit. The cellular components of the unit are: the epithelium, lining the air spaces, and the endothelium, facing the blood compartment.

The epithelium is composed of two types of cells: type I – broad, squamous, highly branched cells occupying ~97% of the total alveolar surface; these cells seem to be involved mostly in exchange of gases; and type II – cuboidal cells containing characteristic osmiophilic lamellar bodies in their cytoplasm. The epithelial cells are connected to one another by tight junctions. A thin layer of a surface-active material – the surfactant – covers the epithelium toward the air space, where its role is to lower the surface tension. Surfactant is a mixture of lipids (~75%) and proteins; dipalmitoyl-phosphatidylcholine is the major lipid component and is synthesized and secreted by type II epithelial cells.

The endothelium is of continuous type and has a large population of plasmalemmal vesicles; the cells are linked together by tight junctions. Morphometric studies indicate that in humans the capillary surface area is ~120 m^2 and the alveolar surface area is ~140 m^2.

Some of the metabolic functions ascribed to the lung have been localized to cellular components. Phospholipids needed for the constantly renewed surfactant are synthesized in type II epithelial cells. Angiotensin-converting enzyme is associated with the endothelial cell membrane and vesicles opening to the blood front. There are indications that pulmonary cells also intervene in the metabolism of circulating vasoactive substances which during their passage through the lung can be activated (angiotensin I), inactivated (bradykinin) or removed from the circulation (5-hydroxytryptamine). The lung is a metabolically active organ where the anabolism and catabolism of pharmacologically active substances and the synthesis of lipids take place and a proper balance for blood homeostasis is maintained.

Metabolic activities of the lung
(Ciba Foundation symposium 78) p 11-36

The normal functioning of multicellular organisms depends on, and is possible as a result of, the maintenance of constant conditions in the internal medium – homeostasis. One component of the internal medium, the blood, circulates continuously within a closed circuit of vessels throughout the body bringing O_2 and nutrients to all cells and taking away CO_2 and other waste products derived from cellular catabolism. At the same time the blood transports hormones from their site of synthesis to the target organs, brings enzymes to various cells, and regulates the water content of the latter. The constancy of the blood composition is ensured by a number of organs and in particular by the lung, as a result of its functional characteristics and its favourable position within the circulatory system. After each passage through the body (systemic circulation) all the blood is pumped through the lungs (pulmonary circulation) before returning to the heart, which propels it throughout the body again. Thus, besides being responsible for the exchange of gases (O_2/CO_2) the lung can screen, monitor and intervene – if needs be – by adjusting the composition of the blood. These roles have been termed the *respiratory* and the *metabolic functions* of the lung respectively. To fulfil these roles the structure of the lung has been differentiated accordingly.

GENERAL STRUCTURE OF THE LUNG

The pulmonary artery carries large volumes of deoxygenated venous blood at low hydrostatic pressure (~40 mmHg) from the right ventricle into the lungs. The artery branches into smaller arteries, arterioles and a very extensive capillary network; from the latter the oxygenated blood is collected into small postcapillary venules which drain into veins. In humans the lung capillaries (~6–15 μm diameter) have a total surface area of ~120 m^2, which offers a large area of contact between the incoming blood and the lining endothelial cells. The capillaries (~1500 miles total length) surround small air spaces of ~250 μm diameter, the alveoli, which are the terminal portion of a branching system of airways (the bronchial tree) (Figs. 1 and 2). The alveoli (300 million in adult man) are lined by a continuous epithelium which, together with the apposed endothelium, constitutes a very thin barrier between the air and the blood: this alveolar-capillary couple represents the functional unit of the lung.

In general, around 40 cell types contribute to the complex structure of the lung. In addition, a system of extracellular fibres (collagen and elastin) organized in a complex network embedded in ground substances forms the backbone which maintains the whole structure of the lung (Weibel & Bachofen 1979).

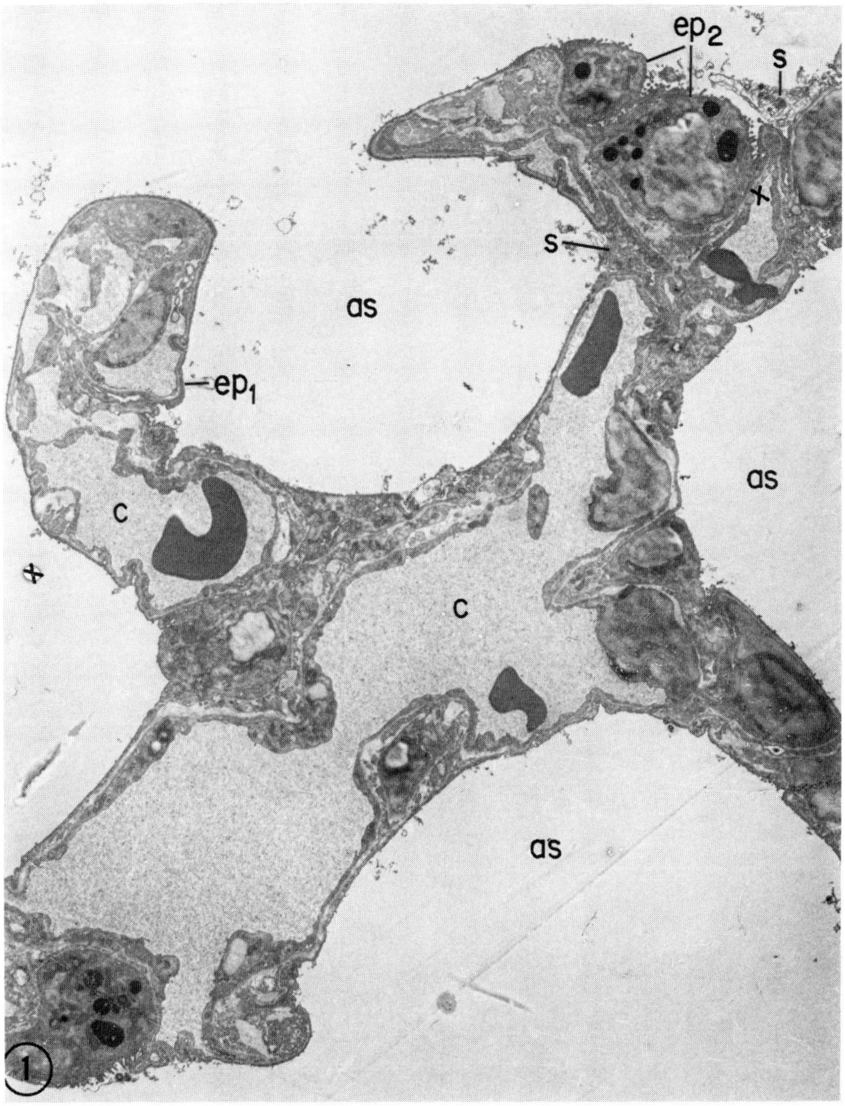

FIG. 1. Longitudinal section through an alveolus of the rat lung. Intercalated in the thin epithelium (ep_1) lining the air space (as) are cuboidal cells distinguished by multilamellar bodies (ep_2). A horizontal plane passing along the x—x plane would give an image comparable to that shown in Fig. 2. Note surfactant deposits (s) in small crevices in the epithelial lining and small bits of probably the same material in the air space. c, capillary. × 2600.

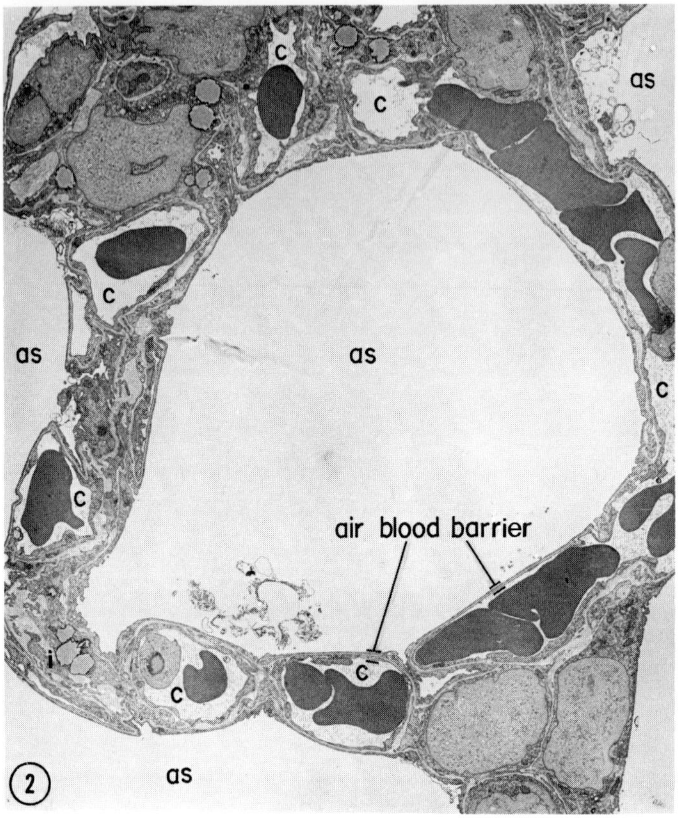

FIG. 2. Cross-section through the base of an alveolus of the rat lung (see Fig. 1). The whole circumference is surrounded by capillaries (c), some of them shared by two air spaces. Some interstitial cells (i) are also present. Note the very thin air–blood barrier. × 3100.

STRUCTURAL–FUNCTIONAL CORRELATIONS OF THE ALVEOLAR-CAPILLARY UNIT

Epithelium

Over its major part the epithelium – of endodermal origin – is formed by simple, flat, broad, squamous cells with long cytoplasmic flaps. These are the epithelial type I cells or agranular pneumonocytes. Intercalated in the epithelial lining are larger, cuboidal cells with the characteristic features of secretory cells; they are the type II epithelial cells or granular pneumonocytes (Fig. 3). Type II epithelial cells are more numerous than type I but the alveolar surface area occupied by the latter is much larger (Weibel et al 1976).

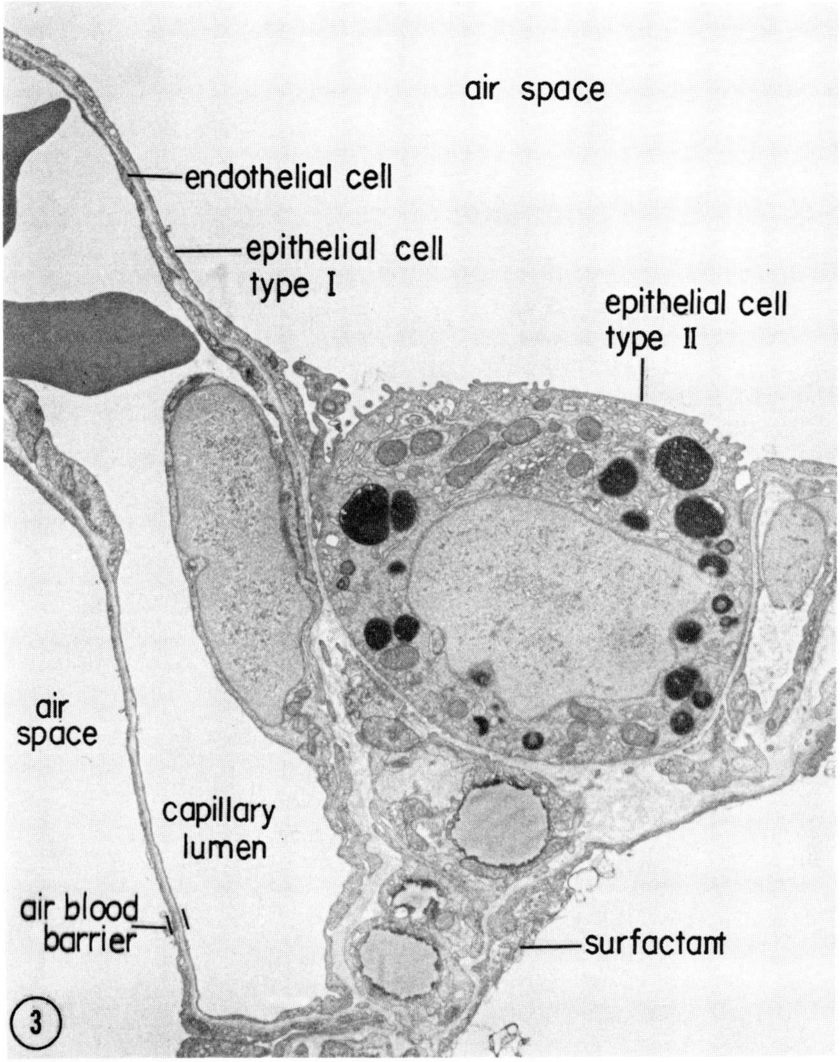

FIG. 3. Cellular components of the alveolar-capillary unit of the rat lung. × 7000.

Kapanci et al (1974) have described contractile interstitial cells (Fig. 2), found at the level of the air–blood barrier and around small vessels. They resemble fibroblasts but contain characteristic bundles of filaments which bind anti-actin antibodies and are assumed to play a role in the autoregulation of the alveoli (see Fig. 7).

Type I epithelial cells occupy ~97% of the alveolar surface area (Weibel et al 1976); they contain very few cytoplasmic organelles, among which are the plasmalemmal vesicles. The presence of such vesicles as well as the results obtained with tracer molecules like horseradish peroxidase suggest that, as in other epithelia, these vesicles are involved in transport across the cell (Schneeberger & Karnovsky 1968). Over large areas the mean thickness of these type I cells does not exceed 0.2 μm. They thus offer only a thin barrier for diffusion (Figs. 3, 9). The cells are linked to one another by tight (occluding) junctions.

Like other epithelia, the alveolar epithelium has a thin, continuous basement membrane.

The main function of type I epithelial cells seems to be gas exchange. The cells are organized in such a way as to provide a very thin barrier to the passive diffusion of gases and to use little O_2 for themselves. Diffusion of gases occurs as a result of the tendency of molecules to move from a region of higher to a region of lower concentration. The concentration gradient from atmospheric pressure (~160 mmHg) to the alveolar air (~100 mmHg) and to the venous blood (~40 mmHg) drives O_2 toward the lung capillaries. Oxygen molecules have to cross the alveolar-capillary unit, the plasma and eventually the red blood cell membrane. About 99% of the O_2 is transported to tissues chemically bound to haemoglobin molecules, bound to the iron atom of each haem group.

Diffusion of CO_2 follows the same rule and takes place from the tissue cells, where it accumulates, to the blood where the CO_2 concentration is lower. CO_2 is transported in solution in the blood plasma (~7%) or as carbamino compounds with the amino group of haemoglobin (~23%). About 70% of the CO_2 combines with water in the red blood cells to form carbonic acid. This reaction is accelerated about 5000 times by carbonic anhydrase (carbonate dehydratase, EC 4.2.1.1). Carbonic acid dissociates into hydrogen ions which react with haemoglobin and bicarbonate ions which diffuse out in the plasma, and are transported to the lungs. Here CO_2 is reformed and diffuses out in the alveolar space.

Una Ryan (personal communication) has recently found that pulmonary endothelial cells in culture are able to synthesize carbonic anhydrase. This suggests that the normal functioning of endothelial cell metabolism might be essential for the respiratory function of the lung.

Type II epithelial cells show a conspicuous polarity; the nucleus is located toward the base of the cell, while the apical domain of the plasmalemma is provided with microvilli. Rough endoplasmic reticulum as well as the Golgi

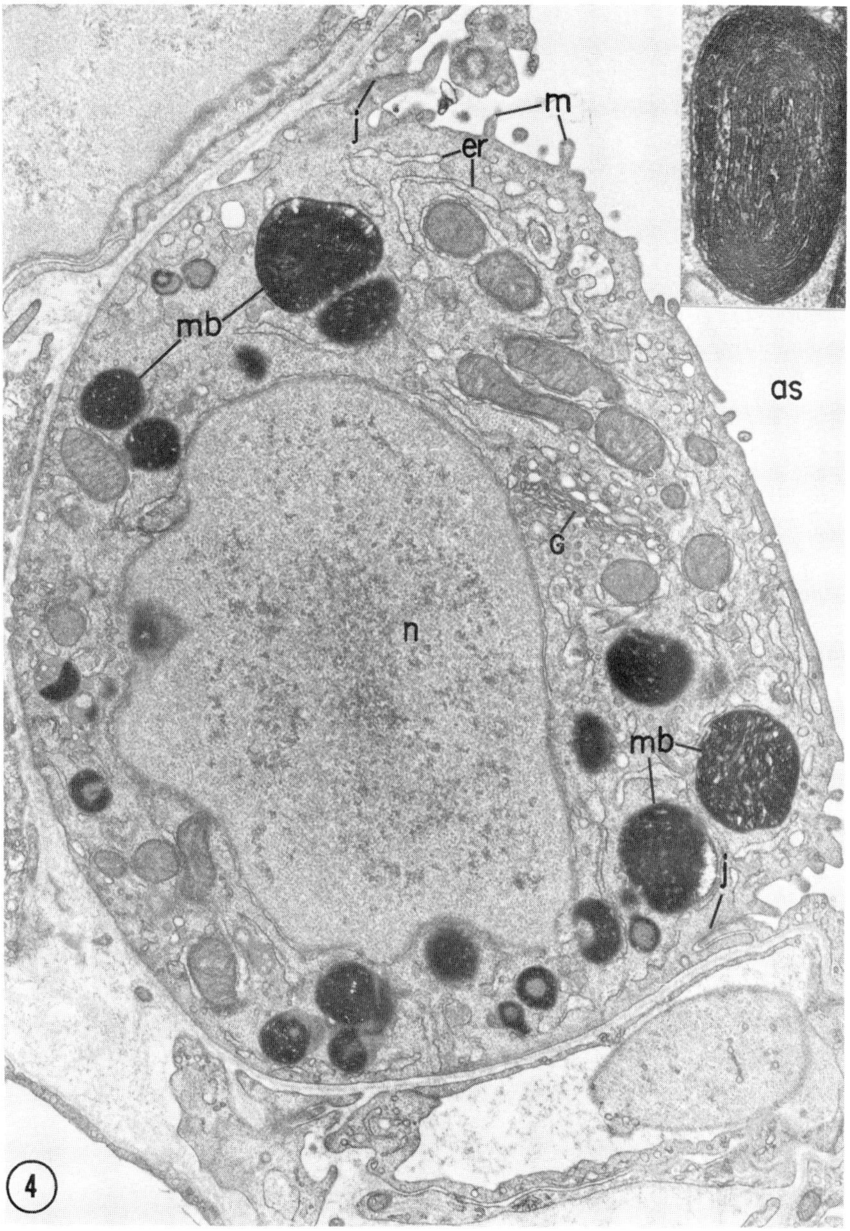

FIG. 4. Enlargement of the type II epithelial cell shown in Fig. 3. Note the microvilli (m), the junction (j) with the neighbouring type I epithelial cells, Golgi complex (G), endoplasmic reticulum (er) and the large number of multilamellar bodies (mb). n, nucleus. × 16 000. *Inset:* higher magnification of a multilamellar body. × 39 000.

apparatus are well represented. The most characteristic features of these cells are membrane-limited structures which, because they look like a series of wrapped-around membranes, have been termed multilamellar bodies (Fig. 4). It has been postulated, but not yet proved, that multilamellar bodies originate from multivesicular bodies by progressive deposition of osmiophilic lamellae between the vesicles of these bodies. When mature and large the lamellae are extruded from the apical part of the cell into the alveolar space by exocytosis: the multilamellar body's membrane becomes contiguous to, and then fuses with, the apical portion of the plasma membrane (Fig. 5). Once freed in the air space the lamellae unravel and spread out in a lattice-like configuration (Fig. 6), named tubular myelin (Weibel et al 1966).

The alveoli are able to maintain their open polyhedral shape (Fig. 1) because of the presence at the tip of each alveolus of a considerable amount of *collagen, elastic fibres* and some *smooth muscle cells* (Fig. 7). In addition the alveolar surface is coated with a thin layer of a surface-tension-lowering material, *surfactant,* which prevents surface tension phenomena at the air–liquid interface. Surfactant is a mixture mostly of phospholipids, probably complexed with a protein; 50% of the total lipids is dipalmitoyl-phosphatidylcholine. Autoradiographic studies with labelled palmitate have shown that surfactant has a relatively short half-life (14 hours). Thus surfactant has to be produced and removed continuously. Surfactant deficiency is lethal, especially in premature newborns. These infants cannot switch from respiration through the maternal placenta to the use of their own lungs because their alveoli, lacking sufficient surfactant, cannot maintain their shape and therefore collapse. Recent experiments have shown that type II epithelial cells store and synthesize at least some of the components of surfactant. Studies by Gil & Reiss (1973) on lung homogenates showed that lamellar bodies, tubular myelin and surfactant have surface-tension-lowering properties and similar lipid composition. Their protein content is different, which suggests that the proteins are added after surfactant is secreted into the alveolar space. Tubular myelin might be the storage form or the breakdown product of surfactant. The formation and extrusion of multilamellar bodies into the alveolar space suggests that the process is related to the synthesis and secretion of tubular myelin and the surfactant monolayer.

Other observations also support the role of type II cells in surfactant production. Isolated type II cells incorporate [^{14}C]palmitate and [^{14}C]glucose (Smith & Kikkawa 1979) and are able to synthesize dipalmitoyl-phosphatidylcholine. In the fetal lung surfactant appears soon after lamellar bodies are present in type II epithelial cells. In humans this takes place at about 6.5 months of gestation.

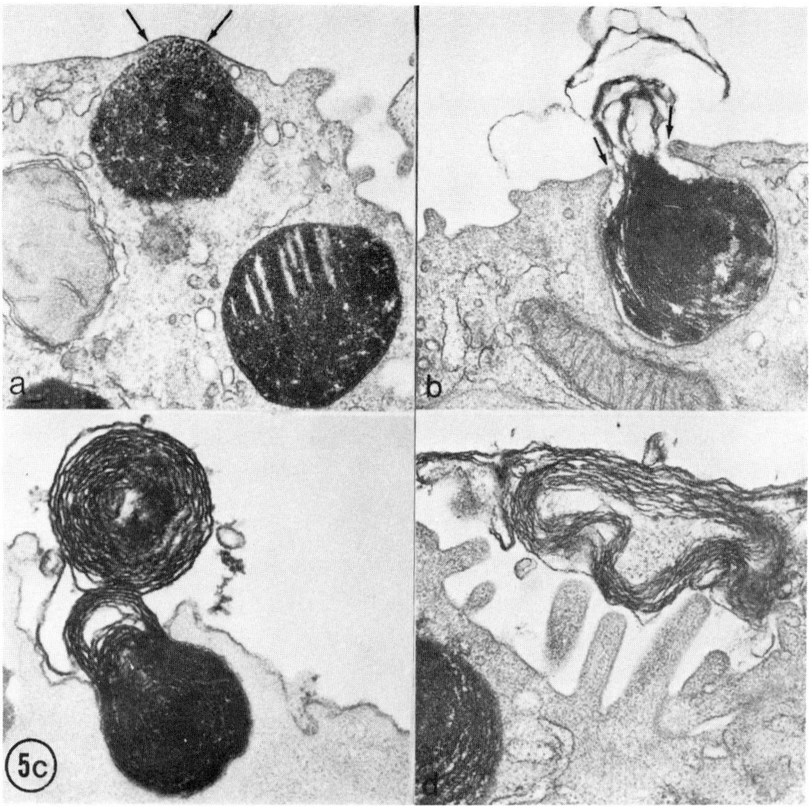

FIG. 5. Multilamellar bodies of type II epithelial cells in different stages of their secretion into the alveolar space by exocytosis. (a) The body is found next to the apical plasmalemma (arrows); (b) the membane surrounding the multilamellar body becomes continuous with the apical plasmalemma (arrows); (c) extrusion of a complex lamellar body; and (d) unravelling of the lamellae over the apical plasmalemma. × 28 000.

Macrophages

Because of their direct contact with the external air, lung epithelial cells are exposed to various risks. Several mechanisms help to prevent damage to these cells, including a mucus layer along the airways, cilia which beat toward the larger airways, and lymphatic cells and vessels. The last line of defence is ensured by alveolar macrophages. These cells patrol the air space along the alveolar surface, sometimes adhering closely to the epithelial layer (Fig. 8). They possess a large spectrum of enzymes (lysozyme, proteases, elastases, etc.) and participate actively in the defence against microorganisms and

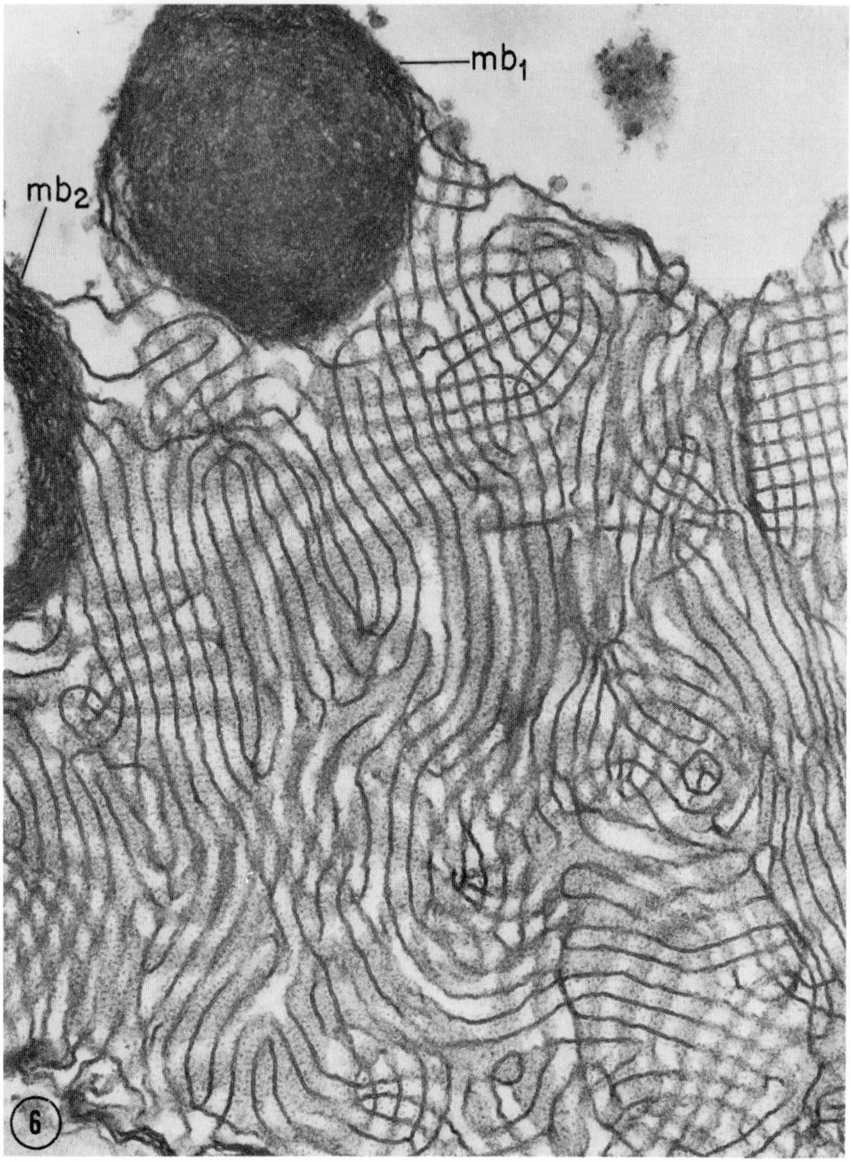

FIG. 6. Tubular myelin. The image suggests the unravelling of the lamellae from two extruded multilamellar bodies, mb_1 and mb_2. × 50 000.

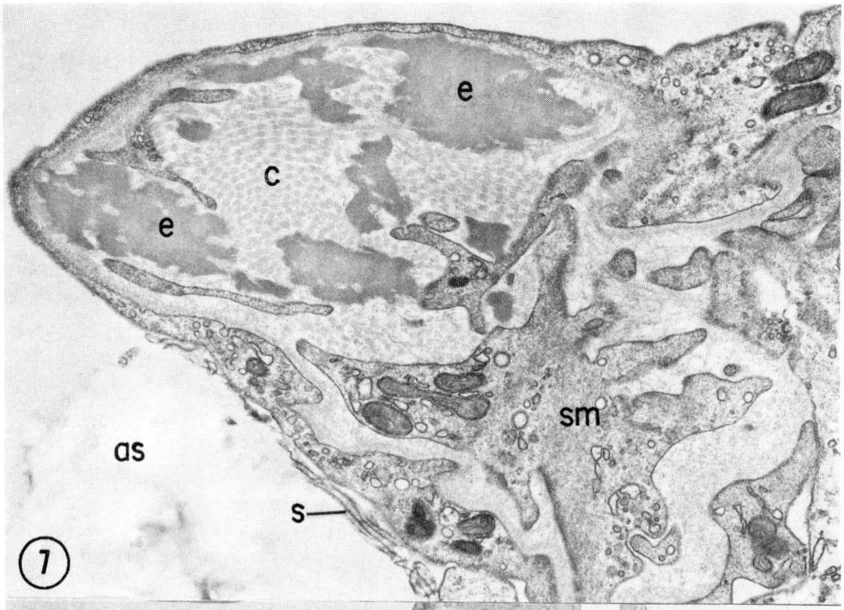

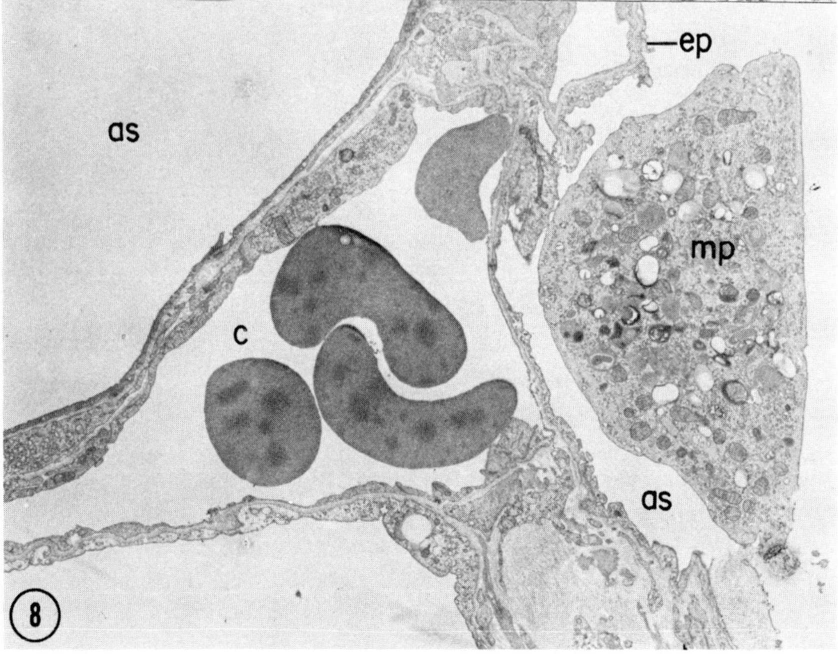

FIG. 7. Tip of an alveolus. Note the large amount of collagen (c), elastin (e) and a smooth muscle-like cell (sm). s, surfactant; as, air space. × 18 000.

FIG. 8. Macrophage (mp) in the alveolar space (as) near the epithelial lining (ep). c, capillary. × 4300.

foreign particles. In addition they contain the enzymic machinery (phospholipases A_1 and A_2) for hydrolysing phospholipids: moreover, it has been shown that the macrophages actively ingest and remove surfactant (Nichols 1976). By their function and their location at the boundary between the external medium and the lung, alveolar macrophages play the role of custodians for the whole organism.

Endothelium

The capillary endothelium – of mesodermal origin – is of continuous type (Fig. 9). The cells have the usual, but not very impressive, equipment of organelles (endoplasmic reticulum, Golgi apparatus, mitochondria, coated vesicles, etc.). The most striking feature is the presence of a large number of vesicles, some provided with diaphragms and some not. Some of these vesicles are open on the blood front (~30%), some on the tissue front (~30%), and about 40% are free in the cytoplasm (Fig. 10). In each endothelial cell large areas subjacent to epithelium are completely devoid of vesicles, thus forming a very thin diffusion barrier (Fig. 10). As in other capillaries (N. Simionescu et al 1975, M. Simionescu 1979), vesicles are involved in the bulk transport of fluid and macromolecules across the endothelial cells (Schneeberger 1978). Neighbouring endothelial cells are linked together by tight junctions. Freeze-fracture studies of the alveolar-capillary unit in the mouse have shown that tight junctions between epithelial cells consist of 3–5 interconnected strands, whereas the junctions between endothelial cells are formed by only 1–3 strands with few interconnections and some discontinuities. Although freeze-fracture studies do not reflect the situation at the level of the true surface of the junctional membranes, but the inner hydrophobic layer of the membrane, this may suggest, according to Schneeberger & Karnovsky (1976), that the main permeability barrier across the alveolar-capillary unit is represented by epithelial cells.

Systematic examination by the freeze-fracture technique of isolated arterioles, capillaries and venules collected from the same vascular units of rat omentum and mesentery (M. Simionescu et al 1975, M. Simionescu 1980) has shown that intercellular junctions vary characteristically from one segment to another. The junctional complex (tight and communicating junctions) of arteriolar endothelium is well developed, the capillary endothelium possesses only occluding junctions made up of 1–3 junctional strands, and the venular endothelium contains the least organized junctional strands with many discontinuities. A similar organization has since been found in random sampling of lung microvessels (Schneeberger & Karnovsky 1976); these junc-

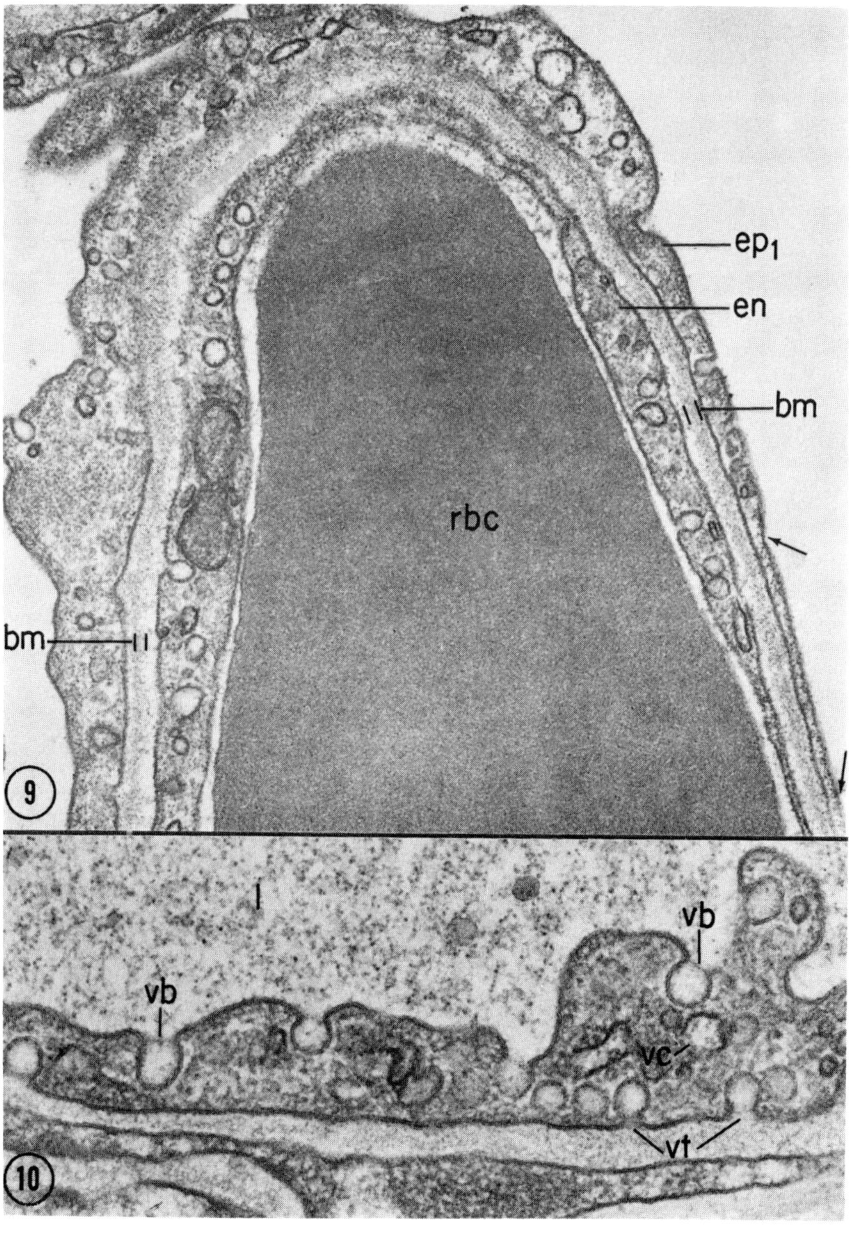

FIG. 9. A type I epithelial cell (ep_I) and the neighbouring endothelial cell (en) have their two basement membranes (bm) fused. In some areas (arrows) the two cell types are extremely thin. rbc, red blood cell. × 41 000.

FIG. 10. Continuous endothelium of lung capillaries. Some vesicles open to the blood front (vb), some to the tissue front (vt), and some are free in the cytoplasm (vc). l, lumen. × 65 000.

tions have been interpreted as of arteriolar, capillary and venular type by extrapolation to the description of these junctions given by M. Simionescu et al (1975). The results suggest that the junctional organization of endothelial cells becomes progressively less developed along the microvasculature from the arteriolar to the venular segment.

In electron microscopic preparations a 'fuzz' is present at the blood vessel wall interface, the cell coat; on the abluminal side there is the basement membrane, which is most probably produced by the cell itself. The endothelial basement membrane is fused over long areas with the apposed epithelial basement membrane (Fig. 9). In such areas the total thickness of the barrier for diffusion of gases is $\sim 0.5\ \mu m$.

Physiological experiments indicated that a large variety of plasma components can be removed, degraded, activated or inactivated during one passage through the lungs. Pulmonary endothelial cells are likely to be responsible for these functions because of their direct and permanent access to the entire cardiac output. Because of their location, number and functional capabilities, lung endothelial cells can control the composition of the arterial blood.

Ryan et al (1976), using immunocytochemical and immunofluorescence techniques, have demonstrated the cellular localization of angiotensin-converting enzyme in endothelial cells of lung. Goat anti-pig lung angiotensin-converting enzyme, coupled to 11-microperoxidase, was localized along the luminal surface of pulmonary endothelial cells and in vesicles opened to the blood front (see Fig. 4a of Dr Bakhle's paper, this volume p 280). The reaction is more prominent at the level of capillaries and venules than on endothelial cells of large vessels. The angiotensin-converting enzyme conjugate reacts specifically with pig lung and aortic endothelial cells in culture. These results corroborate well with and support the physiological results, which showed that in a single passage through the lung angiotensin I is activated to its more potent homologue angiotensin II (Ng & Vane 1967) and that bradykinin is inactivated by an enzyme located on the luminal surface of endothelial cells (Ryan et al 1968). In this way, endothelial cells of the lung may simultaneously regulate the amount of a substance that lowers the blood pressure (bradykinin) and of a substance that raises blood pressure (angiotensin II), both of which enter the arterial circulation, thus contributing to blood homeostasis.

Adenosine triphosphate is almost completely removed in one passage through the lung. By appropriate cytochemical reactions 5′-nucleotidase and ATPase were localized along the vascular lumen and within the vesicles opened on the tissue front (Ryan & Smith 1971). So far the significance of this phenomenon is not completely evident. However, adenosine is one of the metabolic products of ATP and this is known to play a role in vasodilatation (Haddy & Scott 1968). Besides these two enzymes that have been localized on endothelial cell membrane *in situ,* several other enzymes have been identified in the medium of cultured endothelial cells, suggesting that these cells are capable of synthesizing and releasing enzymes of major importance. Lung endothelial cells in culture appear to be able to synthesize prostaglandins and related substances. Ryan & Ryan (1977) showed that four metabolites were detectable in the culture medium of lung endothelial cells incubated with [1-^{14}C]arachidonic acid. These substances co-chromatograph with prostaglandin (PG)E_2, PGB_2, 6-oxo-$PGF_{1\alpha}$ and thromboxane B_2. The exact location of the enzymes involved is yet to be established; cultured type II epithelial cells produce predominantly prostacyclin (Taylor et al 1979). Endothelial cells from other vascular beds seem to be able to produce prostacyclin too. In the arterial wall the intimal surface has the highest capacity for generating prostacyclin (Moncada et al 1977). The exact site of synthesis and the amount of prostacyclin produced by different vascular beds or by other cell types has yet to be determined.

Lung endothelial cells have a remarkable sensitivity and capability for discriminating between and responding to different classes of substances that are carried in the circulating plasma. While prostaglandin A is not affected, prostaglandins E and F are almost completely removed during a single passage through the pulmonary circulation. Histamine is not influenced when it passes through the lung, whereas 5-hydroxytryptamine (serotonin) is almost completely removed. Hormones such as vasopressin and oxytocin pass freely through the lungs towards their target cells.

CONCLUSIONS

Lungs are provided with the necessary cellular constituents for fulfilling their respiratory and metabolic functions. Lung cells have the biochemical and structural equipment to meet the requirement of these demanding functions.

As a result of their number, location and enzymic equipment the endothelial cells of lung capillaries have a direct influence on the maintenance of blood homeostasis. It is not yet understood how endothelial cells can discriminate and react differently to various substances, sometimes closely related, and the limits of their capability for regulating the homeostasis of the plasma have not been defined. It seems reasonable to assume that there is a relationship between respiratory and metabolic functions; malfunctioning of some metabolic activities (e.g. the production of carbonic anhydrase or of surfactant) may interfere with the normal respiratory function.

ACKNOWLEDGEMENT

The author is indebted to Professor Marilyn G. Farquhar of Yale University for stimulating her interest in this subject.

References

Gil J, Reiss OK 1973 Isolation and characterization of lamellar bodies and tubular myelin from rat lung homogenates. J Cell Biol 58:152-171

Haddy FJ, Scott JB 1968 Metabolically linked vasoactive chemicals in local regulation of blood flow. Physiol Rev 48:688-707

Kapanci Y, Assimacopoulos A, Irle C, Zwahlen A, Gabbiani G 1974 'Contractile interstitial cells' in pulmonary alveolar septa: a possible regulator of ventilation/perfusion ratio? J Cell Biol 60:375-392

Moncada S, Herman AG, Higgs EA, Vane JR 1977 Differential formation of prostacyclin (PGX or PGI_2) by layers of the arterial wall. An explanation for the anti-thrombotic properties of vascular endothelium. Thromb Res 11:323-344

Ng KKF, Vane JR 1967 The conversion of angiotensin I to angiotensin II. Nature (Lond) 216:762-766

Nichols BA 1976 Normal rabbit alveolar macrophages. I. The phagocytosis of tubular myelin. J Exp Med 144:906-919

Ryan JW, Ryan US 1977 Pulmonary endothelial cells. Fed Proc 36:2683-2691

Ryan JW, Smith U 1971 Metabolism of adenosine-5′-monophosphate during circulation through the lungs. Trans Assoc Am Physicians 84:297-306

Ryan JW, Roblero J, Stewart JM 1968 Inactivation of bradykinin in the pulmonary circulation. Biochem J 110:795-797

Ryan US, Ryan JW, Whitaker C, Chiu A 1976 Localization of angiotensin converting enzyme (kininase II). II. Immunocytochemistry and immunofluorescence. Tissue & Cell 8:125-145

Schneeberger EE 1978 Structural basis for some permeability properties of the air-blood barrier. Fed Proc 37:2471-2478

Schneeberger EE, Karnovsky MJ 1968 The ultrastructural basis of alveolar-capillary membrane permeability to peroxidase used as a tracer. J Cell Biol 37:781-793

Schneeberger EE, Karnovsky MJ 1976 Substructure of intercellular junctions in freeze-fractured alveolar-capillary membranes of mouse lung. Circ Res 38:404-411

Simionescu M 1979 Transendothelial movement of large molecules in the microvasculature. In: Fishman AP, Renkin EM (eds) Pulmonary edema 1979. Waverley Press, Baltimore, Maryland 2/202, p 21-39

Simionescu M 1980 Structural and functional differentiation of microvascular endothelium. In: Blood cells and vessel walls: functional interactions. Excerpta Medica, Amsterdam (Ciba Found Symp 71) p 39-60

Simionescu M, Simionescu N, Palade GE 1975 Segmental differentiations of cell junctions in the vascular endothelium. The microvasculature. J Cell Biol 67:863-885

Simionescu N, Simionescu M, Palade GE 1975 Permeability of muscle capillaries to small heme-peptides. Evidence for the existence of patent transendothelial channels. J Cell Biol 64:586-607

Smith FB, Kikkawa Y 1979 The type II epithelial cells of the lung. V. Synthesis of phosphatidyl glycerol in isolated type II cells and pulmonary alveolar macrophages. Lab Invest 2:172-177

Taylor L, Polgar P, McAtter JA, Douglas WHJ 1979 Prostaglandin production by type II alveolar epithelial cells. Biochim Biophys Acta 572:502-509
Weibel ER, Bachofen H 1979 Structural design of the alveolar septum and fluid exchange. In: Fishman AP, Renkin EM (eds) Pulmonary edema 1979. Waverley Press, Baltimore, Maryland 2/202, p 1-20
Weibel ER, Kistler GS, Toendury G 1966 Stereologic electron microscope study of 'tubular myelin figures' in alveolar fluids of rat lungs. Z Zellforsch Mikrosk Anat 69:418-427
Weibel ER, Gehr P, Haies D, Gil J, Bachofen M 1976 The cell population of the normal lung. In: Bouhuys A (ed) Lung cells in disease. Elsevier/North-Holland, Amsterdam, p 3-16

Discussion

Vane: Have you compared the amount of angiotensin-converting enzyme in the arteries of the lungs with that in the arteries of other tissues?

Simionescu: I haven't done this myself. Johnson et al (1979) recently compared the amount of converting enzyme in cultured endothelial cells from fetal and adult arteries. They concluded that fetal arteries have less converting enzyme than endothelial cells of adult arteries. However, they found that converting enzyme activity in umbilical arterial endothelial cells is comparable to that in adult pulmonary arterial cells.

Junod: We measured converting enzyme activity in porcine endothelial cells taken from the pulmonary artery and from the aorta, and related it to DNA content (i.e. cell number). On this basis, per cell, activity was the same (Ody & Junod 1977).

Stalcup: We compared converting enzyme activity in endothelial cell tissue cultures from aorta, pulmonary artery, some smaller systemic arteries, and systemic veins, including the vena cava. We also found no difference in activity, normalized to cell number. We also looked at endothelial cells in culture derived from lung by perfusion with collagenase and found no difference in enzyme activity between these cells and cultured endothelial cells from systemic arterial and venous sites. We don't know if these lung cells are from capillaries or larger vessels, of course.

Simionescu: They are probably a mixed population predominantly derived from vessels larger than capillaries. Perfused collagenase loosens endothelial cells along the lung vasculature. Endothelial cells are about 20 μm in length. Freed from their basement membrane, not too many of them will be able to pass through 5–10 μm-diameter capillaries; so the majority of cells obtained in this way probably originate from large vessels.

Aiken: We studied the responses of large blood vessels to angiotensin I (Aiken & Vane 1970). We couldn't normalize the number of endothelial cells for determining the specific activity of converting enzyme. But in terms of ability to form angiotensin II and produce a response, if we compared strips of about the same size, the pulmonary artery produced much more angiotensin II, converting over 50% of angiotensin I, whereas only 3–4% was converted by the aorta.

Reid: Where is the converting enzyme activity within the endothelial cell? Dr Simionescu mentioned that the activity occurs only in the caveolae on the adluminal surface of the cell. These studies are usually done in the intact animal. When one looks at a block of tissue that has been in culture for a short time, I understand that the Ryans have evidence of enzymic activity in all the caveolae, on both sides and throughout the cell. [See also p 286.]

Junod: The question of the presence of angiotensin-converting enzyme on both sides of the cell (adluminal and abluminal) could be answered by comparing the activity of a suspension of cultured endothelial cells to that of similar cells adhering to a Petri dish. An increase in converting enzyme activity of suspended cells could be related to the ubiquitous presence of the enzyme on both sides of the membrane. No systematic study of that sort has been published.

Said: It's a safe premise that from the functional standpoint the endothelial cells of the lung capillary bed are more important than the relatively small area constituted by the pulmonary artery or pulmonary vein endothelium. There have been great advances in the study of endothelial cells in the lung and elsewhere by tissue culture, but for the most part we have been able to study only endothelial cells from the larger vessels, so there may be other features of small-vessel endothelium that we don't know about.

Simionescu: I agree with you. A pure population of endothelial cells of lung capillaries is highly desirable. However, there are some difficulties in obtaining a pure population. There are about 40 types of cells in the lung; that is the first problem. Secondly, the epithelial type I cells and the endothelial cells are morphologically similar. After collagenase perfusion it seems probable that the capillaries (5–10 μm diameter) will quickly be clogged up by cells larger than the lumen. Probably, most studies so far have been done on endothelial cells detached from arterioles and arteries or venules and veins, depending on the perfusion outflow.

A second problem with cultured cells is that we don't know whether the polarity of the cell in the culture dish is the same as it is *in vivo*. We don't know if it settles predominantly with the abluminal side downwards, or not; its detectable polarity is lost. The fate of the vesicles in cultured endothelial cells is also unknown. We have isolated endothelial cells from the rabbit heart microvasculature (Simionescu & Simionescu 1978). Once these cells are isolated and in suspension, most of their vesicles are internalized; very few remain connected with the plasma membrane. So there might be a number of changes in the endothelial cell isolated from its normal environment and grown *in vitro*.

Gryglewski: You mentioned cells in the alveolar-capillary unit which look like smooth muscle cells but differ in their pharmacological reactivity from smooth muscle of large airways. Dr Kapanci and his colleagues (1976) first showed their different reactivity to adrenaline; smooth muscle cells in large airways relax whereas parenchymal contractile cells contract to adrenaline. We have demonstrated that contractile elements of parenchyma generate thromboxane A_2 and they do not generate prostaglandins. On the other hand, smooth muscle cells of large airways do generate prostaglandins and not TXA_2 (Gryglewski et al 1976). Therefore, from a physiological and pharmacological point of view, there are vast differences between the so-called smooth muscles of large airways and those of the parenchyma. Is there any morphological or histochemical difference between these two types of cells?

Simionescu: I referred to the contractile interstitial cells described by Kapanci et al (1974). Like smooth muscle cells, these interstitial cells contain contractile proteins, as shown by electron microscopy and immunocytochemistry. However, they differ in some respects from typical smooth muscle cells: the bundles of filaments do not fill the cytoplasm but are scattered, mostly adjacent to the cell membrane; the cells contain numerous ribosomes and abundant endoplasmic reticulum; more important, they lack a basement membrane.

Reid: Which small airways were you dealing with, Professor Gryglewski, and how did you obtain these parenchymal contractile cells? The alveolar ducts have muscle which is fully differentiated smooth muscle. The so-called contractile interstitial cell (Kapanci et al 1974), or myofibroblast, is a different cell; it is interstitial in position and is very much *pre*-muscle. Also present, still within the alveolar wall, are well-developed vascular smooth muscle cells and precursor vascular muscle cells that contain contractile elements. If you are using strips of the alveolar region, a number of cell types will be present, each with contractile components.

Gryglewski: You are quite right. Using isolated cells one can say little about their spontaneous or drug-modified activity. On the other hand, although the lung parenchymal strip contains a mixture of contractile elements, its contractile response can be easily quantified. I believe that by using various pharmacological agents such as histamine, adrenaline and thromboxane A_2 one can get some information about the contractile elements that are predominantly responsible for the overall response of a strip. The type of substances released during contraction from a strip also offers an interesting insight at the molecular level. For example, during the histamine-induced contraction of a lung parenchymal strip, only thromboxane A_2 is generated. This means that smooth muscle of neither bronchial nor vascular type must be responsible for this particular release reaction. It is known that the strips composed of a single type of smooth muscle (e.g. guinea-pig trachea, human bronchi, bovine coronary artery or rabbit coeliac artery) release prostaglandins and not thromboxane A_2. Therefore, we inferred that other than those contractile elements were responsible for the release of thromboxane A_2 from the guinea-pig lung parenchymal strips. Parenchymal interstitial cells seemed to be good candidates, but I agree that they are not the only ones.

Collier: How do these smooth-muscle-like cells respond to prostanoids?

Gryglewski: We have recently shown that guinea-pig parenchymal strips are contracted by thromboxane A_2, by prostaglandin endoperoxides and by their synthetic analogues, and are relatively insensitive to classical prostaglandins and to prostacyclin. We therefore suggest that a superfused strip of guinea-pig lung would be suitable as the bioassay tissue for thromboxane A_2.

Burri: I agree with Professor Reid: we must distinguish between the smooth muscle cells in the alveolar entrance ring (von Hayek 1970) and the interstitial contractile cells of the alveolar septum (Kapanci et al 1974). The latter have a very clear cytoplasm and contain some filaments.

It may be important to focus more on the interstitial cells, because in terms of their total volume they make up an important part of the lung tissue. As morphologists we have tended to overlook them (the biochemists also), but they may have important metabolic activities besides their ability to contract. The total interstitial tissue mass (cells and intercellular substance) makes up about 3–4 times the total volume of the endothelial cells in the human (Gehr et al 1978): the interstitial cells are more abundant than the endothelial cells in terms of both volume and cell number. In the human lung J.D. Crapo (personal communication 1980) calculated there to be 84 billion (84×10^9) interstitial cells and 68×10^9 endothelial cells, a ratio of about 4:3. In the adult rat lung, by contrast, we find a ratio of almost two endothelial cells to one interstitial cell (Crapo et al 1978). Regarding the epithelial cells, we can say that (taking types I and II together) their number is about equal to that of endothelial cells in the alveolar wall in man.

One should not forget that there are differences not only between species but also with age. In the rat, for example, if we analyse the *volume* of the various components, we find within the first three weeks of life (just taking the parenchymal portion which contributes to gas exchange) a change in the ratio of interstitial to endothelial tissue mass from over 3:1 to less than 2:1 (Burri et al 1974).

Simionescu: Weibel et al (1976) find in adult rat lung that the interstitial cells make up 34.9% of the number of cells in the alveolar wall; epithelial cells type I are 10.5%; type II, 12.9%; and endothelial cells, 41.7%.

Reid: It must be stressed that the figures of both Crapo and Weibel that have been quoted take account of alveolar walls. They do not include the airways cells which are included in the 40 cell types mentioned by Dr Simionescu (Sorokin 1970). Moreover, by 'interstitial cell' Professor Burri means, by definition, any cell in the alveolar wall that is not epithelial or vascular. The interstitium is a *space,* and the cells in it are by his definition 'interstitial cells'. The commonest ones are true fibroblasts. There are also the contractile fibroblasts or myofibroblasts (Kapanci et al 1974), as well as migratory cells.

Burri: In counting cell numbers we rely on counts of nuclei, and the problem is that a shape factor comes into the formula. If one has not established this factor correctly one may get a false result. Crapo has analysed the nuclear shapes of the various cell types by three-dimensional reconstruction; this will help us to obtain more precise numbers.

Reid: It is very important that biochemists and physiologists understand how selective certain morphometric results are, in terms of the lung as a whole. After all, much of the volume of the lung consists of airways, which are not represented in the point counts described. There is also often a selection at the alveolar wall. Not all cell types are separately counted.

Vane: We are told that 50% of the endothelial cells of the body are in the lungs, but nobody says what weight of the *lung* consists of the endothelial cells.

Reid: That is because nobody knows! We don't even know what proportion of the volume of the lung is made up of endothelial cells, because nobody has made the estimates in this way.

Burri: One can calculate this with the available figures, as an approximation at least. If we investigate the lung parenchyma quantitatively we are dealing with about 80 to 90% of the lung volume (not of lung weight: the bronchi and larger vessels make up a larger proportion by weight than by volume). If we take the volume of the human lung as 4.5 litres, we can roughly assume a parenchymal volume of 4.0 litres; of this we can calculate an air volume of 3.5 litres, a capillary blood volume of 200–250 cm^3, and a tissue volume of about 300 cm^3. Improvising here with the data of J.D. Crapo (personal communication 1980) I can calculate from cell numbers and individual cell volumes a total epithelial volume of 70 cm^3, made up of 35 cm^3 each of types I and II cells; a total endothelial volume of 45 cm^3; and an interstitial cell volume of 55 cm^3. These figures comprise the gas exchange region (parenchyma) only.

Vane: If the endothelial cell is one of the most important cells in the lung for metabolism and the activation and inactivation of different substances, it would be useful to know whether it represents a small or large proportion of the total lung mass.

Alberti: It will certainly be helpful for those struggling in the distant corners of the metabolic field to have some concept of where the various cells are and how many of each type there are.

Stubbs: Is the lung more heterogeneous than an accepted 'metabolic' organ like the liver?

Alberti: Yes!

Herbaczyńska-Cedro: It should be stressed that calculations of the volume of a particular tissue or cell type in the lung relate to a static situation – a hypothetical steady state, as it were. We have to keep in mind that the relative contribution of these calculated parameters to the physiological function of the lung will change in relation to the respiratory cycle, degree of lung inflation, status of the bronchial and pulmonary circulation, and other factors known to influence the ventilatory and metabolic function of the lungs.

Reid: Yes, and that is why I am not enthusiastic about thinking of the components in terms of weight.

Alberti: If we want to look at isolated cells it would be helpful to study a cell type that has some numerical relevance in the organ. In overall metabolism, considering for example glucose utilization, it is more likely that a cell comprising 90% of an organ is significant in the total energy economy than one making up 0.5%. This would not apply to aspects such as vasoactivity, obviously.

Vane: Dr Simionescu pointed out that there are about 40 different cell types in the lung; can we specify some of these?

Reid: Concentrating first on the fixed cells, and starting with the alveolus, there are three pneumonocytes. Types I and II are familiar. Dr Meyrick has identified a third type in the rat, making up about 2–5% of the alveolar epithelial cells, depending on the strain (Meyrick & Reid 1968). These cells have also been found in the dog (Weibel 1973) but have not been looked for yet in other species. This type III cell is characterized by a brush border, and is the only cell that, in the adult rat, contains a lot of glycogen. For the first 24–48 hours of exposure, hypoxia causes this cell to lose its brush and to be covered by a process from a type I cell (Meyrick et al 1972). Then it again acquires its characteristic features.

In the airway surface epithelium there are eight cell types: basal, Kulchitsky, ciliated, intermediate or undifferentiated, brush, mucous, serous and Clara; the submucosal gland has its version of mucous and serous cell, duct cell, myoepithelial and clear cell.

In the interstitial space of the alveolar wall are found the fibroblast and myofibroblast. The blood vessels include additionally the endothelial cell, smooth muscle, intermediate cell and pericyte. Lymphatic endothelium should perhaps be considered a separate type of endothelium. Lymphocyte, plasma cell and immunoblast are three more cell types. Bronchial smooth muscle is doubtless a subtype of smooth muscle with different receptors from vascular. The pleural mesothelial cell, fat cell, chondrocyte and glomus cell are additional types. Nervous tissue is represented by ganglion and Schwann cells and satellite cells.

Migratory cells include the mast cell, basophil, eosinophil, macrophage, globule leucocyte, and polymorphonuclear leucocyte.

Moncada: I would like to consider the relationship between the lungs and the homeostatic regulation of the cardiovascular system not from a hormonal point of view but in terms of platelet–endothelium interactions. As you will hear later (p 165–183), we are suggesting that this is another important function of the lung, namely the control of platelet aggregability by prostacyclin either released by, or acting locally in the lung.

In this respect I would like to make several points. We hear very often about megakaryocytes in the lung, but I have never seen a systematic study of this. What are the megakaryocytes doing there? Have their numbers been measured, and do they break down in the lung to produce platelets and, if so, under what conditions? Is there a difference between lung and bone marrow megakaryocytes, and why do they travel from one site to the other?

Simionescu: In the lung we see megakaryocytes only occasionally; I don't think their frequency has been measured.

Burri: It would be difficult to count megakaryocytes in the lung, because they are rare. We would face a difficult problem of sampling.

Mellins: I believe you find differences between the ultrastructure of umbilical and other vessels, Dr Simionescu. Could you tell us what these differences are and of what functional significance you think they may be?

Simionescu: The endothelial cells of human umbilical vessels are quite different from endothelial cells in general and from those of capillaries in particular, including those of the lung. There are three umbilical vessels: two arteries and one vein. From our observations and the studies of Parry & Abramovich (1972) a number of peculiarities are apparent: (1) the peripheral part of the cell is thicker than that of capillary endothelial cells; (2) they contain a large number of contractile myofilaments, especially in the arterial endothelium; (3) their rough endoplasmic reticulum is well developed; (4) it appears that occasionally the intercellular spaces are open, to provide a free pathway for the direct and rapid passage of nutrients; (5) Weibel–Palade bodies are particularly numerous in the umbilical vein (these organelles are not encountered in the endothelium of capillaries); and (6) there is more glycogen present than in ordinary endothelium and there is more in the umbilical arteries than in the vein.

There are also marked differences in the amount of rough endoplasmic reticulum in these endothelial cells at different stages of gestation. At 15 weeks of gestation the rough endoplasmic reticulum is particularly abundant and it decreases substantially later (Parry & Abramovich 1972). There is a progressive increase in the rough endoplasmic reticulum in the arterial endothelium during pregnancy. These findings suggest that functional secretory changes in the endothelium take place during pregnancy. This should be taken into account when umbilical endothelium is cultured.

Bakhle: You said that there are differences among adult endothelial cells from arteries, veins and capillaries; can you specify those differences?

Simionescu: We have examined and compared endothelial cells in well-identified sequential segments in the microvasculature of the mouse diaphragm (N. Simionescu et al 1977). The density of plasmalemmal vesicles per μm^3 of endothelium (counted in the peripheral zone of the endothelial cells) was found to be higher in capillaries ($1000/\mu m^3$) than in arterioles ($\sim 190/\mu m^3$) or venules ($\sim 645/\mu m^3$). The frequency of transendothelial channels is also different, even along the same capillary segment. About half of the total number of channels encountered, especially those made up by single vesicles, are found in the attenuated venular part of the capillaries. Transendothelial channels are problably labile features with a short lifespan; this makes it difficult to count them in tissue processed for electron microscopy.

In addition, as seen in both thin-sectioned and freeze-fractured specimens, intercellular junctions of the vascular endothelium vary characteristically from one segment to another in the microvasculature. The intercellular sealing is strong and elaborate in arterioles and is formed by tight junctions with intercalated communicating (gap) junctions. In capillaries the endothelium is provided with continuous, tight junctions only. In postcapillary (pericytic) venules there are only tight junctions but they differ from capillary junctions in being discontinuous and loosely organized; $\sim 30\%$ of the venular junctions appear in sectioned specimens to be open to a space of 3–6 nm (N. Simionescu et al 1978). This may explain the quick reaction of the venular junctions, which open up under the influence of local mediators like histamine.

Meyrick: Have you found transendothelial channels in pulmonary endothelial cells as well as in the muscle microvasculature?

Simionescu: I have found them occasionally in the lung, but I don't have a morphometric estimate.

Vane: Vesicles are one way of increasing the total surface area of the endothelium. Another way would be to have protrusions from the cells. Scanning electron micrographs show filamentous protrusions from endothelial cells (see Fig. 4b, p 281). Do you see these?

Simionescu: We sometimes see protrusions of the endothelium in thin-sectioned specimens, but fewer than observed in scanning microscopy. In the latter case the high frequency may be related to the method of preparing the tissue.

Datta: You mentioned the lung macrophages and their high content of hydrolytic enzymes, including esterases; alveolar type II cells have all these hydrolytic activities as well, so perhaps they too could be involved in destroying surfactant (Goldfischer et al 1968).

Collier: Surfactant is a mixture of lipids and proteins, and dipalmitoylphosphatidylcholine is the major lipid constituent. Is any appreciable amount of arachidonic acid found in surfactant?

Flower: I don't know for sure.

Said: It is interesting to speculate about a possible link between arachidonic acid and its biosynthetic products on the one hand, and the surfactant system on the other. Arachidonic acid is the precursor of all the prostaglandins and related compounds. For arachidonic acid to be made available an enzyme (phospholipase A_2) has to be activated that acts on phospholipids, presumably including surfactant. The functional implications of this link, to my knowledge, remain unknown.

Vane: Dr Simionescu said that the pulmonary macrophages contain phospholipase A_1 and A_2, so they could be involved in the initiation of this chain of events.

References

Aiken JW, Vane JR 1970 The renin-angiotensin system: Inhibition of converting enzyme in isolated tissues. Nature (Lond) 228:30-34

Burri PH, Dbaly J, Weibel ER 1974 The postnatal growth of the rat lung. I. Morphometry. Anat Rec 178:711-730

Crapo JD, Peters-Golden M, Marsh-Salin J, Shelburne JS 1978 Pathologic changes in the lungs of oxygen-adapted rats. A morphometric analysis. Lab Invest 39:649-653

Gehr P, Bachofen M, Weibel ER 1978 The normal human lung: ultrastructure and morphometric estimation of diffusion capacity. Respir Physiol 32:121-140

Goldfischer S, Kikkawa Y, Hoffman L 1968 The demonstration of acid hydrolase activities in the inclusion bodies of type II alveolar cells and other lysosomes in the rabbit lung. J Histochem Cytochem 16:102-109

Gryglewski RJ, Dembińska-Kieć A, Grodzińska L, Panczenko B 1976 Differential generation of substances with prostaglandin-like and thromboxane-like activities by guinea pig trachea and lung strips. In: Bouhuys A (ed) Lung cells in disease. Elsevier/North-Holland Biomedical Press, Amsterdam, vol 1:289-308

Johnson AR, Nogueira LA, Ervin EG 1979 Biochemical activities associated with vascular endothelial cells cultured from human vessel. Abstracts of the Second World Congress for the Microcirculation, July 22-29, La Jolla, California, p 42

Kapanci Y, Assimacopoulos A, Irle C, Zwahlen A, Gabbiani G 1974 'Contractile interstitial cells' in pulmonary alveolar septa: a possible regulator of ventilation/perfusion ratio? J Cell Biol 60:375-392

Kapanci Y, Mo Costabella P, Gabbiani G 1976 Location and function of contractile interstitial cells of the lungs. In: Bouhuys A (ed) Lung cells in disease. Elsevier/North-Holland Biomedical Press, Amsterdam, vol 1:69-82

Meyrick B, Reid L 1968 The alveolar brush cell in rat lung – a third pneumonocyte. J Ultrastruct Res 23:71-80

Meyrick B, Miller J, Reid L 1972 Pulmonary oedema induced by ANTU, or by high or low oxygen concentrations in rat – an electron microscopic study. Br J Exp Pathol 53:347-358

Ody C, Junod AF 1977 Converting enzyme activity in endothelial cells isolated from pig pulmonary artery and aorta. Am J Physiol 232:C95-C98

Parry EW, Abramovich DR 1972 The ultrastructure of human umbilical vessel endothelium from early pregnancy to full term. J Anat 111:29-42

Simionescu M, Simionescu N 1978 Isolation and characterization of endothelial cell from the heart microvasculature. Microvasc Res 16:426-452

Simionescu N, Simionescu M, Palade GE 1977 Structural basis of permeability in sequential segments of the microvasculature of the diaphragm. II. Pathways followed by microperoxidase across the endothelium. Microvasc Res 15:17-36

Simionescu N, Simionescu M, Palade GE 1978 Open junction in the endothelium of postcapillary venules of the diaphragm. J Cell Biol 79:27-44

Sorokin SP 1970 The cells of the lungs. In: Nettesheim P et al (eds) Morphology of experimental respiratory carcinogenesis. US Atomic Energy Commission, Washington DC. AEC Symposium Series 21:3-43

von Hayek H 1970 Die menschliche Lunge, 2nd edn. Springer, Berlin

Weibel ER 1973 Morphological basis of alveolar-capillary gas exchange. Physiol Rev 53:419-495

Weibel ER, Gehr P, Haies D, Gil J, Bachofen M 1976 The cell population of the normal lung. In: Bouhuys A (ed) Lung cells in disease. Elsevier/North-Holland, Amsterdam, p 3-16

Hypoxia and pulmonary vascular endothelium

LYNNE REID and BARBARA MEYRICK

Department of Pathology, Harvard Medical School, The Children's Hospital Medical Center, 300 Longwood Avenue, Boston, Massachusetts 02115, USA

Abstract The steady development of pulmonary hypertension in the rat between Days 1 and 14 of exposure to hypoxia is based largely on structural remodelling of the pulmonary arterial circulation. The changes induced by hypobaric hypoxia (380 Torr; Pa_{O_2} of 40 mmHg) are different in the pre-acinar muscular arteries from the intra-acinar (alveolar wall) arteries, including the effect on the endothelial cell.

Quantitative analysis of normal lungs has revealed structural features peculiar to the pulmonary microcirculation. The precapillary arterial unit that lies within the alveolar region includes (i) a non-muscular region and (ii) a partially muscular region as well as (iii) a muscular region. The endothelial cells in these segments or 'compartments' appear different from each other in the normal animal and behave differently in disease.

In the various segments the endothelial cell has different neighbours and there are differences in its boundary markers (the basement membrane and elastic lamina). In the normal precapillary arterial unit the neighbour may be a pericyte, intermediate cell or smooth muscle cell. The pericyte and intermediate cell are precursor smooth muscle cells that under the influence of hypoxia develop into mature muscle.

The first contribution to this symposium considered the alveolar-capillary unit (Simionescu p 11–27). Our analysis of the effect of hypoxia on the pulmonary vascular endothelium is concerned with structures upstream and downstream from the capillary but this does not necessarily take us away from the alveolar wall, since this includes muscular arteries and veins. The precapillary and postcapillary alveolar units have structural characteristics peculiar to the lung and, although they resemble each other structurally, their different responses to environmental change – for example, to hypoxia – indicate that they are functionally different.

In the lung within the commonly recognized compartments – arteries, capillaries and veins – a number of additional segments can be identified

Metabolic activities of the lung
(Ciba Foundation symposium 78) p 37-61

(Reid 1979). We shall use the word 'artery' to describe all vessels on the arterial side of the capillary, qualified by reference to structures; the word 'vein' for all on the venous side. The terms 'arteriole' and 'venule' are best avoided since they are commonly given conflicting meanings. The term 'pre-acinar' describes all arteries proximal to the acinus – the respiratory unit supplied by a terminal bronchiolus (Fig. 1).

The variety of segments and their different patterns of response constitute one theme that runs through this analysis of the response of the lung's circulation to hypoxia; another concerns the neighbours of the endothelial cell – the smooth muscle cell and its precursor cells. These neighbours differ in the various segments, as does the communication or contact between the endothelial cell and nearby cells. The 'barriers' of basement membrane and elastic lamina are also different in the various vascular segments. Although superficial inspection of electron micrographs suggests that endothelial cells of the lung are similar at all levels of its circulation and are similar to those in systemic vessels, detailed studies of the normal as well as of pathophysiological states increasingly demonstrate regional differences in structure and function and differences in response to changes in the environment (Tables 1 and 2).

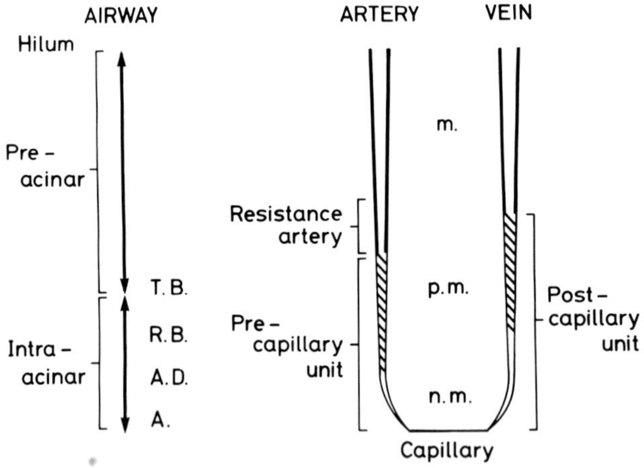

FIG. 1. Diagrammatic representation of a pulmonary vascular pathway (not to scale). The acinus is the respiratory unit of the lung, supplied by a terminal bronchiolus (T.B.). Structures proximal to the terminal bronchiolus are described as pre-acinar and those beyond, within the acinus, as intra-acinar. In the rat the precapillary unit is mainly intra-acinar but it starts in the pre-acinar region (i.e. partially muscular arteries are commonly found with the terminal bronchiolus). R.B., respiratory bronchiolus; A.D., alveolar duct; A., alveolar wall; m., muscular; p.m., partially muscular; and n.m., non-muscular segments of the artery.

TABLE 1

Endothelial cells of normally muscular (pre-acinar) arteries in the rat

	Normal	*Hypoxia*
Diameter (μm)	22	↓
Thickness (μm)	0.85	↑
WPB/cell profile	9–23	↓
Hypertrophy	–	↑
Labelling index	0.8	↑ Days 1–10 (× 3)
Elastic lamina	+ + +	↑↑
Connective tissue superficial to basement membrane	+	+ +

WPB, Weibel–Palade bodies.
Labelling index = % cells labelled with [^{3}H]thymidine.
+, + +, + + +, amount.
↑, increase in amount.
↓, decrease in amount.

TABLE 2

Endothelial cells of normally non-muscular (intra-acinar) arteries in the rat

	Normal	*Hypoxia*
Diameter (μm)	14	↓
Thickness (μm)	0.31	↑
WPB/cell profile	10	↑
Hypertrophy	–	+
Oedema	–	+
Labelling index	1.5	↑ Day 7 (× 3)

Key as in Table 1.

The structure and function of the endothelial cell has been studied mainly in relation to the vascular response of oedema (e.g. Simionescu 1979). This concerns its barrier function in the control of vascular permeability, in relation to water, ions, solutes of small molecular weight, protein and a wide range of mediators. Any discussion of hypoxia highlights another circulatory response in the lung, hypertension, in which it is the interaction of the endothelial cell with its neighbours that is critical. Discussion of the metabolic function of the lung emphasizes enzyme systems and their interaction with substrate to produce or inactivate mediators. Much of this symposium is concerned with the acute or immediate response of the endothelial cell, in seconds, minutes and hours; our paper relates to the structural remodelling that is apparent in hours to days. Much of the present fascination of the endothelial cell lies in its significant modification of substrate as it flows over its surface; the structural remodelling in hypoxic hypertension points to the 'escape' of mediators across the check-point of the endothelial cell to its neighbours.

VASCULAR SEGMENTS OF THE PULMONARY CIRCULATION

The lung's microcirculation has features peculiar to it that are similar in the fetal, infant and adult human lung and in other mammalian species whose

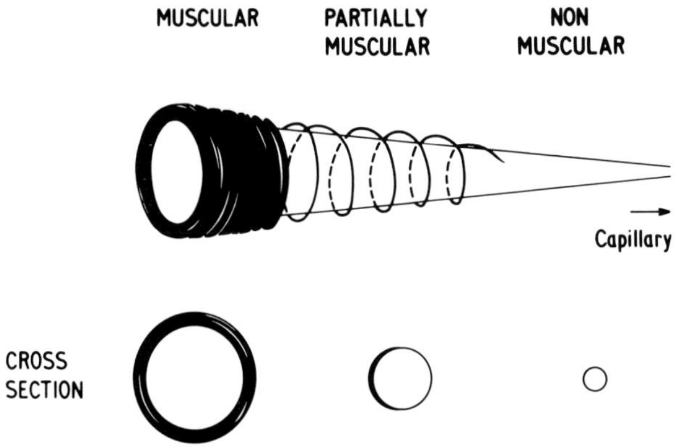

FIG. 2. At the distal end of the arterial pathway the complete muscle coat is replaced by a spiral of muscle, before disappearing in arteries that are still larger in diameter than capillaries.

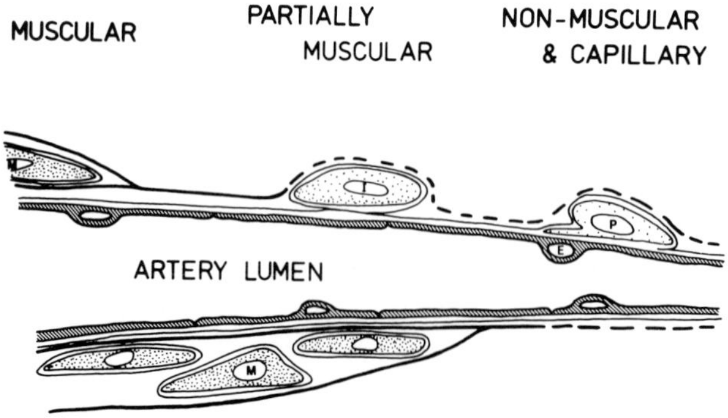

FIG. 3. Additional features of the alveolar precapillary unit demonstrated by electron microscopy. In the muscle-free regions of the wall a pericyte and an intermediate cell are found in the non-muscular and partially muscular artery, respectively.

lungs we have examined – rat, pig, sheep and dog (Rendas et al 1979a, Hislop & Reid 1981, Meyrick & Reid 1979a) (Figs. 1, 2 and 3). By distending the circulation under standard conditions before fixation one can identify an artery by its size. Size or external diameter can be related to structure. An artery can be 'landmarked' by reference to its accompanying airway and thus its level in the branching pattern is established; then one can determine whether its structure and size are appropriate to position or level in the arterial tree. The radio-opaque medium that we use, a barium-gelatin suspension, fills all arteries but does not pass through the capillary bed. By this means the arterial and venous systems can be identified by the presence or lack of medium. If the veins rather than the arteries are injected the venous system can be analysed in the same way. A hypertensive injection pressure is used to provide adequate filling and consistency in the preparation of human and animal lungs, of various ages, and in the normotensive or hypertensive state. A radiograph of the specimen gives an overall assessment of vascular size and filling, particularly of the pre-acinar vessels. This technique offers a satisfactory way of preparing lung for light microscopy.

For ultrastructural studies Dr Meyrick has developed a method that comes close to this in its effect on vessel distension (Meyrick & Reid 1979a). With the veins occluded the trachea and pulmonary artery are simultaneously injected with glutaraldehyde. The effect is to force the red blood cells into the veins and this, as well as position and structure, allows small arteries to be distinguished from veins.

In the rat, the species in which we have mainly studied the effect of hypoxia, the pulmonary artery at the hilum is muscular, as are its large branches. As an indication of their position in the lung the arteries are conveniently 'landmarked' by reference to the airways they accompany. The respiratory unit, the acinus, is defined as the lung supplied by a terminal bronchiolus. (Along any airway this is the bronchiolus immediately proximal to a respiratory bronchiolus, an airway defined in structural terms as one that has alveoli opening into its lumen.) Structures proximal to a terminal bronchiolus are pre-acinar; those within the acinus are intra-acinar (see Fig. 1, p 38).

Toward the periphery of any arterial pathway the muscular artery gives way to a segment where the muscle coat is no longer complete but is represented by a helix or spiral, so that in cross-section muscle is present as a crescent in part of the circumference – a *partially muscular artery.* This gives way to an artery which, although larger than a capillary, has no muscle – a *non-muscular artery* (Fig. 2).

The partially and non-muscular segments constitute a *precapillary unit.* This unit varies in length but can be up to 0.5 mm long. The precapillary unit is found in the alveolar wall; that is to say, it is intra-acinar. In the rat it starts in the pre-acinar region – that is, partially muscular arteries are commonly found with the terminal bronchiolus. (In the adult human the precapillary unit is entirely intra-acinar.) In the adult human and in the rat the largest partially muscular artery is about 150 μm in external diameter; the largest non-muscular artery is about 80 μm. A similar arrangement is seen on the venous side of the capillary bed but, as the response to hypoxia demonstrates, similarity of structure does not imply the same functional behaviour.

Ultrastructural studies reveal additional features of the non-muscular part of the wall of the partially muscular arterial segment, where we have identified a cell that we call an 'intermediate' cell, because it is intermediate in position and structure between a mature vascular smooth muscle cell and a pericyte (Meyrick & Reid 1979a) (Fig. 3). Like a muscle cell it has its own basement membrane and some myofilaments; unlike a mature cell it has no dense bodies and its basement membrane is immediately adjacent to and often fused with the basement membrane of the endothelial cell. Its basement membrane may be incomplete, so that myoendothelial junctions are seen between the endothelial cell and the precursor smooth muscle cell. In the normal lung the smooth muscle layer, even when only one cell thick, lies between an internal and external elastic lamina. The intermediate cell lies internal to a single elastic lamina.

In the non-muscular artery of the precapillary arterial unit pericytes are found (as they are in the capillary) internal to the basement membrane of the endothelial cell – a special relationship indeed – and, of course, internal to the elastic lamina. The pericyte is a stellate cell; it normally has processes that abut on the endothelial cell and run parallel to it within the basement membrane (Fig. 4). Study of the hypoxic response of the precapillary arterial unit has shown that the pericyte and intermediate cell are precursors of the smooth muscle cell (Meyrick & Reid 1978).

The endothelial cell over the pre-acinar muscular arteries has as its nearest cell neighbour a muscle cell or one of its precursors, the intermediate muscle cell or the pericyte. It may be in direct contact with any of these neighbours. Only in some regions is the pericyte separated by a basement membrane; the intermediate muscle cell, by the basement membrane of each cell; and the smooth muscle cell by the two basement membranes and in addition the internal elastic lamina.

In the normal rat, myoendothelial junctions are not seen in the large muscular arteries; any that are present are found in the small muscular arteries (Rhodin 1978).

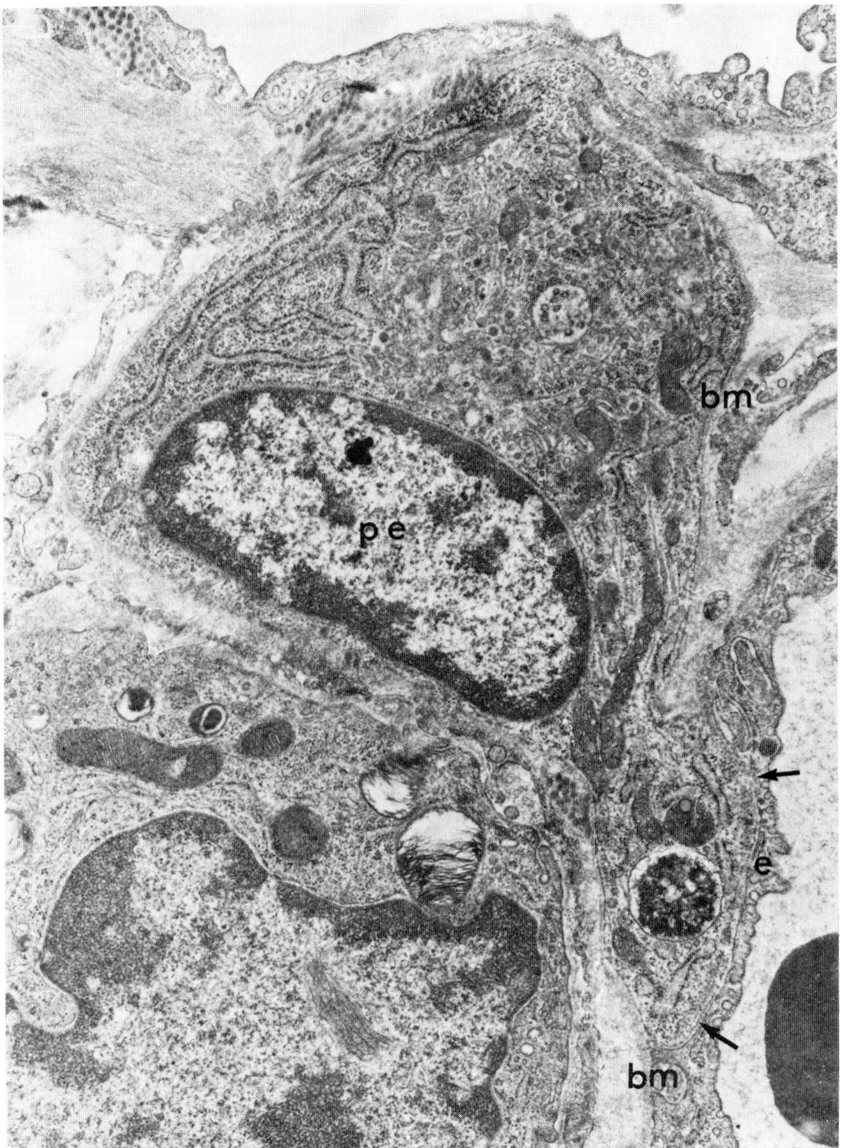

FIG. 4. Pericyte (pe) within the basement membrane (bm) of an endothelial cell (e): a process of the pericyte is lying in close apposition to the endothelial cell (between arrows). × 15 000.

HYPOXIA AND STRUCTURAL REMODELLING OF THE PULMONARY VASCULAR BED

The most studied response to hypoxia is the immediate rise in pulmonary artery pressure and vascular resistance found in most species on exposure to hypoxia (Fishman 1976). The aspect described here is the continuing and increasing elevation in pressure and resistance associated with maintained hypoxia and particularly with the structural remodelling that becomes apparent after just a few days (Hislop & Reid 1976, Meyrick & Reid 1978, Rabinovitch et al 1979). For convenience we describe the Acute Hypoxic Response as within 24 hours; the Early Chronic Response as after 24 hours to Day 14; and the Late Chronic Response from Day 15 (Reid 1979).

We shall use the Early Chronic Response of the rat to hypobaric hypoxia to illustrate the difference in response of the endothelial cell and its neighbours in the various pulmonary vascular segments. Rats have been exposed to half atmospheric pressure – that is, 380 Torr, the equivalent of an altitude of 5800 metres. We use a 'chronically catheterized' rat in which indwelling catheters can be maintained for up to two weeks in the pulmonary artery and aorta. Pressure levels are monitored and, from determinations of oxygen consumption, cardiac output also (Rabinovitch et al 1979). By the third day the pulmonary artery pressure is significantly elevated from normal and continues to rise until it achieves a plateau at 10 to 14 days.

During this period the weight of the right ventricle of the heart increases, as does the thickness of the muscular coat of the normally muscular arteries. In addition to these well-recognized features we have found, in the microcirculation, a remodelling of the alveolar precapillary unit with 'metaplasia' or differentiation of the precursor smooth muscle cells to mature muscle, a burst of mitotic activity, and the development of new basement membranes and elastic laminae. In the pre-acinar, normally muscular arteries, the medial and adventitial coats are remodelled and at all levels of the arterial pathway the endothelial cells are changed, although the pattern differs in the various arterial segments (Tables 1 and 2).

Partially muscular and non-muscular arteries (mainly intra-acinar)

In the non-muscular and partially muscular arteries within two or three days of the start of hypoxia it is apparent by light microscopy that the endothelial cells are swollen and that, in addition, a continuous layer of cells can now be recognized within the single elastic lamina (Fig. 5a, p. 46).

Ultrastructural examination reveals that the pericyte and intermediate cells increase in volume, that the pericyte develops into an intermediate cell, and that the intermediate cells then differentiate to smooth muscle cells (Fig. 5b). Myofilaments increase within the cells and dense bodies appear. After 10 days the new smooth muscle cells begin to lay down an internal elastic lamina, so that the artery is indistinguishable from a normally muscular artery except for its position (Meyrick & Reid 1978). The mitotic activity of these cells has been followed using tritiated thymidine. At Day 5 a burst of mitotic activity occurs in the newly developing muscle cells (Meyrick & Reid 1979b).

What is the biological nature of the pericyte and intermediate cell? In the pericyte tubules and filaments are both striking, the tubules suggesting a relation to nerve rather than to muscle. In collaboration with the Department of Anatomy, Harvard Medical School, we have applied immunofluorescence techniques and have established that the pericyte and intermediate cell, even in the resting state, contain smooth muscle myosin and not platelet myosin. The muscle myosin increases as the cells hypertrophy and differentiate (B. Meyrick & K. Fujiwara, unpublished observations 1980).

The endothelial cells of the newly muscularized arteries also show a burst of mitotic activity, but at Day 7, two days after their muscle cell neighbours. At Day 3, 25% of the alveolar wall (intra-acinar) arteries are newly muscularized; at Day 10, 75%. The mean number of Weibel–Palade bodies per unit length of endothelium is increased (Table 2, p 39). These endothelial cells increase in thickness. Cell hypertrophy as well as a little oedema contribute to a reduction in lumen diameter: the presence of new muscle cells causes further encroachment on the lumen. This leads to a reduction in the number of arteries that fill with radio-opaque medium. The volume of the precapillary circulation is 'restricted'.

The capillary endothelium is also hypertrophied, as are the pericytes in the capillary walls although, at least at the times we have studied, these do not develop into smooth muscle. Weibel–Palade bodies are not found in the capillary segment either normally or after hypoxia.

Muscular arteries (pre-acinar)

With hypoxia, in addition to the increase in the muscle coat (media) of the normally muscular arteries apparent by light microscopy, our ultrastructural studies have shown that adventitia and intima are also increased in thickness and that connective tissues as well as the cells contribute to the increase (Meyrick & Reid 1980b). In the media, muscle cell mitosis increases only slightly with hypoxia (the labelling index is only doubled by Day 14); the increase in thickness is in part due to early and striking muscle cell hypertrophy and to an increase in extracellular ground substance. In the adventitia the

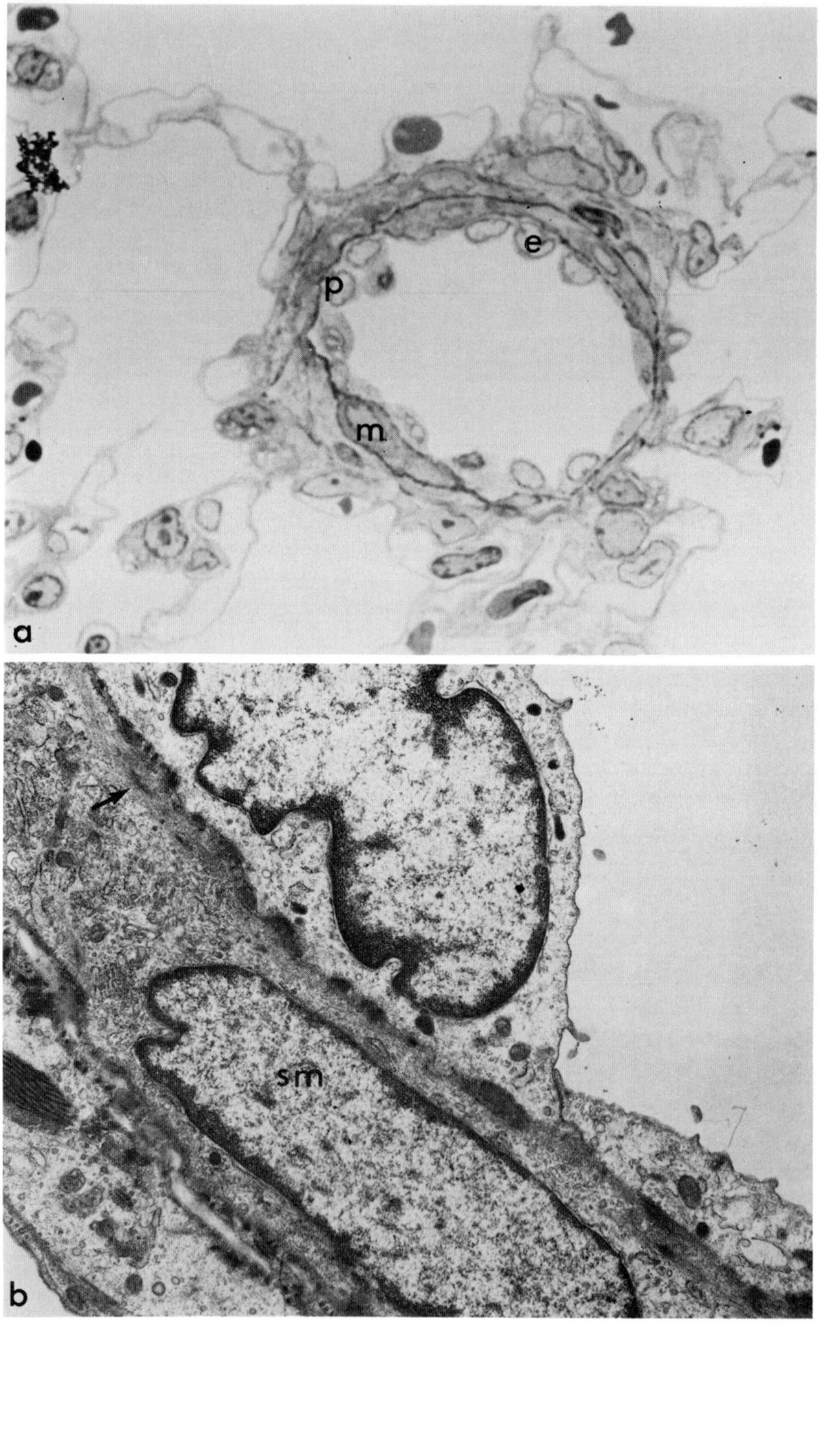
e
p
m
a
sm
b

fibroblasts show a striking early burst of mitosis. After 24 hours the labelling index is increased eightfold, the fibroblasts double in size and extracellular connective tissue increases, particularly collagen.

The endothelial cells of the intima increase in thickness because of hypertrophy. The Weibel–Palade bodies, which in the normal rat are more numerous at the hilum than at the periphery, decrease in areal density and per unit length of endothelium. Over the period of hypoxia between Days 1 and 10 the labelling index shows a threefold increase (Table 1, p 39).

Although the endothelial cell in hypoxia is hypertrophied and not oedematous, subendothelial oedema is striking; the basement membrane disappears in a patchy fashion over about half the surface area of the endothelium (Fig. 6). Although the cells are lifted by the oedema, their junctions are intact save around the rare necrotic cell.

In all the cells of the pre-acinar muscular arteries, whether endothelial, muscle or fibroblast, the hypertrophy affects the organelles responsible for protein synthesis: ribosomes, rough endoplasmic reticulum and Golgi apparatus. In the muscle cell the myofilament concentration is in normal proportion for the increased cell size.

With recovery, in the intima of the pre-acinar muscular artery, the endothelial cell returns to normal thickness and basement membrane re-forms in about 14 days (B. Meyrick, unpublished observation); but not all changes are those of regression. Between the endothelial cell and its basement membrane there is a striking increase in elastin. This is further evidence that the endothelial cell makes not only the collagen type IV of its basement membrane but also other connective tissue fibres.

RECOVERY

After a month's return to normal oxygen tension pulmonary artery pressure has fallen but is still just significantly above normal. The right ventricular weight has returned to within the normal range, while the other structural changes have only partly reversed. A 14-day exposure of rats to half at-

---

←

FIG. 5. (a) Newly muscularized artery after 10 days of hypobaric hypoxia, showing plump endothelial cells (e) and a layer of precursor muscle cells (p) – intermediate cells or pericytes – in process of differentiating to smooth muscle (m) (1 μm section, stained with toluidine blue). × 960.

(b) A 30 μm artery after 10 days of hypoxia, showing a precursor smooth muscle cell (sm) of the new layer, containing numerous myofilaments (arrow) mainly at the adluminal surface. This cell started as a pericyte and now closely resembles an intermediate cell. × 11 250.

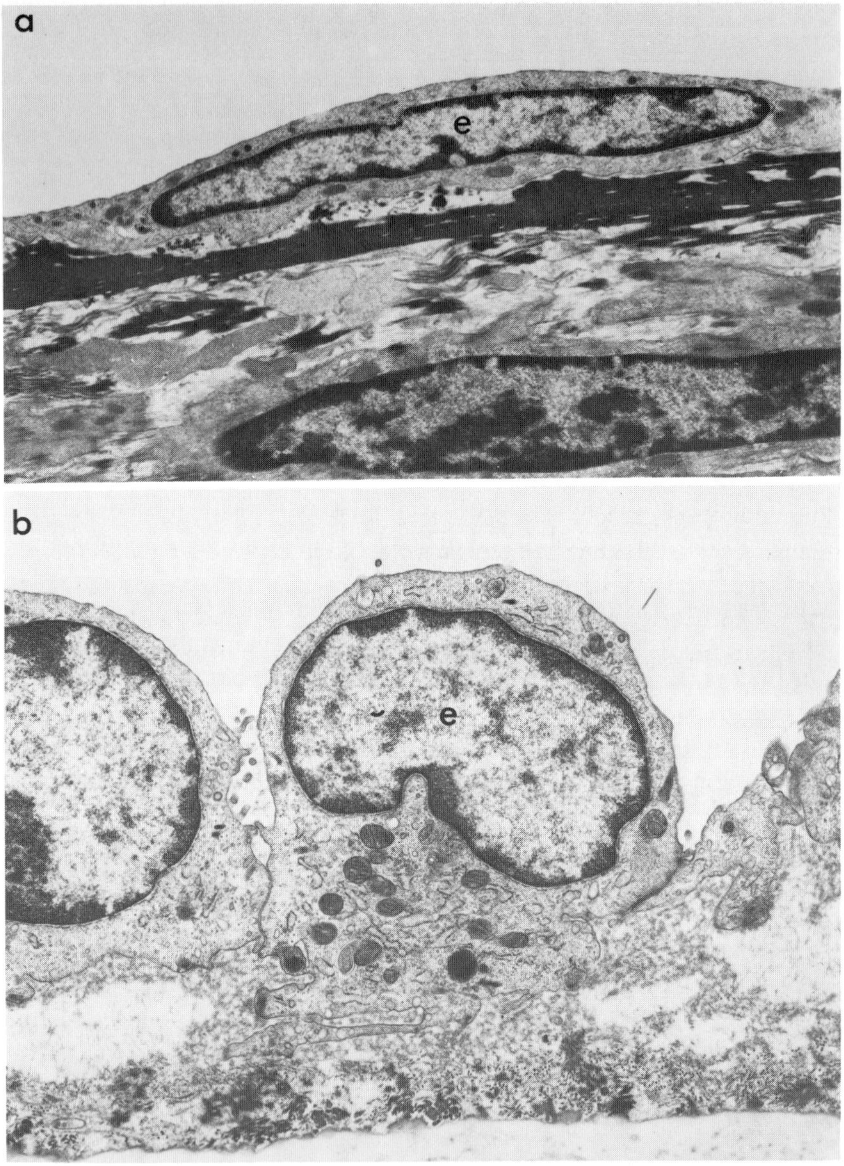

FIG. 6. (a) Endothelial cell (e) from intima of a normal hilar pulmonary artery of rat lung. (b) Endothelial cell after 10 days of hypoxia, showing cell hypertrophy and oedema and basement membrane-like material in the subendothelial layer. × 10 200.

mosphere seems to have permanently altered the microvascular bed, in that some of the newly muscularized arteries persist and the reduction in the volume of the peripheral arteries is still apparent. After a short exposure to hypoxia (three days) the intra-acinar arteries return to normal. It seems that recovery is possible only if it starts before the mitotic burst in the intermediate cell and pericyte (Meyrick & Reid, preliminary unpublished data).

In the pre-acinar muscular arteries 10 days of hypoxia followed by 70 days of recovery leave each of the three coats with stigmata of the remodelling. Although the media and adventitia are each reduced to virtually normal thickness, as are the smooth muscle cells and fibroblasts, the collagen is relatively and significantly increased (Meyrick & Reid 1980b). This fibrosis of the media and adventitia is doubtless the basis for the narrowing of the lumen and external diameter of the pre-acinar arteries seen in the hypoxic rat and also in certain cases of cystic fibrosis (Ryland & Reid 1975, Meyrick & Reid 1980a).

The additional vascular segments that we have identified in the normal pulmonary circulation have a characteristic normal structure but declare their individuality more strongly in response to disease. The remodelling in the precapillary alveolar unit on exposure to hypoxia is concerned with increase in muscle (Meyrick & Reid 1978) while in the pre-acinar arterial segment it is connective tissue that mainly increases, in both the media and adventitia (Meyrick & Reid 1980b). The postcapillary alveolar unit (the venous side) is little changed. The pre-acinar arteries are conditioned to mixed venous blood but, in these rats at half atmospheric pressure, saturation drops from about 75% (Pa_{O_2}, 40 mmHg) to 33% (Pa_{O_2}, 9 mmHg); pulmonary venous blood is 50% saturated (Pv_{O_2}, 40 mmHg) instead of 97% (Pv_{O_2}, 95 mmHg). While change in saturation is great within the venous and arterial structures, it is in the arterial wall that structural adaptation occurs.

It is not yet certain which structural changes represent a direct response to hypoxia and which represent a response to increased arterial pressure. In the aorta, oedema of the subintima has been reported with elevation of pressure (Hüttner et al 1979). We have found structural remodelling in the precapillary alveolar unit similar to that seen after hypobaric hypoxia in two other animal models of pulmonary hypertension: after ingestion of monocrotaline by the rat (Meyrick & Reid 1979c), and as a consequence of the high pulmonary blood flow produced by an aorta–pulmonary shunt in the pig (Rendas et al 1979b). While this would seem to indicate that the structural changes are not specific to hypoxia, hypoxia produces these changes rapidly whereas in the other models it takes weeks. The role of the various mediators that influence the acute response (Said et al 1974, Zakheim et al 1975,

Fishman 1976, Ryan & Ryan 1977, Hales et al 1978, Stalcup et al 1979) has not been established for the subacute and chronic adaptation or for the other models of hypertension. The hypoxic response demonstrates the structural lability of the circulation. Structural remodelling is apparent within hours to days.

The importance of the acute response to hypoxia to the development of the chronic changes we have described is not yet entirely clear. Antagonists are available that suppress the acute rise in pulmonary artery pressure and vascular resistance caused by hypoxia (e.g. McMurtry et al 1976). Their effect on right ventricular hypertrophy and arterial medial thickness has been studied: none has prevented these changes, although they have reduced the effect (e.g. Zakheim et al 1975).

In the chronically catheterized rat model that we have used to study chronic hypoxic hypertension, the animal equilibrates to room air for the serial pulmonary artery pressure measurements. The acute hypoxic pressor response can still be elicited after adaptation to room air (Rabinovitch et al 1979). The structural changes described in this model are those we see in chronic pulmonary hypertension associated with the hypoxaemia of chronic lung diseases such as chronic bronchitis and cystic fibrosis (Ryland & Reid 1975).

The biological advantage of the structural remodelling is not clear. Perhaps as a response to localized hypoxia, vasoconstriction has a 'purpose', that of deflecting blood from a poorly ventilated region. The chronic structural response is much less favourable. Of this it can be said that the response becomes the disease, and so understanding of the mechanisms responsible for the structural remodelling has special functional and practical significance.

ACKNOWLEDGEMENT

The work reported here has been supported by National Institutes of Health Grants HL 19225 and HL 23232.

References

Fishman AP 1976 Hypoxia on the pulmonary circulation. How and where it acts. Circ Res 38:331-231

Hales CA, Rouse ET, Slate JL 1978 Influence of aspirin and indomethacin on variability of alveolar hypoxic vasoconstriction. J Appl Physiol Respirat Environ Exercise Physiol 45:33-39

Hislop A, Reid L 1976 New findings in pulmonary arteries of rats with hypoxia-induced pulmonary hypertension. Br J Exp Pathol 57:542-554

Hislop A, Reid L 1981 Growth and development of the respiratory system. In: Davis JA, Dobbing J (eds) Scientific foundations of paediatrics, 2nd edn. Heinemann, London, in press

Hüttner I, Badonnel MC, Elemer G, Gabbiani G 1979 Aortic intima of the rat in various phases of hypertension. Exp Mol Pathol 31:191-200
McMurtry IF, Davidson AB, Reeves JT, Grover RF 1976 Inhibition of hypoxic pulmonary vasoconstriction by calcium antagonists in isolated rat lungs. Circ Res 38:99-104
Meyrick B, Reid L 1978 The effect of continued hypoxia on rat pulmonary arterial circulation: an ultrastructural study. Lab Invest 38:188-200
Meyrick B, Reid L 1979a Ultrastructural features of the distended pulmonary arteries of the normal rat. Anat Rec 193:71-97
Meyrick B, Reid L 1979b Hypoxia and incorporation of ^{3}H-thymidine by cells of the rat pulmonary arteries and alveolar wall. Am J Pathol 96:51-69
Meyrick B, Reid L 1979c Development of pulmonary arterial changes in rats fed with *Crotalaria spectabilis*. Am J Pathol 94:37-50
Meyrick B, Reid L 1980a Hypoxia-induced structural changes in the media and adventitia of the rat hilar pulmonary artery and their regression. Am J Pathol 100:151–178
Meyrick B, Reid L 1980b Endothelial and subintimal changes in rat hilar pulmonary artery during recovery from hypoxia. Lab Invest 42:603-615
Rabinovitch M, Gamble W, Nadas AS, Miettinen O, Reid L 1979 Rat pulmonary circulation after chronic hypoxia: hemodynamic and structural features. Am J Physiol 236:H818-H827
Reid L 1979 The pulmonary circulation: remodelling in growth and disease. The 1978 J Burns Amberson Lecture. Am Rev Respir Dis 119:531-546
Rendas A, Lennox S, Reid L 1979a Aorta–pulmonary shunts in growing pigs. Functional and structural assessment of the changes in the pulmonary circulation. J Thorac Cardiovasc Surg 77:109-118
Rendas A, Branthwaite M, Reid L 1979b Growth of the pulmonary circulation in normal pig – structural analysis and aspects of cardiopulmonary function. J Appl Physiol 45:806-817
Rhodin JAG 1978 Microscopic anatomy of the pulmonary vascular bed in the cat lung. Microvasc Res 15:169-193
Ryan US, Ryan JW 1977 Correlations between the fine structure of the alveolar capillary unit and its metabolic activities. In: Bakhle YS, Vane JR (eds) Metabolic functions of the lung (Lung biology in health and disease, vol 4) Dekker, New York, p 197-232
Ryland D, Reid L 1975 The pulmonary circulation in cystic fibrosis. Thorax 30:285-292
Said SI, Yoshida T, Kitamura S, Vreim C 1974 Pulmonary alveolar hypoxia: release of prostaglandins and other humoral mediators. Science (Wash DC) 185:1181-1182
Simionescu M 1979 Transendothelial movement of large molecules in the microvasculature. In: Fishman AP, Renkin EM (eds) Pulmonary edema. Williams & Wilkins, Baltimore (American Physiological Society Clin Physiol Ser), p 39-52
Stalcup AS, Lipset JS, Woan JM, Leuenberger P, Mellins RB 1979 Inhibition of angiotensin converting enzyme activity in cultured endothelial cells by hypoxia. J Clin Invest 63:966-976
Zakheim RM, Mattioli L, Molteni A, Mullis KB, Bartley J 1975 Prevention of pulmonary vascular changes of chronic alveolar hypoxia by inhibition of angiotensin I-converting enzyme in the rat. Lab Invest 33:57-61

Discussion

Junod: What is the structure and function of the myoendothelial junctions? Are they involved in the smooth muscle changes induced by hypoxia that you have described?

Reid: We don't know the role of these junctions, although one would expect them to be related to the dialogue between cells. After about four weeks of hypoxic conditions the new muscle makes not only basement membrane but also a new internal elastic lamina (Meyrick & Reid 1978). The new muscle cells reduce the junctions with the endothelial cells.

Collier: We know that human beings adapt to life at 5800 metres and I presume that rats do too. How would these changes help in adaptation to life at that altitude?

Reid: I am not sure they do. A difficult question is the value of this response to hypoxia. Teleologically speaking it may have value as a local response. If part of the lung is hypoxic, a localized constrictor vascular response would divert blood. But when constriction is generalized, then the response becomes disease. It is of course a normal response in the fetus. Before birth the lung's vascular bed is a system of high resistance, and blood is diverted from the lung.

Vane: Of course, the *size* of the blood vessels won't determine the blood flow. Do you know anything about changes in blood flow – total cardiac output – in your experimental situation?

Meyrick: In normal rats cardiac output is 350–400 ml min^{-1} kg^{-1} (Meyrick & Reid 1979). In hypoxic animals it may be as much as halved after 10 days.

Collier: Does it mean that this change is adaptive for localized hypoxia but counteradaptive for generalized hypoxia?

Mellins: The conventional view as indicated by Dr Reid is that from the point of view of curtailing regional blood flow to underventilated portions of lung, hypoxic vasoconstriction is a useful adaptation. On the other hand, generalized vasoconstriction of the pulmonary arteries of the lung in response to generalized hypoxia, for example at high altitude, may prevent oedema at the microvascular level and in this sense would surely still be adaptive by preventing transmission of high vascular pressures to the fluid-exchanging vessels of the lung while still allowing gas exchange.

Reid: I agree. This may be particularly important in the infant. It is possible that it is less forceful in the premature infant, who easily develops oedema. I am thinking more of the child with cystic fibrosis, or such conditions, when hypoxia causes hypertension and remodelling of the vascular bed – cor pulmonale.

Vane: Does respiratory rate alter in your hypoxic rats?

Reid: Yes; the rats hyperventilate. These are rats without airways obstruction, although it is interesting that their lungs enlarge under hypoxia (Hislop & Reid 1976). This seems to arise from a change in compliance, unlike Weibel's findings where young rats show an adaptive hypertrophy to hypoxia (Burri & Weibel 1971). Our rats are older and develop only a reversible change in compliance.

Junod: What are the relative contributions of hypoxia and of hypertension to the changes you showed? If you treated your rats with α-blocking agents, for example, to reduce the hypertensive effect, what would be the effect of hypoxia alone?

Reid: We are studying this now. It has been shown that in cerebral vessels and in systemic vessels, when there is systemic hypertension, the smooth muscle cells make more collagen than normally, so the increased production of connective tissue could be a direct effect of hypertension (Ooshima et al 1975). Also, in the aorta, in certain models of hypertension, oedema of the intimal layer (Hüttner et al 1979) develops. Each of these changes may therefore be due to an increase in pressure. These changes in the periphery occur in conditions where there is no hypoxaemia.

Whether in the lung the effects of pressure and hypoxia are mediated through a common pathway, or whether they are different, we don't know. The difference in our hypoxic model from, say, a high-pressure, high-flow model (Rendas et al 1979) or from the monocrotaline model (Meyrick & Reid 1979) is that the muscle changes are faster with hypoxia.

Antagonists that inhibit the acute hypoxic response (which is probably vasoconstrictive) are available (Fishman 1976). No antagonist prevents the chronic response, either the functional or structural component, although several have been shown to reduce it (Zakheim et al 1975, Oštádal et al 1978).

In our studies we have found similar results: converting enzyme inhibitor (CEI) prevents the acute pressor response and diminishes the chronic response, with some reduction in arterial structural remodelling (Rabinovitch et al 1980). In so far as we can generalize it seems that the structural changes and pressure effects still correlate closely, suggesting that the effects we have been describing are not a direct effect of hypoxia but are caused, indirectly, through its effect on pressure.

Vane: Have you studied the effects of inhibitors of arachidonic acid metabolism?

Meyrick: Not yet. We have injected prostacyclin (PGI_2; donated by Upjohn Co.) as a bolus into rats and find that in the normal rat there is a 2 or 3 mmHg fall in pulmonary artery pressure; in the chronically hypoxic rats we see a fall of 7 or 8 mmHg. This fall is not due to inhibition of the acute vasoconstriction since the animals were acclimatized to room air when the prostacyclin was given and the measurements were taken; it seems that the PGI_2 causes vasodilatation by decreasing muscle tone (B. Meyrick, unpublished observations).

Reid: We have been associated with one case, a child with terminal pulmonary hypertension, in whom tests of different vasodilator agents were justified. Prostacyclin gave the most significant fall in pulmonary artery pressure (Watkins et al 1980).

Woods: Do you know how these changes might affect the uptake and storage of drugs in the lungs?

Reid: No, but in hypoxia we saw an increased concentration of vesicles in arterial endothelial cells, both hilar and peripheral, particularly the latter (Meyrick & Reid 1980a).

Woods: Drug disposition is altered in man in chronic respiratory disease (du Souich et al 1978), but it is difficult to interpret these results because of the possible effects of long-term hypoxia on other drug-metabolizing organs. Your model could be a way of testing these effects.

Alberti: Have you established any metabolic correlates of the morphological changes you have shown – by cytochemical staining, or ATP measurements, for example? You mentioned that various cell components altered; were there any mitochondrial changes?

Meyrick: We have not studied any metabolic correlates. Using quantitative morphometric techniques we have shown that in hypoxic rats the areal density of mitochondria in endothelial and smooth muscle cells, of the hilar and peripheral arteries, is unchanged (Meyrick & Reid 1980a, b). Since both cell types increase in size with exposure to hypoxia, this means that there is hypertrophy of the mitochondria but that it is proportional to increased cell size. In both cell types the organelles that show significant hypertrophy are those associated with protein synthesis – ribosomes, rough endoplasmic reticulum and Golgi apparatus.

Ayuso-Parrilla: We have studied the effect of anoxia on lung metabolism using isolated rat lung cells as experimental model (Pérez-Díaz et al 1977). We found that anoxia does not result in decreased ATP levels. The only metabolic change we could detect was an increased affinity of the system for glucose. However, under normal conditions the apparent K_m for glucose is below its physiological plasma concentration; thus an increased affinity would not have physiological importance. These observations, together with the fact that glucose inhibits oxidative metabolism by the lung cells (Ayuso-Parrilla et al 1978), indicate that in the presence of this sugar the energy used for the metabolic functioning of the lung is mainly derived from the glycolytic pathway and, thus, that lung metabolism is quite independent of the oxygen tension.

Said: Dr Reid, does the rise in pulmonary artery pressure precede the structural changes, or does it follow as a compensatory reaction?

Reid: They go together; the pulmonary artery pressure rise and the remodelling of the periphery parallel each other (Rabinovitch et al 1979).

Ballard: In the newborn baby we sometimes encounter the problem of persistent pulmonary hypertension. Are these structural changes seen in that disease?

Reid: This is an important and interesting question. We say that the fetal or newborn lung is more muscular than the adult lung; it is, in that individual arteries have thicker walls, but it is *less* muscular in that the newborn child has almost no muscular arteries beyond the terminal bronchiolus. So diversion of blood is due to constriction of pre-acinar arteries. The normal fetus or infant has no intra-acinar muscular arteries. In two studies we have found intra-acinar muscular arteries in children with persistent pulmonary hypertension of the idiopathic variety (no cause identified). The first study was of three children, two of whom were more than one week of age (Haworth & Reid 1976). In the recent study there are six children, all under one week of age (Murphy et al 1980). This shifts the question of cause back into the antenatal period. What happened to the mother, which drugs did she take, what went wrong with the mediator system to cause arterial muscle at an abnormal site for age? So there is certainly a group of infants where pulmonary hypertension seems to be based on an unexplained precocious muscularization before birth.

Vane: When you prolong the period of hypoxia in your animals, does the remodelling become irreversible?

Reid: I cannot tell you the effect of periods of hypoxia of longer than four weeks. After three months of recovery, although we see fairly good regression of muscle changes, some loss of vessels remains (M. Rabinovitch, personal communication 1979). One might predict that the animals would show reduced functional reserve. Moreover, if we expose infant rats, eight days old, to hypoxia, we are left with a more serious degree of remodelling and higher pulmonary artery pressure. So the young animal is worse off than the adult for the same period of exposure to hypoxia (Rabinovitch et al 1979).

Vane: Can you predict what will happen in chronic hypoxia from what you have observed in acute hypoxia?

Reid: No. The acute hypoxic response is essentially a functional response that is measured in terms of pressure. Until recently the chronic response had been assessed in structural terms of right ventricular weight increase with only rarely a measurement of right ventricular or pulmonary artery pressure. Our results provide continuous monitoring of the haemodynamic state as well as some new structural end-points.

The important feature of the acute response is the rapidity with which it develops and its complete reversibility, and that it is vasoconstrictive (Fishman 1976). It has been prevented experimentally in a variety of ways, by attacking the metabolism of the muscle cell, or by inhibition either of movement of calcium into the cell or of the liberation of calcium within the cell. It can be prevented by vasodilators. In some species the acute response can be prevented by verapamil, SKF-525A, indomethacin and perhaps aspirin. In our chronic hypoxic model we can still elicit an acute hypoxic response.

If we consider intermittent hypoxia, we are obtaining rather different results from others (Unger et al 1977). They found, in the dog, with 15 minutes in and 15 minutes out of hypoxia, potentiation of the pressor effect with complete reversal on return to room air.

In rats we have used intermittent hypoxia in 30-minute periods separated by 30 minutes of room air for a total of up to eight hours and compared it with a continuous exposure of this duration (M. Rabinovitch & L. Reid, unpublished observations 1980). The potentiation is not as striking as in the dog. In fact, the later periods of exposure to hypoxia produced less effect than the earlier. In both groups, on return to room air, pressure fell — in most to baseline values. This intermittent response is probably different from the acute or chronic one and no study with antagonists has yet been made of it. This of course may be important clinically, if one thinks about the intermittent periods of hypoxia associated with anaesthesia, airways obstruction, or sleep apnoea.

Almost any agent that has been investigated in the acute response has been applied to the chronic and its effect assessed structurally by the amount of increase in heart weight or artery muscle. In no case has the chronic response been completely prevented. For example, CEI (Zakheim et al 1975), hexoprenaline (McMurtry et al 1977a), dopamine (Naeye 1965, Suggett & Herget 1977), verapamil (Davidson et al 1978) and aspirin (Kentera et al 1979) have all reduced the hypertension, the right ventricular hypertrophy and the increase in medial thickness of the muscular artery, but nothing is yet known of their effect on the peripheral remodelling we describe.

Among our inbred rats we find an occasional non-responder to acute hypoxia, just as in humans. If we study the responders to hypoxia and prevent the acute response with verapamil we frequently pick up rats whose pressor response is not inhibited by this drug. In those that respond to verapamil, about three days after hypoxia we see a potentiation of their chronic hypoxic response, with the highest pulmonary artery pressures at three days that we have seen after this period of hypoxia (M. Konstam & M. Rabinovitch, personal communication 1980).

Vane: It seems that the mediators of the acute response, whatever they may be, are not necessarily the mediators of the chronic response, since when you obtain the chronic hypoxic response, the change with a further acute exposure is not the same as the initial one.

Reid: Originally we thought they were the same. Now it seems that the muscle cell has really been altered.

Soffer: Is it clear that the signal for the hypoxic response is coming through the alveoli of the lung, and not through the capillary circulation? If the response were mediated through the blood, would you not expect the same kind of structural change in some other organ?

Reid: This effect is obtained through the alveoli. The work on heart muscle (Stere & Anthony 1977) shows that in hypoxia, at this site, the trend is to get an increase in blood vessel concentration rather than a decrease, as in the lung.

Soffer: Is this structural pathological parameter specifically related to hypoxia or is it generated in response to other injurious stimuli as well?

Reid: For the structural changes hypoxaemia does not seem to be necessary. I mentioned the two further models of pulmonary hypertension that do not involve hypoxaemia, and in each we find the same structural change. In the first we use monocrotaline, a toxic alkaloid, given to rats either by feeding or by injection. This gives a similar structural change in the pulmonary arterial circulation, a similar increase in pulmonary artery pressure and similar hypertrophy of the right ventricle, but there is no hypoxaemia, except in the last hours of life. So the trigger is not necessarily hypoxaemia (Meyrick & Reid 1979). This compound is broken down to active metabolites in the liver and appears to be an endothelial toxin, which can ultimately cause pulmonary arteritis and necrosis. But we use a smaller dose than this.

In our second non-hypoxic model we induce increased pulmonary artery pressure without hypoxaemia by producing a shunt from aorta to pulmonary artery in a young piglet (Rendas et al 1979). We obtain a rise in pulmonary artery pressure and we see the same structural changes in the pulmonary vessels.

Soffer: Is there something specific about these structural changes, then, or would they perhaps develop after doing anything harmful to the lung? Is there any reason to think that monocrotaline, for example, has anything in common with lack of oxygen, apart from being damaging to the lung?

Reid: I don't think this structural change is specific for hypoxia; it *is* specific for hypertension.

Vane: What then are the mediators of the acute hypoxic response? Is it the removal of a vasodilator during hypoxia or the appearance of a vasoconstrictor?

Stubbs: Sole et al (1979) showed that the clearance of noradrenaline was decreased from 25% to 0.02% in patients with primary pulmonary hypertension. I don't know whether this holds for pulmonary hypertension secondary to hypoxia. There is also decreased conversion of angiotensin I to II by the lungs of dogs exposed to acute hypoxia, although systemic blood pressure is unaffected (Leuenberger et al 1978). Hypoxia is accompanied by changes in circulating hormones and metabolites with, for example, rises in circulating levels of noradrenaline, cortisol, glucagon, insulin and glucose (Bloom et al 1977) which may themselves produce direct effects on lung metabolism. When looking at the mechanism by which agents protect the lung from hypoxia one must ask whether this is due to a direct structural or metabolic effect on the lung itself, or secondary to a reversal of the changes in circulating hormones and metabolites accompanying hypoxia.

Vane: You can resolve that question partially by using an isolated lung preparation where there are no circulating hormones other than those which originate in the lung itself. Do we know what the local hormonal contribution of the lung is, during hypoxia?

Said: I don't think anybody knows the mediators responsible for the hypoxic pressor response of the pulmonary circulation. In the cat, vasoconstrictor prostaglandin-like substances may be released in acute hypoxia (Said et al 1974) but in other species vasodilator prostaglandin-like compounds may be released and might modulate or reduce rather than bring about the pressor response (Vaage et al 1975, Weir et al 1976, Hales et al 1977).

Vane: We did not obtain an effect on blood-perfused lungs of the cat with indomethacin (an inhibitor of prostaglandin synthesis) (H. Duke & J.R. Vane, unpublished observations).

Soffer: I am impressed by how rapidly Dr Stalcup sees an effect of hypoxia on angiotensin I conversion in the dog (p 293–311). This suggests that the initial physiological event is a disruption of the endothelial membrane. If so, one can ask what kind of structure or physiological activity there is in the endothelial membrane through which a systemic effect could be exerted, by virtue of a change in membrane configuration. For example, if the particulate fraction of pulmonary guanylate cyclase were localized in this membrane, it might provide a mechanism by which one could expect a global event from a membrane change. Conceivably also there may be enzymes concerned with prostaglandin metabolism that fit into the membrane in such a way that a change in its structure causes a change in their activities. This might be one way to think about the question.

Stalcup: When we were trying to make sense of the vast literature on pharmacological approaches to the hypoxic pressor responses we concluded that, basically, everybody who has suggested a putative mediator was probably right, and that a more useful approach was to try to understand how one type of mediator system (whether it be circulating peptide or amine) was articulated with local mediator systems and how those local systems (such as prostanoids and cyclic nucleotides) were stimulated to achieve a new balance between vasoconstriction and vasodilatation. The question then becomes: how does a change in P_{O_2} affect the balance among a whole cascade of relationships, including blood-borne substances, the autonomic nervous system, local regulating substances, and intracellular factors? We wanted to link this with the idea that there would first have to be a cell that senses a change in P_{O_2}, transduces that change to adjacent cells and sends a signal to tell smooth muscle in the body to relax or in the lung to constrict. I don't find it productive to think of *a* mediator, but it seems helpful to think of *all* the mediators, and the challenge is to put them together into a scheme of constricting and dilating and a new balance between them.

Bakhle: Is it still thought to be true that the hypoxic response does not develop in lungs that are not perfused with blood (McMurtry et al 1977b)?

Reid: No. The hypoxic response can occur without blood if a sub-pressor amount of angiotensin II is available (Berkov 1974).

References

Ayuso-Parrilla MS, Pérez Díaz J, Martin A, Parrilla R 1978 Glucose inhibition of oxygen utilization by isolated rat lung cells. Biochimie (Paris) 60:823-826

Berkov S 1974 Hypoxic pulmonary vasoconstriction in the rat. The necessary role of angiotensin II. Circ Res 35:256-261

Bloom SR, Edwards AV, Hardy RN 1977 Adrenal and pancreatic endocrine responses to hypoxia and hypercapnia in the calf. J Physiol (Lond) 269:131-154

Burri PH, Weibel ER 1971 Morphometric estimation of pulmonary diffusion capacity. II. Effect of environmental PO_2 on the growing lung. Respir Physiol 11:247-264

Davidson A, McMurtry I, Reeves JT 1978 Pulmonary vascular effects of verapamil. Am Heart J 95:810-811

du Souich P, McLean AU, Lalka D, Erill S, Gibaldi M 1978 Pulmonary disease and drug kinetics. Clin Pharmacokinet 3:257-266

Fishman AP 1976 Hypoxia on the pulmonary circulation. How and where it acts. Circ Res 38:221-231

Hales CA, Rouse E, Buchwald IA, Kazemi H 1977 Role of prostaglandins in alveolar hypoxic vasoconstriction. Respir Physiol 29:151-162

Haworth SG, Reid L 1976 Persistent fetal circulation – newly recognized structural features. J Pediatr 88:614-620

Hislop A, Reid L 1976 New findings in pulmonary arteries of rats with hypoxia-induced pulmonary hypertension. Br J Exp Pathol 57:542-554

Hüttner I, Badonnel M-C, Elemer G, Gabbiani G 1979 Aortic intima of the rat in various phases of hypertension. Exp Mol Pathol 31:191-200

Kentera D, Sušić D, Zdrarković M 1979 Effects of verapamil and aspirin on experimental chronic hypoxic pulmonary hypertension and right ventricular hypertrophy in rats. Respiration 37:192-196

Leuenberger PJ, Stalcup SA, Mellins RB, Greenbaum LM, Turino GM 1978 Decrease in angiotensin I conversion by acute hypoxia in dogs. Proc Soc Exp Biol Med 158:586-589

McMurtry IF, Reeves JT, Will DH, Grover RF 1977a Reduction of bovine pulmonary hypertension by normoxia, verapamil and hexoprenaline. Experientia (Basel) 33:1192-1194

McMurtry IF, Hookway BW, Roos G 1977b Red blood cells play a crucial role in maintaining vascular reactivity to hypoxia in isolated rat lungs. Chest 71S:253S-256S

Meyrick B, Reid L 1978 The effect of continued hypoxia on rat pulmonary arterial circulation. An ultrastructural study. Lab Invest 38:188-200

Meyrick B, Reid L 1979 Development of pulmonary arterial changes in rats fed with *Crotalaria spectabilis*. Am J Pathol 94:37-50

Meyrick B, Reid L 1980a Endothelial and subintimal changes in rat hilar pulmonary artery during recovery from hypoxia. A quantitative ultrastructural study. Lab Invest 42:603-615

Meyrick B, Reid L 1980b Hypoxia-induced structural changes in the media and adventitia of rat hilar pulmonary artery, and their regression. Am J Pathol 100:151–178

Murphy JD, Rabinovitch M, Goldstein J, Reid L 1980 The structural basis of neonatal persistent pulmonary hypertension. Pediatr Res, in press

Naeye RL 1965 Effect of alpha-methyl-dopa on heart and pulmonary arteries of hypoxic mice. Am J Physiol 209:702-704

Ooshima A, Fuller G, Cardinale E, Spector S, Udenfriend S 1975 Collagen biosynthesis in blood vessels of brain and other tissues of the hypertensive rat. Science (Wash DC) 190:898-900

Oštádal B, Ressl J, Urbanová D, Widimsky J, Procházka J, Pelouch V 1978 The effect of beta adrenergic blockade on pulmonary hypertension, right ventricular hypertrophy and polycythemia, induced in rats by intermittent high altitude hypoxia. Basic Res Cardiol 73:422-432

Pérez-Díaz J, Martín-Requero A, Parrilla R, Ayuso Parrilla MS 1977 Relationship between cellular energy production and rate of glucose utilization by lung cells. Pflügers Arch Eur J Physiol 371:19-24

Rabinovitch M, Gamble W, Nadas AS, Miettinen O, Reid L 1979 Rat pulmonary circulation after chronic hypoxia: hemodynamic and structural features. Am J Physiol 236:H818-H827

Rabinovitch M, Gamble WJ, Williams G, Reid L 1980 SQ 14,225 converting enzyme inhibitor diminishes pulmonary artery hypertension secondary to chronic hypoxia in rat. Fed Proc 39:765

Rendas A, Lennox S, Reid L 1979 Aorta-pulmonary shunts in growing pigs. Functional and structural assessment of the changes in the pulmonary circulation. J Thorac Cardiovasc Surg 77:109-118

Said SI, Yoshida T, Kitamura S, Vreim C 1974 Pulmonary alveolar hypoxia: release of prostaglandins and other humoral mediators. Science (Wash DC) 185:1181-1183

Sole MJ, Drobac M, Schwartz L, Hussain MN, Vaughan-Neil EF 1979 The extraction of circulating catecholamines by the lungs in normal man and in patients with pulmonary hypertension. Circulation 60:160-163

Stere AJ, Anthony A 1977 Myocardial Feulgen-DNA levels and capillary vascularization in hypoxia-exposed rats. J Appl Physiol 42:501-507

Suggett AJ, Herget J 1977 Effect of α-methyldopa on the pulmonary vascular changes induced by chronic hypoxia in rats. Clin Sci Mol Med 53:397-400

Unger M, Atkins M, Briscoe WA, King TK 1977 Potentiation of pulmonary vasoconstrictor response with repeated intermittent hypoxia. J Appl Physiol 43:662-667

Vaage J, Bjertnaes L, Hauge A 1975 The pulmonary vasoconstrictor response to hypoxia: effects of inhibitors of prostaglandin biosynthesis. Acta Physiol Scand 95:95-101

Watkins WD, Peterson MB, Crone RK, Shannon DC, Levine L 1980 Prostacyclin and prostaglandin E_1, for severe idiopathic pulmonary artery hypertension. Lancet 1:1083

Weir EK, McMurtry IF, Tucker A, Reeves JT, Grover RF 1976 Prostaglandin synthetase inhibitors do not decrease hypoxic pulmonary vasoconstriction. J Appl Physiol 41:714-718

Zakheim RM, Mattioli L, Molteni A, Mullis KB, Bartley J 1975 Prevention of pulmonary vascular changes of chronic alveolar hypoxia by inhibition of angiotensin I-converting enzyme in the rat. Lab Invest 33:57-61

Methods for the study of lung metabolism

H.F. WOODS, A. MEREDITH, G.T. TUCKER and J.R. SHORTLAND*

*University Departments of Clinical Pharmacology, Therapeutics and *Pathology, The Royal Hallamshire Hospital, Sheffield, S10 2JF, UK*

Abstract The recognition of the non-respiratory functions of the lung has led to an increased interest in pulmonary metabolism. The practical methods used to study metabolism in other tissues have all been applied to the investigation of lung metabolism. Methods fall into two groups: those used *in vivo* and those used *in vitro* after disrupting the organ or isolating it from other tissues and perfusing its circulation.

Some of the methods used *in vitro* disturb the tissue environment in such a way as to introduce experimental artifacts which make the interpretation of results difficult. There are advantages to the use of the isolated perfused organ technique which, although it has been established for many years, has recently been improved. This method lends itself particularly well to studies of the intermediary metabolism and uptake of drugs by lung tissue. These improvements are described and the application to pulmonary drug uptake is illustrated by reference to the drug mexiletine.

The relative advantages of the various methods and their applications are discussed.

The investigation of the physiological functions and responses of lung has been the main object of pulmonary research. Thus the published information on the metabolic activities of lung tissue is sparse when compared with that relating to pulmonary physiology in both health and disease. In recent years the non-respiratory functions of the lung have been identified and this has led to a considerable interest in the metabolism of lung tissue. This includes intermediary metabolism and the metabolism of naturally occurring compounds, drugs and toxic chemicals.

The methods that have been applied to the study of metabolism in other organs have all been applied to the lung and to a large extent it is the nature of the main thrust of pulmonary research rather than the availability of practical

Metabolic activities of the lung
(Ciba Foundation symposium 78) p 61-83

methodology which accounts for the relative shortage of metabolic information.

In this chapter we review the methods used for the study of lung metabolism and discuss their applications. In addition to a general survey, special consideration will be given to the influence of the type of preparation used on the results obtained and to the use of isolated perfused lung preparations.

If conclusions about the properties of metabolic pathways and the enzymes which comprise those pathways *in vivo* are to be drawn from experiments performed *in vitro,* it is essential to consider the influence of the type of preparation used upon the results obtained. This stricture arises from a consideration of the influence of tissue environment on metabolic processes. The problem has been reviewed by Youdim & Woods (1975) and before individual methods are described the relevance of the tissue environment will be discussed.

Within an organ cells are arranged in juxtaposition with other cell types, blood vessels and extracellular fluid, each component making up the structure which is characteristic of a particular organ. At a finer anatomical level within the cells there exists what has been described as the 'catalytic organization' (Dixon & Webb 1971) which parallels the cell morphology. Thus the subcellular organelles which have both common and specific metabolic functions are arranged within the cell in a pattern such that there exist numerous physical and metabolic compartments.

The question to be answered concerns how the disturbances of the organ and cellular environment which inevitably occur during the preparation of tissue samples for metabolic studies places limitations upon the investigator, in terms of the application of the methods and the interpretation of the results.

The methods available can be divided into two main groups, those used to study lung metabolism in the whole organism *in vivo* and those used *in vitro*

TABLE 1

Methods for the study of lung metabolism

In vivo	*In vitro*	*Perfused organ*
Arterio-venous differences across the organ		Isolated perfused lung *In situ* perfused lung
(Tissue biopsy) →	Tissue slices Tissue homogenates Tissue minces Isolated cells Subcellular fractions	
	Cells in culture	

after either disrupting the organ in some way or isolating it as a whole from all connections with other organs and perfusing it.

Table 1 shows a classification of the methods that have been used. In general these have all been employed in the study of the metabolism of other organs and it would be wrong to assume that their application to lung tissue has always been recent: slice techniques and homogenates were used over 40 years ago to study the lung.

The classification used in Table 1 takes into consideration the use of methods to obtain tissue samples which can be further treated and their metabolism studied at a lower level of anatomical organization.

METHODS USED IN VIVO

Whole-organ arterio-venous differences

The measurement of the uptake or production of a substance by an organ by determining the arterio-venous difference in concentration of that substance across the organ together with the blood flow through it is an established method in physiology and biochemistry. It has been successfully applied to the lung in a number of mammalian species including man. There are, however, problems of interpretation when it is used, although these do not apply equally to all types of substrate studied. The lungs have a large blood flow, receiving, as they do, the whole cardiac output, and it is this that leads to problems of application and interpretation. The large blood flow will hide concentration differences resulting from substrate uptake or production. Thus, there could be a substantial production or removal of a compound which would result in only a small change in the concentration gradient across the lung.

An example is the uptake of glucose by the rat lung. Tierney et al (1977) calculated, on the basis of isolated lung experiments, that the expected arterio-venous concentration differences for this substrate in the whole animal would be about 0.02 mmol/l. This concentration difference is so small as to be difficult to detect reliably and reproducibly using the available specific assay methods. Added to this difficulty are the problems of sampling where, because of the flow characteristics within the sampling blood vessels, there may be streaming of the blood, resulting in a sample being not necessarily representative of the concentration of compound in all of the blood entering or leaving the organ.

Although the concentration gradient may be too small to detect with accuracy and reproducibility it should not be supposed that this means that the lung is unimportant in the overall economy of the compound being studied. This is best illustrated by comparing the pulmonary and hepatic clearance of 5-hydroxytryptamine from the blood perfusing the lung and liver. Some 90% is removed by the lung when the organ is perfused at a rate of 10 ml/min (Alabaster & Bakhle 1970). The amine is then metabolized by the tissue monoamine oxidase.

The two variables to be considered when calculating the relative contributions of organs such as lung and liver to total 5-hydroxytryptamine clearance are the total activity of monoamine oxidase (metabolic capacity) in the organs and the blood flow to the organs.

The relationship between the rate of organ perfusion and hepatic clearance for certain drugs is well established. For drugs that are almost or completely removed from the blood during one passage through the liver (i.e. those with a high extraction ratio) the hepatic clearance depends on the magnitude of blood flow to the liver. Perfusion-limited models for the hepatic clearance of drugs have been described (e.g. Wilkinson & Shand 1975). These models include the intrinsic organ clearance, which is a measure of the maximal ability of an organ to remove a drug present in the blood perfusing the organ under conditions when there is no flow limitation. Rane et al (1977) showed that this quantity can be predicted from enzyme kinetic data obtained *in vitro* and used to predict the clearance of a drug in the whole animal. These concepts and methods have been applied to the problem of assessing the contribution of the lung to total drug clearance by Roth & Wiersma (1979). They determined 5-hydroxytryptamine clearance in both isolated perfused rat liver and lung and showed that although the monoamine oxidase content of lung is only 8% of that of the liver the total clearance of the compound by lung is three times larger than that by the liver. This arises in part from the fact that the lung receives the full cardiac output, the liver blood flow being 25% of that to the lung. If the clearance is perfusion limited, the lower enzyme activity of lung is compensated for by the larger lung blood flow.

Tissue biopsy

Biopsy of the lung during thoracotomy and percutaneous lung biopsy (Steel & Winstanley 1969) could both be applied to the study of lung metabolism. Although their place in diagnosis is well established their usefulness for metabolic studies is limited. If biopsies are obtained at thoracotomy there is the influence of underlying disease and its therapy, together with that of anaesthesia. Once obtained the biopsy tissue has to be studied at a lower level of tissue organization.

METHODS USED IN VITRO

The majority of metabolic studies of lung have been done using *in vitro* methods and there is considerable information on the limitations of each technique. These are best discussed individually.

Lung slices

The use of a tissue slice is a fundamental method in metabolic experiments and has been the commonest way of studying lung metabolism. Disruption of the tissue is inherent in the technique even if a standard slicing apparatus is used. This arises because of the lateral shear forces that are applied.

Once the slice has been prepared certain factors alter its metabolic capabilities. The slice has two cut surfaces and thus can lose intracellular contents such as enzymes, cofactors and ions by leakage. Some lysosomal enzymes may be activated, causing further cellular damage or death. When a slice is incubated the supply of substrates and the removal of metabolic products are abnormal, being through the cut surfaces rather than via the capillaries. Substrates can also enter via the alveolar surfaces. It is not clear whether this latter route may influence substrate supply or product removal through selective permeability or transport. Thus in the slice the normal concentration gradients may be destroyed and abnormal concentration differences become established.

We have mentioned the damage caused by tissue slicing. To this factor must be added the influence of slice thickness, because it is a determinant of both gas and metabolite diffusion. The limiting thickness of a tissue slice is determined by the metabolic rate of that tissue and the diffusion constraints of the reactants in the metabolic process being studied. Umbreit et al (1964) found that, in general, the limiting thickness is 0.5 mm or less when the tissues are exposed to oxygen at a pressure of one atmosphere. Levy & Harvey (1974) investigated these factors in relation to the metabolism of rat lung. When slices of varying thickness were prepared with a McIlwain tissue slicer the oxygen consumption was maximal when the slice thickness was between 0.6 and 1.0 mm. Slices less than 0.6 mm thick had a much lower oxygen consumption. These results are shown graphically in Fig. 1. Also shown are the results obtained when the lung tissue was sliced with a Stadie–Riggs microtome. These results were surprising in that, at the lower slice thickness, limitation of metabolism by substrate diffusion would not be expected. It was calculated that the lower respiratory rate of the thinner slices reflected tissue damage, particularly to the mitochondria. Similar findings have been reported for rat

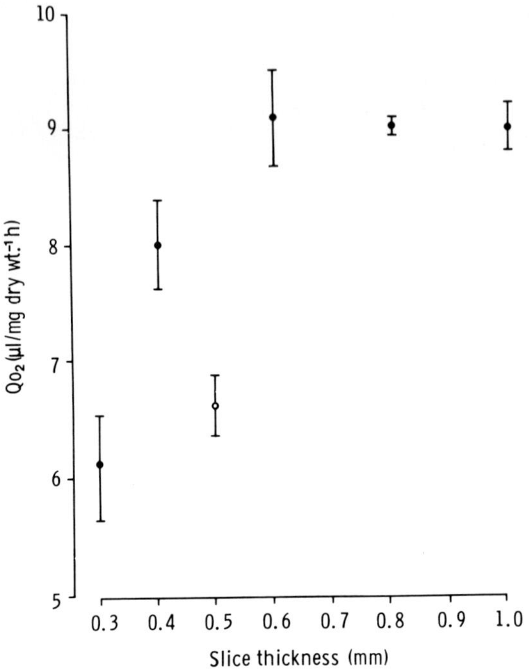

FIG. 1. The influence of slice thickness on oxygen consumption by lung slices from rats (Sprague-Dawley strain). The data have been plotted using the results of Levy & Harvey (1974). The closed circles represent mean (± SEM) values for lung slices cut with a McIlwain slicer. The open circle represents values (mean ± SEM) for slices cut with a Stadie–Riggs slicer. The oxygen consumption by slices of 0.5 mm thickness or less was significantly different from that of slices 1.00 mm thick.

liver slices by Fuhrman & Field (1945) and were predicted by Shorr (1942).

However, the maximal rates of respiration in slices may not represent the rate in the whole lung, because Faridy & Naimark (1971) found that the oxygen consumption of the isolated unperfused lung was lower than that of lung slices. A further factor investigated by these authors was that of tissue distention. In isolated lobes of dog lung the oxygen consumption was directly dependent upon the extent of inflation. This effect of mechanical distention was reversible.

A final modifying influence is that of temperature. Scholz & Rhoades (1971) found that lung slices were sensitive to the lowered temperature during the process of preparing the slices.

Tissue minces and homogenates

These preparations have been among the most unsatisfactory. The oxygen uptake of ground-up lung tissue is very low compared with that of tissue slices and it has been suggested that this is due to the leakage of intracellular metabolites, particularly adenine nucleotides (Ryan & Smith 1971).

The process of homogenization may expose to substrates enzymes that may not be accessible to substrates when the tissue is intact. The drugs chlorcyclizine and imipramine are oxidized by broken cell preparations from lung but not when they are delivered via the vascular system to the intact lung (Orton et al 1973, Eling et al 1975, Law et al 1974).

Isolated cells

The separation of single cell types in bulk has been applied very effectively in the study of metabolism in organs such as liver. The technique has been described for the lung by Gould et al (1972), but there remains the problem posed by the large variety of cell types within the organ.

Culture of single cell types has been used by Smith et al (1975) for the study of the lung and found to be useful.

Cell fractions

The use of cell fractions has not added much to knowledge of lung metabolism. The yield of structures such as mitochondria is low and again the multiplicity of cell types in lung leads to the possibility that the material obtained may be derived from only certain lung cells, as described by Reiss (1966).

General conclusions on organ fragments

The information presented so far demonstrates how experimental results can depend on the type of preparation used. The main points are summarized in Table 2. The interpretation of such results in relation to lung function *in vivo* must be made with caution. In particular it should always be remembered that *in vivo* a circulating compound may never come into contact with lung structures which *in vitro* either bind it or react with it in some other way.

TABLE 2

Problems with organ 'fragments'
Slices
1. Damage during preparation (mechanical/temperature)
2. Thickness of slice
3. Selective permeability
Minces and homogenates
1. Release of essential cofactors
Isolated cells
1. Difficult technique
2. Cell death
3. Change in cell characteristics
4. Cell selection
5. Substrate supply
Subcellular fractions
1. Low yield

WHOLE-ORGAN PREPARATIONS

The respiratory functions of lung have been studied using the perfused lungs of animals since Knowlton & Starling (1912) developed the heart–lung preparation. The importance of whole-organ preparations in pulmonary research is thus well established. This type of preparation has advantages which make it particularly suitable for the investigation of tissue metabolism (Table 3). However, it has not been widely used because of practical problems which arise because the lung is not an ideal organ for isolated perfusion studies. In order to conform with the 'ideal' described by Ross (1972, p 15) an organ should be easily accessible, have a single arterial supply and venous drainage, and consist of a single cell type. In practice, isolated perfused lung

TABLE 3

Advantages of the perfused lung
1. Anatomical relationships are maintained
2. The organ is isolated from other metabolically active tissues and organs
3. Avoidance of chemical modulators of lung perfusion and metabolism
4. Lends itself particularly to the study of excretion and detoxification
5. Gives the investigator considerable experimental flexibility

preparations in small animals have until recently been difficult to use because of lengthy operative procedures, subsequent low rates of perfusion, and pulmonary oedema. The whole lung has not been uniformly perfused and the time of perfusions has been short. Improved methods for small animals have recently been described. In this section these will be discussed, together with examples of their application to the investigation of drug uptake and metabolism.

Methods for lung perfusion

There are two main methods of perfusion. The first is that in which the lungs are removed intact from the thoracic cavity and either perfused via the attached vessels or superfused. The second method involves leaving the lungs within the thoracic cavity. The bulk of the whole-organ work has been done using the first of these methods, for example with the preparation used by Bakhle et al (1969). This method has been modified by using various types of ventilation and flow, as summarized in Table 4. The preparations usually have low flow rates (< 10 ml per minute) which may result from the considerable tissue manipulation involved and the subsequent release of vasoactive substances such as prostaglandins (Piper & Vane 1971).

Considerable improvements have been made to the second type of preparation (Table 4). Leary & Ledingham (1969) described a method in which the lungs remained intact within the thoracic cavity and were perfused by using

TABLE 4

Methods for lung perfusion

Isolated lung perfusion	
(a) Without ventilation	Bakhle et al (1969)
(b) With ventilation	
1. *Positive pressure*	
Pulsatile perfusion	Hauge (1968)
Hydrostatic perfusion	Levey & Gast (1966)
2. *Negative pressure*	Delaunois (1964)
	Niemeier & Bingham (1972)
In situ	
(a) Without ventilation	Leary & Ledingham (1969)
(b) With ventilation	Ross (1972, p 439)
	Stubbs (1979)
	Wolfe et al (1979)

the heart as a conduit after inserting cannulae into the left ventricle and right atrium. Flow rates greater than 30 ml per minute were achieved, which are comparable with those found in the rat by Spector (1956) (17–76 ml per minute). The method was used for short-term experiments and a major criticism of its use for studies of intermediary metabolism is the possible contribution of myocardial metabolism to any measured metabolic changes, because the heart is used as a conduit and is still beating.

This method forms the basis for that described by Stubbs (1979) and Wolfe et al (1979), and that used in our laboratory. A detailed description of this improved method can be found in the original literature. The advantages stem from two factors: the method of cannulation, which makes it rapid to set up, and the use of a semi-synthetic perfusion medium which does not include red cells. The cannulation is shown schematically in Fig. 2. The inflow cannula is inserted into the pulmonary artery through an incision in the right ventricle and the outflow cannula is then placed through a transverse incision in the tip of the left ventricle, being tied into position where the pulmonary veins enter the atrium.

The perfusion medium consists of bicarbonate-buffered saline (Krebs & Henseleit 1932) and dialysed bovine serum albumin (40 g/l), the mixture being gassed with a carbon dioxide–oxygen mixture (5% CO_2:95% O_2). The apparatus used is a modification of that described by Hems et al (1966) for perfusing the isolated liver and is housed in a thermostatically controlled heated cabinet. The perfusion circuit is shown in Fig. 3 (p. 72).

The viability of perfused lung preparations

The best way to judge the viability of an isolated perfused organ is a matter for discussion (Woods & Youdim 1977). Some authors have argued that the ability to carry out metabolic processes at a rate close to that observed *in vivo* is sufficient proof of viability. An alternative is to look upon the maintenance of lung structure at the gross and microscopic levels as an important test of viability.

The rat lung perfused *in situ* using the method outlined above has a creamy-white appearance and is perfused uniformly. This latter observation can be confirmed by adding dyes to the perfusion medium. A further simple test is to determine the ratio of dry weight to wet weight, which gives a good indication of water uptake. This ratio for unperfused lungs was 0.217 ± 0.013 (SD) and after 60 minutes of perfusion was 0.196 ± 0.016 (SD) (n = 32), suggesting a small water uptake during perfusion. When perfused lungs were examined by light microscopy and compared with unperfused lungs no gross changes were

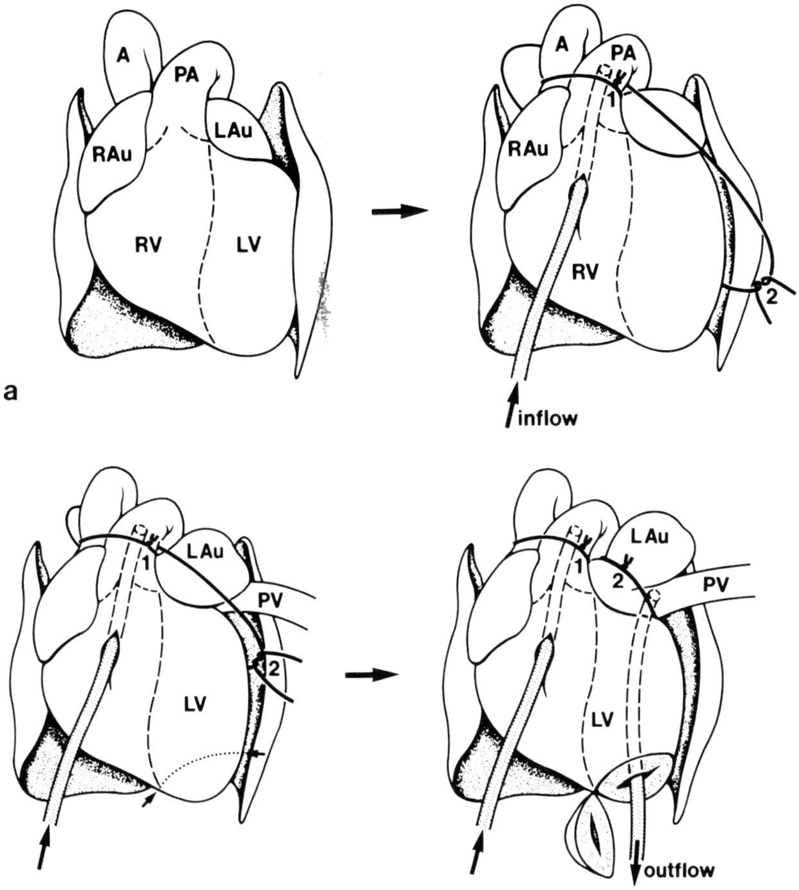

FIG. 2. The cannula positions and ligature placement necessary for perfusion of the isolated lung of the rat. (a) Inflow cannula. (b) Outflow cannula. A, Aorta; PA, pulmonary artery; PV, pulmonary vein; RV, right ventricle; LV, left ventricle; R Au, right auricle; L Au, left auricle.

detected. However, electron microscopy revealed changes comparable with the small increase in the ratio of dry weight to wet weight. The most characteristic feature was lifting of the endothelium away from the basement membrane (Fig. 4). These changes were not seen throughout the lung and were detected only after perfusions lasting 60 minutes or more.

Applications of the method to lung metabolism

The use of the preparation in the study of the intermediary metabolism of

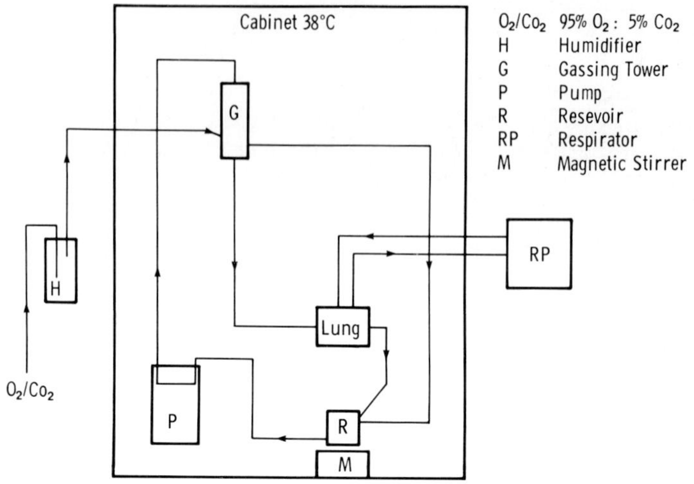

FIG. 3. Schematic diagram of the perfusion circuit for the isolated rat lung. The apparatus is shown in the form used for a constant pressure perfusion with ventilation of the lungs. In experiments where constant flow is needed a second pump is placed in the 'inflow' part of the circuit between the gassing tower and the lung.

lung has been described by Stubbs et al (1977) and is discussed elsewhere in this volume (Datta et al, p 85–104). We have used it to investigate uptake of drugs by the lung. This can be studied in two ways (Fig. 5). In the first the lung is perfused with a medium containing the drug which is recycled continuously. Serial determinations of the drug concentration in the medium are made and the uptake is determined. Fig. 5b shows such an experiment using the anti-arrhythmic drug mexiletine, which is a primary amine. It is rapidly taken up from the medium by the lung tissue.

The efflux of the drug can be studied by substituting a new medium, as shown in Fig. 5b. In this case the efflux is small and does not account for all the drug removed from the medium in the first part of the experiment. The tissue concentration can be measured after freeze-clamping the lung. These experiments show the flexibility of the method.

A second method for studying drug uptake is by simultaneous estimation of arterial and venous concentrations across the organ during a 'once through' perfusion (Fig. 5c). In this case the drug concentration in the efflux from the lung rises towards that in the medium entering the lung. When the uptake of mexiletine is studied in this way the efflux concentration does not reach that of the input. This may represent either a 'slow' component of the uptake system, or alternatively drug metabolism.

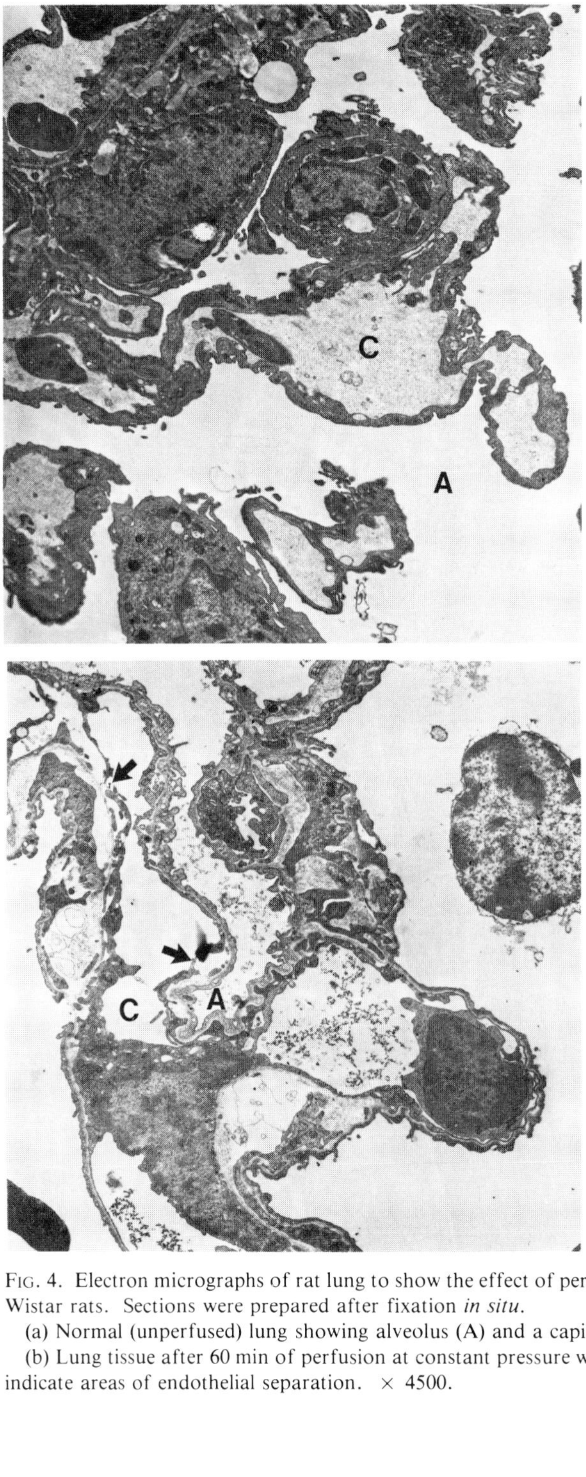

a

b

FIG. 4. Electron micrographs of rat lung to show the effect of perfusion. The animals were male Wistar rats. Sections were prepared after fixation *in situ*.

(a) Normal (unperfused) lung showing alveolus (A) and a capillary (C). × 3700.

(b) Lung tissue after 60 min of perfusion at constant pressure without ventilation. The arrows indicate areas of endothelial separation. × 4500.

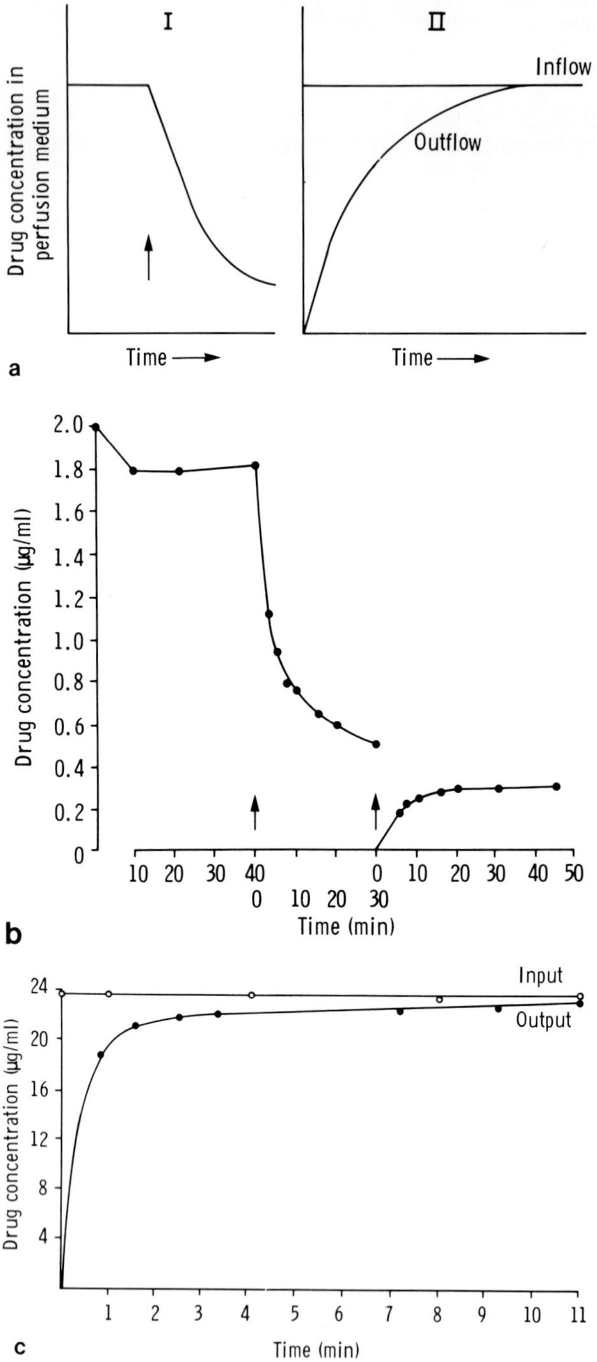
I
II
Inflow
Outflow
Drug concentration in perfusion medium
Time
a
2.0
1.8
1.6
1.4
1.2
1.0
0.8
0.6
0.4
0.2
0
Drug concentration (μg/ml)
10 20 30 40
0 10 20 30
0 10 20 30 40 50
Time (min)
b
24
20
16
12
8
4
Drug concentration (μg/ml)
Input
Output
1 2 3 4 5 6 7 8 9 10 11
Time (min)
c

General conclusions on whole-organ preparations

The newer perfusion methods for the lungs of small animals have the advantage of providing a stable preparation that can be used for long periods. The cannulation technique means that preparations can be set up rapidly, thus avoiding tissue anoxia. There are, however, the possible adverse effects of the high oxygen tension in the perfusion medium. The toxic effects of oxygen on the lung have been described by many authors (e.g. Fisher 1978), and these are difficult to avoid with the red-cell-free medium.

It would thus be wrong to assume that 'perfusion is best' for all experimental situations. The simple lung slice technique can yield important results with a simple experimental system. A good example of this is the work of Smith et al (1974) on the uptake of paraquat by lung.

The perfused lung is, however, at an early stage of use when compared to other methods, and has already yielded important results in the field of drug disposition in both normal and abnormal lung (Junod 1976, Roth 1979, Dollery & Junod 1976, Gardiner et al 1979).

ACKNOWLEDGEMENTS

The data in Fig. 1 are reproduced with permission. A. Meredith is a Medical Research Council research student. The authors wish to thank Dr W.A. Stubbs for his invaluable advice when developing the method of lung perfusion for drug studies.

References

Alabaster VA, Bakhle YS 1970 Removal of 5-hydroxytryptamine by rat isolated lung. Br J Pharmacol 38:440-441P

Bakhle YS, Reynard AM, Vane JR 1969 Metabolism of the angiotensins in isolated perfused tissues. Nature (Lond) 222:956-959

Delaunois AL 1964 A new isolated lung apparatus. Arch Int Pharmacodyn Ther 148:597-606

Dixon M, Webb EC 1971 Enzymes, 2nd edn. Longman, London, p 621

Dollery CT, Junod AF 1976 Concentration of (±)-propranolol in isolated perfused lungs of rat. Br J Pharmacol 57:67-71

Eling TE, Pickett RD, Orton TC, Anderson MW 1975 A study of the dynamics of imipramine accumulation in the isolated perfused rabbit lung. Drug Metab Dispos 3:389-399

Faridy EE, Naimark A 1971 Effect of distention on metabolism of excised dog lung. J Appl Physiol 31:31-37

←

FIG. 5. Uptake of drugs by the isolated perfused rat lung. (a) The two methods of studying drug uptake in the perfusion system: by recycling (I) and by a 'once through' perfusion (II). These are illustrated in (b) and (c), which show the uptake of mexiletine by the perfused rat lung by the two methods. In (b) the vertical arrows show when the lung was placed in the circuit and when subsequently the perfusion medium was replaced by one free of drug. (Male Wistar rat.)

Fisher AB 1978 Energy status of the rat lung after exposure to elevated Po_2. J Appl Physiol 45:56-59

Fuhrman FA, Field J 1945 Factors determining the metabolic rate of excised liver tissue. Arch Biochem 6:337-349

Gardiner TH, McAnally BH, Heaton J, Reynolds RC 1979 Changes in pulmonary uptake and binding of drugs in an experimental model of lung fibrosis. Toxicol Appl Pharmacol 49:487-496

Gould KG, Clements JA, Jones AL, Felts JM 1972 Dispersal of rabbit lung into individual viable cells. A new model for the study of lung metabolism. Science (Wash DC) 178:1209-1210

Hauge A 1968 Conditions governing the pressor response to ventilation hypoxia in isolated perfused rat lungs. Acta Physiol Scand 72:33-34

Hems R, Ross BD, Berry MN, Krebs HA 1966 Gluconeogenesis in the perfused rat liver. Biochem J 101:284-292

Junod AF 1976 Uptake, release and metabolism of drugs in the lungs. Pharmacol Ther 2:511-521

Knowlton FP, Starling EH 1912 The influence of variations in temperature and blood pressure on the performance of the isolated heart. J Physiol (Lond) 44:208-219

Krebs HA, Henseleit K 1932 Untersuchungen über die Harnstoffbildung im Tierkörper. Hoppe-Seylers Z Physiol Chem 210:33-66

Law FCP, Eling TE, Bend JR, Fouts JR 1974 Metabolism of xenobiotics by the isolated perfused lung. Comparison with *in vitro* incubations. Drug Metab Dispos 2:433-442

Leary WP, Ledingham GG 1969 Removal of angiotensins by isolated perfused organs of the rat. Nature (Lond) 222:959-960

Levey S, Gast R 1966 Isolated perfused rat lung preparation. J Appl Physiol 21:313-316

Levy SE, Harvey E 1974 Effect of tissue slicing on rat lung metabolism. J Appl Physiol 37:239-240

Niemeier RW, Bingham E 1972 An isolated perfused lung preparation for metabolic studies. Life Sci 2:807-820

Orton TC, Anderson MW, Pickett RD, Eling TE, Fonts JR 1973 Xenobiotic accumulation and metabolism by isolated perfused rabbit lungs. J Pharmacol Exp Ther 186:482-497

Piper PJ, Vane JR 1971 The release of prostaglandins from lung and other tissues. Ann N Y Acad Sci 180:363-385

Rane A, Wilkinson GR, Shand DG 1977 Prediction of hepatic extraction ratio from *in vitro* measurements of intrinsic clearance. J Pharmacol Exp Ther 203:377-387

Reiss OF 1966 Studies of lung metabolism. I. Isolation and properties of sub-cellular fractions from rabbit lung. J Cell Biol 30:45-57

Ross BD 1972 Perfusion techniques in biochemistry – a laboratory manual. The Clarendon Press, Oxford

Roth JA 1979 Use of isolated perfused lung in biochemical technology. In: Hodgson E et al (eds) Reviews in biochemical toxicology. Elsevier, Amsterdam

Roth RA, Wiersma DA 1979 Role of the lung in total body clearance of circulating drugs. Clin Pharmacokinet 4:355-367

Ryan JW, Smith V 1971 Metabolism of adenine 5-monophosphate during circulation through the lungs. Trans Assoc Am Physicians 84:297-306

Scholz RW, Rhoades RA 1971 Lipid metabolism of rat lung *in vitro*. Effect of starvation and refeeding on utilisation of [U-^{14}C]glucose by lung slice. Biochem J 124:257-264

Shorr E 1942 Factors affecting the preparation of tissue for metabolic studies. In: Symposium on respiratory enzymes. University of Wisconsin Press, Madison, Wisconsin, p 268

Smith BT, Girond CPJ, Robert M, Avery M 1975 Insulin antagonism of cortisol action on lecithin synthesis by cultured foetal lung cells. J Pediatr 87:953-955

Smith LL, Wright A, Wyatt I, Rose MS 1974 Effective treatment for paraquat poisoning in rats and its relevance to treatment of paraquat poisoning in man. Br Med J 4:569-571

Spector WS 1956 In: Handbook of physiological data. Saunders, Philadelphia, p 279

Steel SJ, Winstanley DP 1969 Trephine biopsy of the lung and pleura. Thorax 24:516-584

Stubbs WA 1979 Metabolic studies of the lung. PhD Thesis, University of Southampton
Stubbs WA, Morgan I, Lloyd B, Alberti KGMM 1977 The effect of insulin on lung metabolism in the rat. Clin Endocrinol 7:181-184
Tierney DF, Young SL, O'Neil JJ, Abe M 1977 Isolated perfused lung – substrate utilization. Fed Proc 36:161-165
Umbreit WWR, Borris RH, Stauffer JF 1964 Manometric techniques. Burgess, Minneapolis, p 132
Wilkinson GR, Shand DG 1975 A physiological approach to hepatic drug clearance. Clin Pharmacol Ther 18:377-390
Wolfe RR, Hochachka PW, Trelstad RL, Burke JF 1979 Lactate oxidation in perfused rat lung. Am J Physiol 236:276-282
Woods HF, Youdim MBH 1977 The isolated perfused rat brain preparation – a critical assessment. In: Youdim MBH et al (eds) Essays in neuropharmacology. Wiley, Chichester, vol 12:46-69
Youdim MBH, Woods HF 1975 The influence of tissue environment on the rates of metabolic processes and the properties of enzymes. Biochem Pharmacol 24:317-323

Discussion

Alberti: What is your view about the usefulness of isolated cells in the study of pulmonary metabolism?

Woods: I have no experience of this myself, but we have heard already about the problems of harvesting lung cells by perfusion techniques with, for example, collagenase (p 27). I think it would be difficult to separate the cells shed in this way to give sufficient numbers to study. It has been used successfully for obtaining cells for culture and for studying the metabolism of those cells after a period in culture.

Ayuso-Parrilla: We have been working with a preparation of isolated rat lung cells that appears to be a very convenient experimental model for studies on lung metabolism (Pérez-Díaz et al 1977a). The whole procedure for obtaining the isolated cells is very rapid and consists in perfusing the vascular system of the lungs *in situ* with buffer in order to remove the blood. After about five minutes' perfusion, buffer containing collagenase is injected through the trachea and the lung is taken out of the chest. The tissue is then finely minced and incubated with collagenase.

The functional viability of the lung cells isolated by this procedure is shown by the following criteria: (1) more than 95% of the cells exclude vital dyes like eosin or nigrosine; (2) the rate of oxygen utilization is constant for several hours; (3) substrates are utilized and metabolites produced at constant rates for long periods of incubation; and (4) added ADP is unable to alter the rate of respiration.

The efficiency of the lung cell isolation procedure is about 25%. This can be considered as optimal, taking into account the large number of non-cellular supporting structures contributing to the total fresh weight.

Alberti: Which cell types are you actually dealing with?

Ayuso-Parrilla: We obtain a mixture of cells in which we can identify the different types of alveolar cells present in the lung tissue by their staining or ultrastructural organization characteristics. Of course, we cannot be sure that the proportions of the different cell types are the same as in the whole lung, but at least we know that the different cell types are present, and the metabolic parameters studied so far (Pérez-Díaz et al 1977b) compared rather well with those reported for the perfused organ (Rhoades et al 1975, Stubbs et al 1977b).

Woods: I don't want to give the impression that perfusion is best; there are very good examples of the use of, for example, tissue slices. In terms of medical application, the work of Rose et al (1974) on the uptake of paraquat by human lung slices has led to interesting suggestions about the treatment of paraquat poisoning.

Morishige: When you are studying the metabolism of agents passing through the perfused lung, how do you account for the retention of the substance within the lung cells?

Woods: There is information on this. Dr Junod has published work on the uptake of propranolol by the isolated perfused lung (Dollery & Junod 1976). Our own work also suggests that for some drugs this must be an active process, perhaps dependent upon energy metabolism.

Piper: Have you any evidence that if the perfusion rate is not the physiological rate, you get misleading results on metabolism in the lung?

Woods: I can't answer that directly. Some of the problems of the earlier studies on the isolated perfused lung did arise because it was not possible to obtain rates of flow anywhere near the rate seen in the living rat. One advantage of the methods derived from Leary's work (Leary & Ledingham 1969) is that we can get rates of flow up to and beyond 20 ml/min through the whole lung preparation. I don't know how that affects metabolism. One could postulate that with particularly low rates of flow, if products that were inhibitory were not being removed from the organ rapidly enough, as does happen in perfused liver, one might alter the rates of metabolism.

Piper: You would however have longer contact between the drug to be metabolized and the tissue and this might give erroneously high values.

Alberti: Most of the published metabolic studies have used flow rates of about 4–15 ml/min. We, like you, have been using the perhaps more physiological range of 20–30 ml/min. The differences in metabolic response are not large, and are unlikely to affect intermediary metabolism, in a gross sense, although I am always more comfortable using more physiological flow rates.

Vane: One difference between the ventilated and unventilated lung could be in the amount of oedema. In the non-ventilated lung most people clamp off the trachea, so they don't see what oedema is formed. Do you see any in your preparation?

Woods: No, not in our preparation, either ventilated or unventilated. This brings up the subject of viability and how you judge it in this system. We evaluate this using histology and electron microscopy and on simple measures like wet/dry weight ratios. This ratio after one hour in our non-ventilated and ventilated preparations is no different from that measured in lungs taken straight out of the animal. Electron microscopy shows certain changes; there is some stripping and separation of the endothelial layer (Fig. 4, p 73) but no gross oedema. We do not find ventilation-dependent differences in rates of drug uptake. It doesn't matter whether you ventilate the lung or not, the uptake mechanism for drugs seems to be working at the same rate and in the same way. That may not apply to other processes.

Ballard: Do you envisage any special problems in perfusing the fetal lung?

Woods: We have perfused some organs such as brain where the vessels to be cannulated were very small (Woods et al 1976). I can imagine that there would be problems in some species, simply because of size.

Stalcup: We have perfused fetal rabbit lungs from 20 days' gestation, when the fetus weighs 4–7 g, up to term, when it reaches 45–50 g (Stalcup et al 1978). We were able to cannulate the pulmonary vessels; we had to perfuse *in situ,* since isolated fetal rabbit lungs become desiccated. One can use these techniques in the fetal lung; ligating the ductus arteriosus is the most difficult part.

Junod: The main advantage of perfusing the lung *in situ* is the maintenance of lymphatic drainage. What is the P_{O_2} of your perfusion medium? Do you use 95% oxygen, as most people do? Would hyperoxia affect the results you obtain?

Woods: That is an important point. The P_{O_2} in this sort of preparation is very high, about 200 mmHg in the perfusion medium. This may have some relevance to the results. It may also affect the rates of metabolism measured, if high oxygen concentrations influence metabolic pathways.

Stubbs: Over a four-hour perfusion period, pulmonary oedema isn't a problem with the *in situ* preparation. Histologically we found interstitial oedema, although we don't know whether this is due to the use of non-pulsatile flow, the high P_{O_2}, or some other cause.

The use of pulsatile or non-pulsatile flow may affect vasomotor tone, interstitial fluid flow and the cellular metabolism of the lung and other organs (Withers et al 1962, Trinkle et al 1969).

On the question of oxygen tension, Bassett & Fisher (1979) found that oxygen at one atmosphere produced no detectable changes in lung metabolism, although oxygen at five atmospheres for 80 minutes did. Watkins & Rannels (1979) showed that lung perfusion over four hours with 20% and 95% oxygen gave similar results in terms of tissue ATP and glycogen and glucose uptake. I don't think that the 'high' P_{O_2} (around 500 mmHg) we use is influencing lung metabolism over four hours, although I think we could reduce the O_2 tension.

Ventilation produces another variable when lung metabolism is examined, since it affects glucose uptake (Gassenheimer & Rhoades 1974, Tierney et al 1977), metabolite production (Stubbs et al 1977a) and the clearance of drugs (Roth & Gillis 1977). It is obviously necessary to pay close attention to ventilation characteristics when examining lung metabolism. Most lung preparations have an absolute requirement for ventilation if one is to prevent pulmonary oedema. Our *in situ* system has the advantage that ventilation can, if you wish, be omitted. Incidentally, these comments may also have clinical relevance in designing the best ventilation characteristics for patients.

In general, the choice of preparation really depends on the questions being asked. If you want to investigate basic biochemical mechanisms, for example, isolated cells can provide an acceptable technique.

Aiken: Is the inclusion of albumin in the perfusion medium important for the viability of the preparation and, if so, doesn't binding of drugs by this protein complicate the interpretation of data?

Woods: It *is* essential; unless we have about 4 g/100 ml of albumin we find rapidly developing oedema in our perfused lungs. In drug studies, binding is certainly a factor. If you use a drug that is highly protein bound and you don't have a physiological concentration of albumin, you alter the kinetics of that drug in the system. Equally, of course, this is an example of flexibility of the system, because it provides a way of looking at the effect of protein concentration on the handling of a drug.

Said: Does the addition of blood elements make the situation easier or more complicated?

Woods: Much more complicated. We have used aged human red cells with bovine serum albumin and Krebs–Henseleit buffer; but it caused problems, because there is no pump which does not cause haemolysis.

Said: Would plasma alone be better?

Woods: Perhaps, but it will contain various small molecular weight substances that are vasoactive and thus alter the rate and pattern of perfusion in the tissue.

Slater: Some liver perfusion procedures (for example, see Bullock et al 1974) have used a circulating pump based on a pulsating rubber diaphragm. In general, this reduces the extent of haemolysis compared to what happens with peristaltic pumps, and satisfactory perfusions have been regularly performed over 6–8 hours. Has such a pumping arrangement been used with lung perfusions?

Woods: It has been tried in the lung and found to be effective.

Slater: When the perfusate in isolated liver perfusions is gassed with 95% O_2:5% CO_2, significant and early changes occur in the lysosome population (Abraham et al 1968). In particular, there is a rapid increase in the number of secondary lysosomes, indicative of some cellular injury. Does the same happen in lungs during perfusion experiments?

Woods: I can't answer that; we haven't looked for it.

Ferreira: May I comment on the cardiac output in the non-anaesthetized rat? The dye dilution technique gives a value of about 40 ml per 100 g; thus a 250 g rat has a cardiac output of 100 ml/min (Salgado & Krieger 1976). In fact, all the perfusion experiments are being done in far from physiological conditions.

Stubbs: We obtained flow rates of about 20–30 ml/min in the rat lung perfusion *in situ*. How frightened are your rats?

Ferreira: They are quite all right!

Reid: Our rats are conditioned to the procedure, which is repeated each day, so they are *not* terrified. We find a value of 35 ml/min per 100 g, or about 90–100 ml/min per 250 g rat.

Bakhle: The problem of flow may not be as important as it sounds because, for instance in dogs *in vivo,* you can increase the flow rate five times and not change the conversion of angiotensin I to II (Fanburg & Glazier 1973). Surely,when you increase or decrease flow you merely recruit or lose vessels, so perhaps even at the lowest rates you are fully perfusing just one vessel, whereas at a higher rate more vessels are perfused. The point is that flow rate doesn't change metabolism in perfusion experiments.

Stubbs: Certainly in our *in situ* system and that of Watkins & Rannels (1979) the concentrations of indicators of tissue metabolism such as ATP were similar at the beginning and end of the perfusion. This suggests that, despite the experimental limitations, including the flow rate, the preparation remains reasonably intact.

Alberti: Since the preparation also has no red blood cells, and no innervation, one can't really consider it a physiological preparation anyway!

Woods: We are always arguing about this. Let me turn it back on you: one application of such a preparation, whether liver or lung or any perfused organ, is that it enables you to separate out individual variables.

Junod: I think that flow *does* matter in some respects, because the results (uptake, extraction rates etc.) are generally related to lung weight. If you use a flow of 20 ml/min for a lung weighing 1 g and perfuse only 20% of the units, you should relate values to 0.2 g of lung, rather than 1 g. Otherwise, the correlation you try to establish with the weight of lung is not correct. It is important in kinetic studies. We should be aware that we are still dealing with a very crude method.

Stubbs: It is crude, but when dye is introduced into the perfusate of the *in situ* preparation, serial sections of the lung show it to be evenly distributed.

Alberti: In other words, it is slower perfusion rather than regional perfusion. That would agree with the fact that you don't see much difference in glucose metabolism with variations between flow of 6 or 7 ml/min and 30 ml/min. I do, however, accept Dr Junod's comment, and we need to go on looking for other ways to establish whether flow is or is not physiologically important.

Reid: It is extremely important to know whether or not, with perfusion, there really is maximum opening up of the vascular bed, as Dr Junod indicates. How do you measure uniformity of distribution, Dr Stubbs? Is the whole lung, grossly, stained blue? Or have you some way of knowing that every capillary is dilated?

Stubbs: No, I suspect that not every capillary is perfused.

References

Abraham R, Dawson W, Grasso P, Goldberg L 1968 Lysosomal changes associated with hyperoxia in the isolated perfused rat liver. Exp Mol Pathol 8:370-387

Bassett DJP, Fisher AB 1979 Glucose metabolism in rat lung during exposure to hyperbaric O_2. J Appl Physiol 46:943-949

Bullock G, Eakins MN, Sawyer BC, Slater TF 1974 Studies on bile secretion with the aid of isolated perfused rat liver. I. Inhibitory action of sporidesmin and icterogenin. Proc R Soc Lond B Biol Sci 186:333-356

Dollery CT, Junod AF 1976 Concentration of (±)propranolol in isolated, perfused lungs of rat. Br J Pharmacol 57:67-71

Fanburg BL, Glazier JB 1973 Conversion of angiotensin I to angiotensin II in the isolated perfused dog lung. J Appl Physiol 35:325-331

Gassenheimer LN, Rhoades RA 1974 Influence of forced ventilation on substrate metabolism in the perfused rat lung. J Appl Physiol 37:224-247

Leary WP, Ledingham JG 1969 Removal of angiotensin by isolated perfused organs of the rat. Nature (Lond) 222:959-960

Pérez-Díaz J, Carballo B, Ayuso-Parrilla MS, Parrilla R 1977a Preparation and metabolic characterization of isolated rat lung cells. Biochimie (Paris) 59:411-416

Pérez-Díaz J, Martin-Requero A, Parrilla R, Ayuso-Parrilla MS 1977b Relationship between cellular energy production and rates of glucose utilization by lung cells. Pflügers Arch Eur J Physiol 371:19-24

Rhoades RA, Shaw ME, Eskew ML 1975 Influence of altered O_2 tension on substrate metabolism in perfused rat lung. Am J Physiol 229:1476-1479

Rose MR, Smith LL, Wyatt J 1974 Evidence for energy dependent accumulation of paraquat into rat lung. Nature (Lond) 252:314-315

Roth RA, Gillis CN 1977 Effect of ventilation on removal of [^{14}C]mescaline by perfused rabbit lung. Biochem Pharmacol 26:325-329

Salgado MCO, Krieger EM 1976 Cardiac output in unrestrained conscious rats. Clin Exp Pharmacol Physiol (Suppl 3):165-167

Stalcup SA, Pang LM, Lipset JS, Odya CE, Goodfriend TL, Mellins RB 1978 Gestational changes in pulmonary converting enzyme activity in the fetal rabbit. Circ Res 43:705-711

Stubbs WA, Kelly DM, Walters FJ, Alberti KGMM 1977a The metabolic characteristics of the ventilated and non-ventilated perfused rat lung. Biochem Soc Trans 5:1312-1314

Stubbs WA, Morgan I, Lloyd B, Alberti KGMM 1977b The effect of insulin on lung metabolism in the rat. Clin Endocrinol 7:181-184

Tierney DF, Young SL, O'Neil JJ, Abe M 1977 Isolated perfused lung–substrate utilization. Fed Proc 36:161-165

Trinkle JK, Helton NE, Wood RE, Bryandt LR 1969 Metabolic comparison of a new pulsatile pump and a roller pump for cardiopulmonary bypass. J Thorac Cardiovasc Surg 58:562-569

Watkins CA, Rannels DE 1979 *In situ* perfusion of rat lungs: stability and effects of oxygen tension. J Appl Physiol 47:325-329

Withers H, Regelson W, Hoffmeister F 1962 The physiologic importance of pulsatile blood flow. N Engl J Med 267:443-446

Woods HF, Graham CW, Green AR, Youdim MBH, Grahame-Smith DG, Hughes JT 1976 Some histological and metabolic properties of an isolated perfused rat brain preparation with special reference to monoamine metabolism. Neuroscience 1:313-323

Substrate utilization by the lung

H. DATTA, W.A. STUBBS* and K.G.M.M. ALBERTI

*Department of Clinical Biochemistry and Metabolic Medicine, Royal Victoria Infirmary, Newcastle upon Tyne, NE1 4LP, and * Department of Medicine, St. Bartholomew's Hospital, West Smithfield, London EC1, UK*

Abstract Intermediary metabolism of the lung and its regulation have received relatively little attention in the past, partly because of difficulty in producing suitable models for study. An *in situ* perfused rat lung preparation is described which remains viable for four hours or more. Concentration-dependent glucose utilization has been found with this model, associated with marked lactate production. More than half the glucose used appears as lactate, despite the high Po_2 and maintenance of normal ATP concentrations. The high rates of glycolysis may be related to glycerol-3-phosphate requirements for lipid synthesis. Glucose clearance from the perfusion medium is dependent on nutritional status, clearance by lungs from 48-hour starved animals being decreased by comparison with lungs of fed controls. Lactate is taken up actively at concentrations of 2 mmol/l or above but is produced at an initial lactate concentration of 0.4 mmol/l. Non-esterified fatty acids (1 mmol/l in the perfusate) are also cleared by lung and may be important as an energy source even though 80% is used for synthetic reactions. Alanine, glycerol and 3-hydroxybutyrate are unimportant as substrates.

The lung responds to metabolically important hormones. Insulin and adrenaline cause an acute increase in glucose utilization whereas corticosterone and noradrenaline are inhibitory. Utilization of glucose is also diminished in lungs from diabetic ketoacidotic rats.

Further work is required to establish the relative importance of oxidative and synthetic routes for added substrates and the mechanisms of hormonal regulation.

'... the lung is not only the place of excretion of carbonic acid ... and of the absorption of oxygen. This organ is also at the same time, to a variable degree, the place of the converse phenomenon; that is to say, a process in which oxygen is consumed and carbonic acid formed' (Bohr & Henriques 1897).

Despite the comments of Bohr and Henriques more than 80 years ago relatively little attention has been paid to the metabolism of the lung with respect to either its own energy requirements or its possible contribution to

Metabolic activities of the lung
(Ciba Foundation symposium 78) p 85-104

whole-body metabolism. Sporadic reports have appeared but only in the past 15 years have serious attempts been made to delineate the metabolic requirements of the lung.

Glucose has been the most widely investigated of the possible oxidative substrates (Table 1). However, glucose may have a more important role, in that it provides the glycerol moiety for phospholipid synthesis and, via the pentose phosphate pathway, the NADPH needed for fatty acid synthesis (Felts 1964). Indeed it has recently been suggested that the lung may preferentially oxidize other substrates in the presence of glucose (Wolfe et al 1979), again emphasizing the non-oxidative roles of glucose.

The substrates other than glucose reported to be used by lung are shown in Table 1. Discrepant results have been reported for lactate. Mitchell & Cournand (1955) were unable to demonstrate utilization although Eppinger & Wagner (1920) and Tierney (1971) reported definite clearance and metabolism of lactate by lung. The physiological importance of the utilization of some of the other substrates listed remains questionable in view of the unphysiological concentrations tested.

The main problem in assessing and interpreting previous work relates primarily to the many different methods and tissue preparations used. There has been considerable difficulty in obtaining satisfactory well-validated preparations for studying the lung. Lung slices, the isolated lung, isolated alveolar cells and arterio-venous (A-V) differences have all been used with varying degrees of success. A-V differences, based on the Fick principle, have been applied successfully to many organs and appear to be ideal for studying lung *in vivo*. Eventually, however, it was realized that even a relatively high substrate clearance produces only a small difference in substrate concentra-

TABLE 1

Substrates utilized by lung

Substrate	*Reference*
Glucose	Tierney 1974
NEFA }	Van Golde 1976
Glycerol }	Rhoades 1974
Lactate	Eppinger & Wagner 1920
	Tierney 1971
	Wolfe et al 1979
Pyruvate	Lochner et al 1957
Acetate	Salisbury-Murphy et al 1966
Citrate	Scholz 1972
Amino acids	Massaro et al 1971
	Gacad et al 1972

tion between artery and vein because of the large blood flow of lung. O'Neil & Tierney (1974) calculated that the expected A-V difference in glucose concentration would be only 0.02 mmol/l, which is less than the variability of most methods used to measure glucose.

Studies using slices, technically the easiest preparation, present the greatest problems, including diffusional problems, the release of proteolytic enzymes, which cause tissue damage, and depressed metabolic rates. Krebs (1970) showed that liver tissue slices lost 72% of their ATP after 10 minutes and ketogenesis was tenfold less than in the isolated perfused organ. In contrast, isolated cells and cell fractions yield useful information on the metabolism and characteristics of the cell studied. The lung, however, contains many different cell types and the influence of the delicate morphological relationship of one cell type to another will be lost.

The most satisfactory model available for studying lúng metabolism is the isolated perfused lung, although its use is obviously restricted to animal investigation. The possible advantages are:

(1) Substrate supply takes place through capillaries – that is, the physiological route;

(2) The metabolism of the whole organ with the spatial arrangement of its constituent cells undisturbed can be studied;

(3) There is minimal damage to the organ;

(4) Neurohumoral factors are removed, allowing easier interpretation of data, although metabolic regulation may thereby be changed from the *in vivo* state.

Despite these obvious advantages relatively little use has been made of the perfused lung, with studies restricted mainly to dog and rat. The major reason is that preparing the isolated organ is difficult and time-consuming, with many preparations remaining viable for only short periods.

In our own laboratory we have been able to produce an isolated rat lung that can be maintained for four hours or more. We have used this preparation to re-investigate and extend previous work on substrate utilization, and have gone on to examine the effects of metabolically important hormones on substrate utilization. The results of these investigations are reported here and compared with results obtained by other workers.

METHOD

The method is described in detail elsewhere (Stubbs 1979). In brief, Wistar rats (300–450 g) with free access to water and standard laboratory chow, except where stated, are anaesthetized with sodium pentobarbital. After thoracotomy the animals are heparinized and a polythene tube is inserted into the pulmonary artery through the right ventricle. The ventricles are cut transversely and a second cannula is inserted into the left atrium. Care is taken to trim off excess cardiac tissue so that diffusion from myocardium does not contribute to any observed metabolic changes. The lungs are left *in situ* and are perfused by a system similar to that used for liver (Hems et al 1966).

There are several advantages of this system. Since the lung is left *in situ,* as suggested by Leary & Smith (1970), the operation can be performed rapidly (5–10 minutes) and there is relatively little handling of the lung tissue itself. This could be important, in that Piper & Vane (1971) have suggested that handling of lung may release vasoactive substances, particularly prostaglandins, which could influence lung metabolism.

The second benefit is that a medium free of red blood cells is used. This is obviously unphysiological but eases interpretation of metabolic data. Even aged red cells, classically used in perfusion systems, produce enough lactate from glucose to conceal the relatively small metabolic changes observed with lung. Thus after two hours' circulation of an appropriate amount of red cells we have calculated that 150 μmol glucose/g dry weight of lung would be apparently used and 220 μmol lactate/g dry weight produced. Instead a buffer containing albumin is used and sufficient oxygen is carried in solution to supply the requirements of the lung. We have found a P_{O_2} of 547 $\pm$ 10 mmHg at the beginning of perfusion and 493 $\pm$ 16 mmHg after four hours' perfusion. Equivalent figures for P_{CO_2} were 28 $\pm$ 1 and 26 $\pm$ 1 mmHg and for pH, 7.3 $\pm$ 0.01 and 7.4 $\pm$ 0.01. The criticism could be made that the P_{O_2} is supraphysiological (Clark & Lambertsen 1971) and that this could have deleterious effects.

On histological examination the perfused lungs show some perivascular oedema which may be due either to the high P_{O_2} or to the use of non-pulsatile flow, as suggested by others (O'Neil & Tierney 1974, Bassett & Fisher 1976). On the other hand, lung water content did not increase detectably during four hours' perfusion in most cases. The problem of whether the perfused lung should or should not be ventilated is difficult. Our own studies suggest that it may not be necessary (Stubbs & Alberti 1980).

Finally, we use flow rates of 20–30 ml/min which are within the range reported for pulmonary blood flow in the normal rat (17–76 ml/min), this being achieved with a hydrostatic pressure of about 25 cm. These values are higher than the 4–16 ml/min reported by many others (Levey & Gast 1966, Fisher et al 1974, Rhoades 1974, O'Neil & Tierney 1974, Bassett & Fisher 1976).

RESULTS AND DISCUSSION

Glucose utilization and lactate production by perfused rat lung

Initially we studied lungs from fed rats. Glucose clearance from the perfusion medium was concentration dependent (Table 2), as previously shown by Weber & Visscher (1969) and Shaw & Rhoades (1975), with a threefold increase in clearance when the concentration in the perfusate was increased from 1.5 to 8 mmol/l (Stubbs 1979). Lactate production was high, with lactate/glucose ratios between 1 and 2.

Table 2 shows glucose clearance rates and lactate production reported by other workers for perfused lung from rat, dog and rabbit. The values obtained are similar to our own. It is also evident that lactate production represents a significant proportion of glucose utilization, 50% or more. 'Utilization' as used in this paper implies clearance from the perfusion medium and not necessarily metabolism. However, using lung slices Yeager & Massaro (1972) have shown directly that of the glucose consumed, 30% was recovered as lactic acid; while Longmore & Mourning (1976) found that 60–80% of the lactate produced is derived from glucose. It is not known why there should be such a preponderance of glycolysis; perhaps it is required to generate glycerol-3-phosphate for phospholipid production.

We next investigated the effects of the nutritional status of the rat on lung metabolism. Lungs were perfused after 48 hours of starvation. Glucose utilization (Fig. 1, Table 3) was clearly decreased in lungs from the starved

TABLE 2

Glucose utilization and lactate production by perfused lung of fed rats

Reference	*Species*	*Perfusate glucose concentration (mmol/l)*	*Glucose utilization* (μ*mol/g dry wt per h)*	*Lactate production*
Evans et al 1934	Dog	5.5 – 11	35	35
Koga 1956	Rabbit	5.5	44 – 78	32 – 37
Lochner & Nasseri 1960	Dog	5.3	212	250
Levey & Gast 1966	Rat	8.3	45	83
Weber & Visscher 1969	Dog	4.8	41	25
		15.3	69	41
O'Neil & Tierney 1974	Rat	4.2	70	75
Rhoades 1974	Rat	5.0	131	101
Stubbs 1979	Rat (fed)	1.5	30	43
		4.0	57	76
		8.0	91	131
This study	Rat (fed)	5.0	101	115

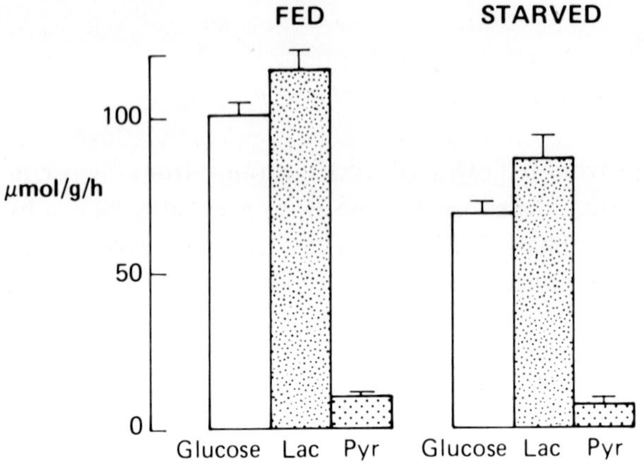

FIG. 1. Glucose utilization and lactate and pyruvate production by lungs from fed and 48-hour starved rats. Glucose was present at 5 mmol/l in the perfusion medium. Perfusions were for 4 h and uptake and production rates are calculated from the change in substrate concentration in the medium during the entire perfusion (30 min equilibration, followed by 3½ h experimental period). *n* = 5 or more.

TABLE 3

Glucose utilization and lactate production (means ± SEM) by lungs from fed and starved rats perfused for four hours

Reference	*n*	*Perfusate glucose concentration (mmol/l)*	*Glucose utilization* (*μmol/g dry wt per h*)	*Lactate production* (*μmol/g dry wt per h*)
Rhoades 1974				
Fed	12	5.0	132 ± 10.5	102 ± 7.10
72-h starved	12	5.0	123 ± 10.0	105 ± 4.70
Stubbs 1979				
Fed	5	4.0	57 ± 3	76 ± 4
48-h starved	5	4.0	40 ± 2	63 ± 6
This study				
Fed	10	5.0	101 ± 3.0	115 ± 6.0
48-h starved	8	5.0	68 ± 3.0	86 ± 7.0

rats. Lactate production was decreased relatively less, as reflected by a rise in the lactate/glucose ratio. These results are in contrast to those of Rhoades (1974) who found no effect of starvation, but was using a different perfusion system. Other workers have, however, found changes in lung metabolism with starvation: incorporation of glucose into lung lipids was decreased by 40% in starved compared with fed rats (Scholz & Rhoades 1971), and the activity of enzymes of pulmonary fatty acid and phospholipid synthesis is markedly decreased by fasting (Gross et al 1975).

In general the lung seems to behave like other tissues in contributing to overall glucose conservation during starvation (Cahill 1976). The predominance of lactate production in the starved state could be due to decreased pyruvate dehydrogenase activity, as found in other tissues. This hypothesis is supported by the finding of increased amounts of pyruvate in freeze-clamped lung of starved rats.

Unlike many other tissues lung contains little glycogen, although the amount does show a significant decrease in the starved state (4.0 ± 0.1 versus 2.7 ± 0.1 μmol/g wet weight). Similarly, triglyceride levels are relatively low (12.5 ± 1.5 versus 6.9 ± 0.9 μmol/g wet weight; $P < 0.01$). The lung must therefore depend largely on exogenous substrates, although we have found that even with no added substrates in the perfusion medium the lung maintains its morphological integrity over a four-hour period and continues to produce lactate. This lactate could arise from endogenous amino acid metabolism although, as described below, alanine, a major amino acid found in many tissues, is poorly catabolized by lung.

Utilization of other substrates by perfused rat lung

Lactate has received more attention as a product of glycolysis in the lung than as a substrate in its own right. In the absence of glucose the lung from fed rats takes up lactate in a concentration-dependent fashion from concentrations of 2 mmol/l (Datta & Alberti 1979) (Fig. 2). At 0.4 mmol/l, significant amounts of lactate are produced. Utilization was not influenced by nutritional state. Wolfe et al (1979) studied the relative contributions of lactate and glucose to CO_2 production when both substrates were present. They found, as we did (Datta & Alberti 1979), that at high lactate concentrations (10 mmol/l) there was substantial oxidation of lactate. More important, when both substrates were present in physiological concentration (5 mmol/l glucose and 1 mmol/l lactate) there was preferential oxidation of lactate. Lactate may therefore be an important fuel for lung in situations such as exercise where circulating lactate levels are raised. It should be emphasized that the lactate level must be somewhat elevated for it to contribute significantly to oxidative metabolism.

We have also examined the non-lipid substrates alanine and glycerol. As Fig. 2 shows there is a small but significant clearance of alanine and of glycerol by the lung. This was achieved, however, at supraphysiological concentrations and neither is likely to be important as a substrate *in vivo*.

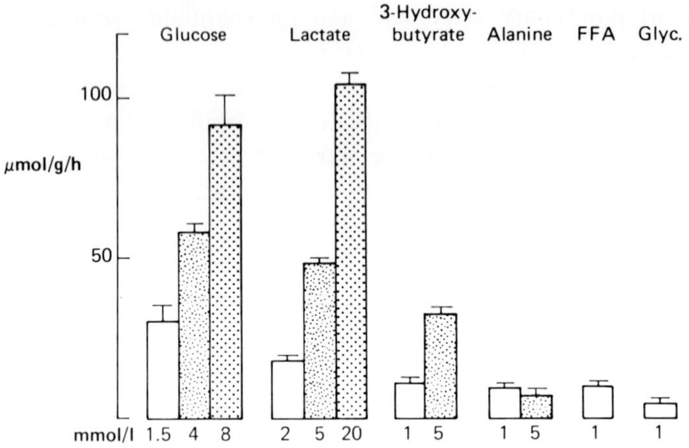

FIG. 2. Utilization of different substrates by perfused lung from fed rats. FFA, non-esterified fatty acid (palmitate); Glyc., glycerol. Conditions as described in legend to Fig. 1. Results are given as µmol/g dry weight per h. Substrate concentrations in the perfusion medium are shown below the bars.

The lipid metabolites 3-hydroxybutyrate and non-esterified fatty acids (NEFA) have also been investigated. Relatively small amounts of the ketone body are used (Fig. 2), but clearance is increased threefold by increasing the perfusate concentration from 1 to 5 mmol/l. Interestingly, values were 50% higher in lungs from fed than from starved rats. NEFA were also taken up by perfused lung (Fig. 2). At the physiological concentration of 1 mmol/l, utilization was only one-fifth of that of glucose at 5 mmol/l. However, the ATP yield per mole from the oxidation of fatty acid is much greater than that from glucose, particularly as much of the glucose is metabolized only as far as lactate. At 30% oxidation of glucose only 12 moles of ATP would be formed per mole of glucose used. NEFA could therefore be relatively important as a substrate. Fatty acids are, however, also incorporated into triglyceride and phospholipids. Felts (1964) has nonetheless shown that the rate of oxidation of palmitic acid by the lung is second only to that in the kidney, up to 20% being recovered as CO_2. This would still yield 26 moles ATP per mole palmitic acid used. Our results differ from those of Rhoades (1974), who found twice as much NEFA utilization as we did and no dependence on nutritional status, wheras we again found lower clearance rates by lung from fasted rats. Rhoades (1975) later showed increased fatty acid oxidation in lung slices from starved rats, but decreased fatty acid incorporation into lipids.

Several broad conclusions can be drawn from these results. On a molar

TABLE 4

Preferred substrates for lung

Molar basis	*Physiological basis*
Glucose	Glucose
Lactate	Fatty acid
Fatty acid	Lactate
3-Hydroxybutyrate	3-Hydroxybutyrate
Alanine	Alanine
Glycerol	Glycerol

basis glucose is the most important substrate for lung with fatty acid and lactate coming next (Table 4). Physiologically – that is, on the basis of normal circulating concentrations – glucose is probably still the most important substrate, although fatty acids are also important, and lactate may be. Account must be taken of other disposal routes for these substrates. We have measured only clearance or total utilization, not oxidation. Thus glucose is obviously important in the generation of glycerol-3-phosphate and fatty acids in lipid metabolism, while lactate is largely oxidized. On the other hand, with lactate at low normal concentration (0.4 mmol/l) the lung produces rather than takes up lactate. Further experiments are necessary with quantitative estimation of carbon disposal to establish the preferred substrates for lung *in vivo*.

Effect of hormones on glucose utilization by lung

In receiving the whole of the circulation of the body the lung is constantly bathed by a hormone-rich medium. It would be surprising if some of these hormones did not influence lung metabolism. In terms of the whole animal the most important hormones influencing metabolism are the anabolic hormone insulin, and the catabolic hormones cortisol (corticosterone in the rat), adrenaline, noradrenaline and glucagon.

Insulin. Although Salisbury-Murphy et al (1966) and Felts (1964) were unable to show acute effects of insulin on glucose utilization, other workers such as Weber & Visscher (1969) and Moxley & Longmore (1977) have found positive effects of insulin on glucose disposal. More recently, Morishige et al (1977) have demonstrated insulin receptors in rat lung, while Fricke & Longmore (1979) have shown that insulin enhances 2-deoxyglucose transport into lung. Conversely, glucose utilization is diminished in lungs from diabetic rats (Stubbs 1979).

We have examined both the acute and chronic effects of insulin on glucose disposal. In the acute experiments insulin was added to the perfusion medium at physiological (50 mU/l) and supraphysiological (500 mU/l) concentrations. Glucose utilization was increased by 50 mU/l insulin in lungs from fed but not starved rats (Table 5). In fed rats there was no further increase with 500 mU/insulin but a significant increase was now found in lungs from starved animals.

In chronic experiments rats were made diabetic with streptozotocin and maintained on insulin for one week as previously described (Blackshear & Alberti 1974). Insulin treatment was then withdrawn from one group and the lungs were perfused in insulin-treated and insulin-deficient rats. Glucose utilization was significantly increased (+ 30%) in lungs from insulin-treated rats by comparison with control values (non-diabetic rats) and little further effect was noted when insulin was added to the perfusion medium. Lungs from ketoacidotic animals cleared significantly less glucose than lungs from either control or insulin-treated rats. Again no effect was noted when insulin was added to the perfusion medium. Lactate production/glucose clearance ratios were also markedly increased in ketoacidotic rat lungs.

Lungs were freeze-clamped after perfusion with and without insulin in addition to 5 mmol/l glucose. With insulin at 50 mU/l there were significant decreases in the concentration of glucose, lactate and ADP, while levels of glucose-6-phosphate and citrate and the ATP/ADP ratio rose. Triglyceride and citrate levels were unchanged.

Our findings in the diabetic rats confirm those of Morishige et al (1977) and

TABLE 5

Acute effect of insulin on glucose utilization and lactate production by lung from fed and 48-hour starved rats

Addition to perfusion medium	*Fed*		*Fasted*	
	Glucose utilization	*Lactate production*	*Glucose utilization*	*Lactate production*
	(μmol/h per g dry weight)			
4 mM-glucose	57 ± 3	76 ± 4	40 ± 2	63 ± 6
4 mM-glucose + 50 mU/ml insulin	73 ± 5	98 ± 1	37 ± 5	72 ± 3
4 mM-glucose + 500 mU/ml insulin	74 ± 4	87 ± 1	50 ± 3	70 ± 4

Conditions as in Fig. 1.
Data from Stubbs et al (1977) and Stubbs (1979).

Moxley & Longmore (1977). The acute effect of insulin on glucose clearance has not previously been described, presumably because of the shorter perfusion times used by others or the use of different lung preparations. It seems clear, however, that insulin plays a role in regulating carbohydrate as well as lipid metabolism in the lung.

Glucocorticoids. Acute and chronic effects of glucocorticoids were investigated (Alberti et al 1978). In the acute experiments corticosterone was added to the perfusion medium to give a final concentration of 100 μg/100 ml. At this concentration there was a 28% decrease in glucose uptake and lactate production by lungs from fed rats. Glucose clearance was decreased by 18% when lungs from starved rats were perfused with corticosterone. This decrease in glucose clearance or uptake caused by glucocorticoids has been described in several other tissues (Alberti & Johnston 1977).

In the chronic experiments rats were given 'Synacthen depot' (a synthetic ACTH-like preparation) 36 and 12 hours before lung perfusion. Glucose utilization was unchanged but lactate and glycerol production was decreased in lungs from fed rats.

There has been considerable interest in the effects of glucocorticoids on lung metabolism, directed mainly at surfactant production. Glucocorticoid receptors have been identified (Ballard 1977, Iacobelli et al 1978) but little attention has been paid to the effects of glucocorticoids on substrate utilization. Further studies using labelled and diverse substrates are necessary.

Catecholamines. We have also looked at the effects of the catecholamines adrenaline and noradrenaline on glucose metabolism in the perfused lung. Noradrenaline is cleared rapidly by lung, so it was added to the perfusate initially and again after 90 minutes of perfusion. Care was taken to use concentrations of the hormones which might be encountered *in vivo*. All studies were done on lungs from fed rats, with 5 mmol/l glucose in the perfusing medium.

Adrenaline at 400 pg/ml caused a 30% increase in glucose clearance but no significant rise in lactate production (Fig. 3). Interestingly, at a supraphysiological concentration of adrenaline (10 ng/ml), the increase of glucose clearance was not significant after four hours of perfusion although increases were significant at several time points up to four hours. Again lactate production was unchanged. By contrast noradrenaline (10 ng/ml) inhibited glucose utilization by 40% and lactate production by 30%.

A possible mechanism of action of catecholamines is through changes in perfusate flow. Total flow was unaltered but there may have been a

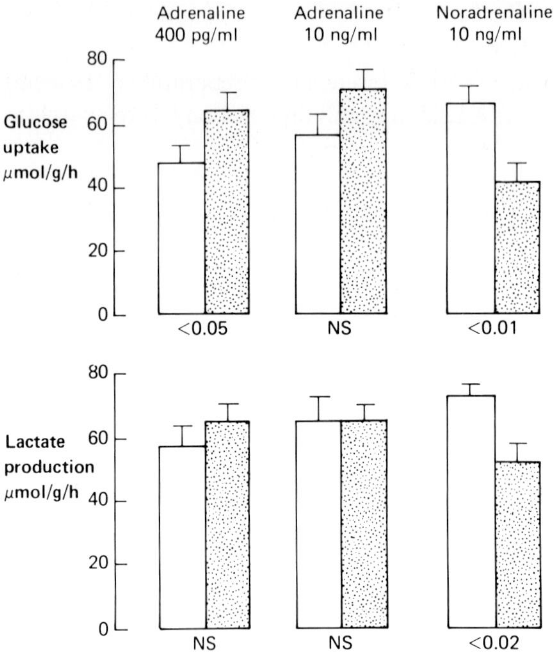

FIG. 3. Effect of adrenaline and noradrenaline in the perfusion medium on glucose utilization and lactate production by lung from fed rats. Open columns, control values. Stippled columns, values with catecholamine. Initial concentrations of catecholamines are shown. Further noradrenaline was given at 90 min in the noradrenaline experiments. Glucose present at 5 mmol/l in the perfusion medium. *P* values are shown: NS, not significant; $P < 0.05$.

redistribution of flow within the lung. The smaller apparent effect of high doses of adrenaline may have been due to stimulation of α-receptors as well as β-receptors. The exact mechanisms remain to be elucidated.

CONCLUSIONS

The studies summarized here, together with recent work from other groups, show that the lung is able to use a wide variety of substrates, with glucose, lactate and non-esterified fatty acids the most important. More information is needed on the interplay between these substrates and the relative amounts used for synthetic purposes and energy production. The lung responds to a variety of metabolically important hormones and shows variation in substrate utilization with nutritional status. It would be interesting to know what effect other hormones, such as glucagon, have on pulmonary metabolism, and whether there are any metabolic effects of the many peptide hormones that can be taken up and metabolized by lung.

Finally, it should be stressed that the lung contains many different types of cell. The perfused preparation by its very nature gives no information on the metabolism of individual cell types. The studies of Plopper & Morishige (1978) suggest that granular (type II) pneumonocytes are most affected morphologically by experimental diabetes, while others have described methods for preparing free lung cells (Gould et al 1972). Studies with isolated cells need to proceed in close juxtaposition to those of the whole organ and to *in vivo* studies if we are to establish in more detail the use of substrates by the lung and the regulation of their metabolism.

ACKNOWLEDGEMENTS

We gratefully acknowledge the financial assistance of Southampton University, Newcastle Area Health Authority (T) and the British Diabetic Association. W.A.S. was in receipt of an MRC Training Fellowship during part of this work. We are also grateful to Dr I. Morgan and Dr D. Kelly for their assistance.

References

Alberti KGMM, Datta H, Kelly DM, Morgan I, Stubbs WA 1978 Carbohydrate metabolism in the lung. Biochem Soc Trans 6:527-530

Alberti KGMM, Johnston DG 1977 Cortisol and catabolism: a new perspective. Clin Sci Mol Med 52:333-336

Ballard PL 1977 Glucocorticoid receptors in the lung. Fed Proc 36:2660-2665

Bassett DJP, Fisher AB 1976 Metabolic response to carbon monoxide by isolated rat lungs. Am J Physiol 230:658-663

Blackshear PJ, Alberti KGMM 1974 Experimental diabetic ketoacidosis. Biochem J 138:107-117

Bohr CH, Henriques V 1897 Comparison des quotients respiratoires déterminés simultanément dans le sang et dans l'air expiré. Arch Physiol 9:819-831

Cahill GF Jr 1976 Starvation in man. Clin Endocrinol Metab 5:397-415

Clark JM, Lambertsen CJ 1971 Pulmonary oxygen toxicity: a review. Pharmacol Rev 23:37-133

Datta H, Alberti KGMM 1979 Substrate utilization by the isolated perfused rat lung. Biochem Soc Trans 7:1026-1028

Eppinger H, Wagner R 1920 Zur Pathologie der Lunge. Wien Arch Inn Med 1:83-146

Evans CL, Hsu FY, Kosaka T 1934 Utilisation of blood sugar and formation of lactic acid by lungs. J Physiol (Lond) 82:41-61

Felts JM 1964 Biochemistry of the lung. Health Phys 10:973-979

Fisher AB, Steinberg H, Bassett DJP 1974 Energy utilization by the lung. Am J Med 57:437-446

Fricke RF, Longmore WJ 1979 Effects of insulin and diabetes on 2-deoxy-D-glucose uptake by the isolated perfused rat lung. J Biol Chem 254:5092-5098

Gacad G, Dickie K, Massaro D 1972 Protein synthesis in lung; influence of starvation on amino acid incorporation into protein. J Appl Physiol 33:281-284

Gould KG, Clements JA, Jones AL, Felts JM 1972 Dispersal of rabbit lung into individual viable cells. A new model for the study of lung metabolism. Science (Wash DC) 178:1209-1210

Gross I, Rooney SA, Warshaw JB 1975 The inhibition of enzymes related to pulmonary fatty acid and phospholipid synthesis by dietary deprivation in the rat. Biochem Biophys Res Commun 64:59-63

Hems R, Ross BD, Berry MN, Krebs HA 1966 Gluconeogenesis in the perfused rat liver. Biochem J 101:284-292

Iacobelli S, Ranelletti F, Sica G, Basile G 1978 Glucocorticoid receptors in human fetal lung. J Endocrinol Invest 1:209-213

Koga H 1956 Studies on the function of isolated perfused mammalian lung. II. Carbohydrate metabolism of rabbit lung. Kumamoto Med J 9:182-187

Krebs HA 1970 Rate control of the tricarboxylic acid cycle. Adv Enz Regul 8:335-353

Leary WP, Smith U 1970 *In situ* perfusion of rat lung. Life Sci 9:1321-1326

Levey S, Gast R 1966 Isolated perfused rat lung preparation. J Appl Physiol 21:313-316

Lochner W, Nasseri M 1960 Weitere Untersuchungen über den Eigenstoffwechsel der Lunge, insbesondere eine Freisetzung unveresterten Fettsaüren. Arch Ges Physiol Mens Tiere (Pflugers) 272:180-186

Lochner W, Piiper J, Schumeyer E, Bostrom B 1957 Über die Grosse eines Milchsaüreschwundes in der Lunge narkotisierter Hunde. Arch Ges Physiol Mens Tiere (Pflugers) 264:549-560

Longmore WJ, Mourning JT 1976 Lactate production in isolated perfused rat lung. Am J Physiol 231:351-354

Massaro D, Simon MR, Steinkamp H 1971 Metabolic factors affecting protein synthesis by lung *in vitro.* J Appl Physiol 30:1-6

Mitchell AM, Cournand A 1955 The fate of circulating lactic acid in the human lung. J Clin Invest 34:471-476

Morishige WK, Uetake CA, Greenwood FC, Akaka J 1977 Pulmonary insulin responsivity: *in vivo* effects of insulin on the diabetic rat lung and specific insulin binding to lung receptors in normal rat. Endocrinology 100:1710-1722

Moxley MA, Longmore WJ 1977 Effect of experimental diabetes and insulin on lipid metabolism in the isolated perfused rat lung. Biochim Biophys Acta 488:218-224

O'Neil JJ, Tierney DF 1974 Rat lung metabolism: glucose utilization by isolated perfused lungs and tissue slices. Am J Physiol 226:867-873

Piper PJ, Vane JR 1971 The release of prostaglandins from lung and other tissues. Ann NY Acad Sci 180:363-385

Plopper CG, Morishige WK 1978 Alterations in granular (type II) pneumocyte ultrastructure by streptozotocin-induced diabetes in the rat. Lab Invest 38:143-148

Rhoades RA 1974 Net uptake of glucose, glycerol and fatty acids by the isolated perfused rat lung. Am J Physiol 226:144-149

Rhoades RA 1975 Influence of starvation on the lung: effect on glucose and palmitate utilization. J Appl Physiol 38:513-516

Salisbury-Murphy S, Rubenstein D, Beck JC 1966 Lipid metabolism in lung slices. Am J Physiol 211:988-992

Scholz RW 1972 Lipid metabolism by rat lung *in vitro:* utilisation of citrate by normal and starved rats. Biochem J 126:1219-1224

Scholz RW, Rhoades RA 1971 Lipid metabolism by rat lung *in vitro.* Biochem J 124:257-264

Shaw ME, Rhoades RA 1975 Influence of hypoglycemia on glucose metabolism in perfused lung. Fed Proc 34:427

Stubbs WA 1979 Metabolic studies of the lung. PhD thesis, University of Southampton

Stubbs WA, Alberti KGMM 1980 The lung, whole-body metabolism and disease. This volume, p 351-368

Stubbs WA, Morgan I, Lloyd B, Alberti KGMM 1977 The effect of insulin on lung metabolism in the rat. Clin Endocrinol 7:181-184

Tierney DF 1971 Lactate metabolism in rat lung tissue. Arch Intern Med 127:858-860

Tierney DF 1974 Lung metabolism and biochemistry. Annu Rev Physiol 36:209-231

Van Golde LMG 1976 Metabolism of phospholipids by the lung. Am Rev Respir Dis 114:977-1000
Weber KC, Visscher MB 1969 Metabolism of the isolated canine lung. Am J Physiol 217:1044-1052
Wolfe RR, Hochachka PW, Trelstad RL, Burke JF 1979 Lactate oxidation in perfused rat lung. Am J Physiol 236:E276-E282
Yeager H, Massaro D 1972 Glucose metabolism and glycoprotein synthesis by lung slices. J Appl Physiol 32:477-482

Discussion

Parrilla: You have shown that the perfused lung can use lactate as a substrate. However, the fact that lung tissue relies heavily on glucose as a fuel (Pérez-Díaz et al 1977a), converting 65% of it into lactate, seems to be in conflict with the idea of lung cells as lactate users.

Alberti: It depends on concentration, as in any other tissue. With little lactate in the medium, both liver and lung tissue produce lactate. We obtained significant lactate production only at a low lactate concentration of 0.4 mmol/l.

Parrilla: Lung cells under physiological conditions always receive lactate in conjunction with glucose (with an approximate glucose/lactate ratio of 10). I agree that if lactate alone is added to a lung or isolated lung cell preparation, some lactate may be 'used', since the system is being forced to do that. In order to maintain equilibrium between lactate dehydrogenase reactants, about a tenth of the lactate will be converted to pyruvate and a rise in the steady-state levels of pyruvate will favour its transamination or its oxidation in the Krebs cycle. My point is not whether lung cells could eventually use lactate but whether this utilization has any physiological significance since, as I said, lung cells are never exposed to lactate alone but in combination with much higher concentrations of glucose which is used preferentially by lung cells.

Alberti: When Wolfe et al (1979) used a higher lactate concentration than our 0.4 mmol/l, namely 1 mmol/l, together with 5 mmol/l glucose, they obtained preferential oxidation of lactate, so presumably if it is available it will be oxidized. It makes sense to use whatever substrate is most available, whether fatty acids, lactate or glucose, so that metabolism doesn't stop. If skeletal muscle 'stops' for a bit it doesn't matter; if heart or lung stop metabolizing actively, there would be immediate problems. That is a teleological argument!

Parrilla: From a teleological point of view also, lactate production is important because it seems to be the main way of reoxidizing NADH; from our findings we believe that NADH shuttles probably cannot translocate reducing equivalents across the inner mitochondrial membrane efficiently, so *in vivo* apparently the lung cell must be a producer rather than a consumer of lactate in order to reoxidize the NADH produced in glycolysis.

Alberti: We know from Wolfe that at high lactate concentrations (10 mmol/l) lactate is oxidized; it is still energetically more sensible to regenerate NAD from NADH by going into the Krebs cycle, because ATP is produced. Higher lactate concentrations force lactate through the system, and produce oxidation *per se*.

Parrilla: I agree that it would be more sensible to reoxidize NADH in the Krebs cycle; however, for some still unclear reason, lung cells do not do that, since they prefer to convert 65% of the glucose utilized into lactate rather than oxidizing pyruvate in the Krebs cycle, obtaining a more beneficial energetic balance. On the other hand, when you add small amounts of glucose to isolated lung cells the rate of oxygen consumption falls by 40–60% (Ayuso-Parrilla et al 1978). This suggests that when glucose is present the main method of reoxidizing NADH is by the conversion of pyruvate into lactate.

Datta: We don't know how all the NADH is oxidized; lactate production may not be the only way of regenerating NAD from NADH. Lung mitochondria actively synthesize fatty acids (Tombropoulos 1964), unlike the mitochondria in liver and adipose tissue, and will probably be dependent on a shuttle system to transfer the reducing equivalent since the mitochondrial membrane is impermeable to pyridine nucleotides. The malate–aspartate shuttle system could serve this function, and its activity will be high in type II alveolar cells, where most of the mitochondria in lung are found (Fisher 1976).

Parrilla: Actually, it doesn't matter whether NADH enters the mitochondria or not, because in the presence of glucose the rate of the respiratory chain has been decreased by 60%; in our experience these shuttles are not efficient enough in these cells but, even if they were, the respiratory chain would be unable to reoxidize an increased supply of NADH.

Datta: You are using isolated lung cells; it depends which cells you have taken. You may have left out cells that have a more active shuttle system, such as alveolar type II cells.

Parrilla: We used a mixed population of lung cells (Pérez-Díaz et al 1977b) which behaves similarly to whole lung from a metabolic point of view.

Alberti: This is a theoretical argument where further data will resolve the issue. I think we agree that glycolysis is an efficient way of regenerating NAD but that if lactate is available in high concentration, it is used for that purpose and oxidized.

Gryglewski: Using 0.4 mmol/l of lactate you appear to have a decrease in lactate consumption by the lungs. What does this imply? Is lactate not used, or does the endogenous lactate stimulate endogenous lactate production?

Alberti: It means that endogenous lactate production is continuing. With a higher concentration of lactate, such as 2 mmol/l, production is blocked and there is a net uptake of lactate. In most situations the lung will be producing rather than taking up lactate but there are physiological situations, such as exercise, where blood lactate levels are higher. In these conditions the lung will tend to take lactate up.

Gryglewski: So the low concentration of exogenous lactate does not stimulate lung tissue to generate *extra* lactate. The lung is continuing to generate lactate at the same level.

Woods: It has been said that the dependence of the lung on glycolysis as a major source of energy gives it an advantage over other tissues. Have you studied the maximum glycolytic capacity of your system? From the proportion of glucose taken up going to lactate one could calculate the maximal ATP production; what is the upper limit of the capacity of the system? Have you tried making the preparation hypoxic?

Alberti: No, and we haven't gone to the upper limits of glucose concentration. Some recent results on anaerobic metabolism showed that lactate output increases only a little with hypoxia, suggesting that normally the lung is relying on glycolysis, equivalent to a slightly anaerobic state (Longmore & Mourning 1976).

Bakhle: Is the fact that the lung gets a lot of oxygen 'free' reflected in its biochemistry in any direct way?

Alberti: No; in fact Bill Stubbs thinks that, on the contrary, this reliance on glycolysis rather than oxidative metabolism may be a way of *preventing* the lung from getting into a state of oxygen toxicity, because oxygen is so much more readily available than in other tissues.

Said: Two of the most metabolically active cells in the lung, namely the alveolar macrophages and the type II alveolar cells, are known to depend on oxidative phosphorylation (Said et al 1966), so the overall reliance of the lung on glycolysis seems surprising. Do we know which cell types are responsible for the glycolysis?

Alberti: It doesn't have to be glycolysis alone; fatty acids are a good substrate for oxidative metabolism and are well used by the lung. What is the percentage of lung mass made up by the type II cells and the alveolar macrophages? The macrophages may not be so abundant but the type II cell will make up a considerable mass. This is one place where we have to bring together results from work on isolated cells and on perfused organs.

Ayuso-Parrilla: We have some observations that allow us to compare the relative importance of glucose and fatty acids as energy-producing substrates for lung tissue. We have determined the rate of glucose utilization by isolated rat lung cells as about 250 nmol/10^6 cells per hour. This rate compares well with the results reported by others (Rhoades et al 1975, Stubbs et al 1977). Approximately 60% of the glucose utilized is converted into lactate. Regarding long-chain fatty acid utilization, only about 500 pmol of oleate/10^6 cells per hour are oxidized to CO_2. Assuming that the total rate of long-chain fatty acid utilization was about the same order of magnitude as already reported (Rhoades 1974), this means that less than 1% of the total fatty acid utilized is converted to CO_2. These observations suggest that most of the fatty acid utilized is used for lipid synthesis rather than as an energy-producing substrate. On the other hand, when we added a long-chain fatty acid (such as oleic acid) to the incubation medium of isolated lung cells, the ATP levels decreased dramatically (Table 1). However, when glucose was present, the ATP levels remained close to those in the control conditions. These results suggest that under physiological conditions where the lung is receiving both substrates (glucose and fatty acids), energy is mostly derived from substrate-level phosphorylation during glucose breakdown, while fatty acids are mostly spared for lipid synthesis.

TABLE 1 (Ayuso-Parrilla)

Effect of oleate and glucose on the ATP levels of isolated rat lung cells

Substrate present	*ATP levels (nmol/10^6 cells)*
None	4.1 ± 0.54
Glucose (5 mM)	5.5 ± 0.47
Oleate (0.6 mM)	0.74 ± 0.1
Oleate (0.6 mM) + glucose (5 mM)	3.1 ± 0.23

Soffer: As a more general point about this type of experiment on carbohydrate metabolism and hormonal responsiveness, I have been intrigued to learn that insulin is present in every tissue in the body (Rosenzweig et al 1980). It may or may not be of pancreatic origin; I suspect that it is not. In a study of hormone responsiveness and glucose utilization in the lung, should one not consider the pulmonary content of insulin and whether it changes during starvation? Can it account for metabolic fluxes, for example? And is there any evidence that endogenous insulin in extra-pancreatic organs is localized in specific cell types?

Alberti: The glucose values after freeze-clamping were somewhat higher in the lung in fed than in starved rats, 1.8 ± 0.4 μmol/g dry weight as against 1.4

± 0.1 μmol in the starved ones, so there is rather little glucose in the tissue in either state. I think the evidence for the extra-pancreatic production of insulin is weak. I don't know how much insulin is present in lung tissue.

Morishige: Our results in diabetic rats indicate that two cell types are affected morphologically, the Clara cell and the type II epithelial cell (Plopper & Morishige 1978, 1979). The ultrastructural changes are reversed by insulin in both cell types. I think one could probably demonstrate immunoreactive insulin in lung tissue.

Soffer: It might be useful in studying intermediary metabolism to investigate how much insulin there is under varying conditions in the organ in question.

Alberti: It would not be difficult to do an acid ethanol extraction.

Morishige: We didn't measure the amount of insulin in lung tissue, because it is not really meaningful to measure a hormone in an organ as such without distinguishing the location of the hormone in different cell types and in the subcellular compartments.

Stubbs: Wahlqvist et al (1972) and more recently we ourselves (unpublished observations) have found insulin production from the human heart *in vivo*, but whether it is produced in the tissue or adsorbed to heart and then released isn't known.

Vane: Removal of the pancreas would answer this question.

Said: The local presence of insulin in tissues may have special significance, but insulin is a circulating hormone. It gets wherever it wants in the bloodstream, so even if it weren't present in the lung it could still get there as a blood-borne hormone.

Soffer: Is there a possibility that it could be both a local and a systemic hormone and that there is some anatomical compartmentalization? This is speculative, but I have been surprised to read that insulin is found everywhere, and that nobody knows its function (Rosenzweig et al 1980).

Parrilla: In starvation do you see an increase in glucose utilization, Dr Alberti, whereas plasma insulin levels decrease?

Alberti: No; in starvation we see a rather rapid fall in glucose uptake, within two hours.

Parrilla: We could not see any significant differences in glucose utilization by lung cells isolated from fed or starved rats, perhaps because they were incubated for only 60 minutes.

Alberti: We have seen earlier effects; in fact more often we see effects of starvation on substrate uptake in the first 60–90 minutes of perfusion which then reach a plateau.

Bakhle: You were perfusing the pulmonary circulation only; is it possible that many of the metabolically most active cells in the lung are normally perfused by the bronchial circulation? In your perfused lung, is the substrate reaching those comparatively distant cells?

Alberti: This is certainly a possibility. We may be missing some cells by perfusing through one part of the circulation only. I don't know the answer to that.

Bakhle: There is no reason why the substrate shouldn't be able to diffuse through the entire tissue.

Alberti: One would expect glucose to do this. Perhaps this is why we have to wait four hours to see major effects.

References

Ayuso-Parrilla MS, Pérez-Díaz J, Martin A, Parrilla R 1978 Glucose inhibition of oxygen utilization by isolated rat lung cells. Biochimie (Paris) 60:823-826

Fisher AB 1976 Oxygen utilisation and energy production. In: Crystal RG (ed) The biochemical basis of pulmonary function. (Lung biology in health and disease, vol 2) Dekker, New York, p 75-104

Longmore WJ, Mourning JT 1976 Lactate production in isolated perfused rat lung. Am J Physiol 231:351-354

Pérez-Díaz J, Martin A, Ayuso-Parrilla MS, Parrilla R 1977a Metabolic features of isolated rat lung cells. I. Factors controlling glucose utilization. Am J Physiol 232:E394-E401

Pérez-Díaz J, Carballo B, Ayuso-Parrilla MS, Parrilla R 1977b Preparation and metabolic characterization of isolated rat lung cells. Biochimie (Paris) 59:411-416

Plopper CG, Morishige WK 1978 Alterations in granular (type II) pneumocyte ultrastructure by streptozotocin-induced diabetes in the rat. Lab Invest 38:143-148

Plopper CG, Morishige WK 1979 Alterations in the ultrastructure of non-ciliated bronchiolar epithelial (Clara) cells by streptozotocin-induced diabetes in rats. Am Rev Respir Dis 120:1137-1143

Rhoades RA 1974 Net uptake of glucose, glycerol, and fatty acids by the isolated perfused rat lung. Am J Physiol 226:144-149

Rhoades RA, Shaw ME, Eskew ML 1975 Influence of altered O_2 tension on substrate metabolism in perfused rat lung. Am J Physiol 229:1476-1479

Rosenzweig JL, Havrankova J, Lesniak MA, Brownstein M, Roth J 1980 Insulin is ubiquitous in extrapancreatic tissues of rats and humans. Proc Natl Acad Sci USA 77:572-576

Said SI, Klein RM, Norrell LW, Maddox YT 1966 Metabolism of alveolar cells: histochemical evidence and relation to pulmonary surfactant. Science (Wash DC) 152:657-659

Stubbs WA, Morgan I, Lloyd B, Alberti KGMM 1977 The effect of insulin on lung metabolism in the rat. Clin Endocrinol 7:181-184

Tombropoulos EG 1964 Fatty acid synthesis by subcellular fractions of lung tissue. Science (Wash DC) 146:1180-1181

Wahlqvist ML, Kaijser L, Lassers BW, Löw H, Carlson LA 1972 Release of immunoreactive insulin from the human heart. Eur J Clin Invest 2:407-411

Wolfe RR, Hochachka PW, Trelstad RL, Burke JF 1979 Lactate oxidation in perfused rat lung. Am J Physiol 236:E276-E282

Inactivation of monoamines by the lung

M.B.H. YOUDIM, Y.S. BAKHLE* and R.R. BEN-HARARI*

*Department of Pharmacology, Technion School of Medicine, Haifa, Israel and *Department of Pharmacology, Institute of Basic Medical Sciences, Royal College of Surgeons, Lincoln's Inn Fields, London WC2A 3PN, UK*

Abstract Inactivation of monoamines was the first pharmacokinetic property of lung to be identified. For some amines inactivation in perfused lung but not in liver is limited by uptake. Inactivation of β-phenylethylamine in lung is limited not by uptake but by the activity of intracellular monoamine oxidase. The uptake of this amine is like that of basic drugs such as amphetamine and propranolol.

Changes in the external environment of the lung (exposure *in vivo* to gaseous anaesthetics or to high concentrations of oxygen, > 95%) change amine inactivation processes in lung. The oestrous cycle and administration of ovarian steroids also affect the inactivation of 5-hydroxytryptamine and phenylethylamine. Monoamine oxidase activity in lung homogenates is highest at met- and lowest at pro-oestrus for both substrates. However, in perfused lung, inactivation is better correlated with variations in uptake. Therefore the main effect of the oestrous cycle is on uptake rather than on enzymic activity.

Uptake processes are thus crucial determinants of monoamine activation in lung and the pharmacokinetic properties of lung are capable of responding to changes in its internal or external environment.

The first indication of what has become known as the 'pharmacokinetic function' of the lung was provided by the observation of Starling & Verney (1925) that 'a serum vasoconstrictor substance was detoxicated' on passage through a heart–lung preparation. Several years later this was shown to be due to the inactivation of 5-hydroxytryptamine (5-HT) as it passed through the pulmonary circulation (Gaddum et al 1953). Now, some fifty years later, we are still discovering new features of monoamine inactivation in lung. The lung metabolizes a wide range of substrates including monoamines, peptides, fatty acids and nucleotides. A constant feature of this whole range of enzymic activities is that the enzymic properties of lung homogenates are not a reliable guide to the enzymic properties shown by the perfused lung in isolation or *in vivo* (Bakhle & Vane 1974). This characteristic is clearly demonstrated by the

Metabolic activities of the lung
(Ciba Foundation symposium 78) p 105-128

inactivation of monoamines and in this case derives from the intracellular location of the inactivating enzyme, mitochondrial monoamine oxidase (MAO; amine:oxygen oxidoreductase [deaminating]; EC 1.4.3.4). Because of this location, substrates have to cross the cell membrane and it is at this stage – uptake of substrate – that the lung exerts a crucial control over the inactivation process.

IMPORTANCE OF UPTAKE IN LUNG

We have characterized the mitochondrial MAO from rat lung (Bakhle & Youdim 1979) and shown it to have substrate specificities and pH optima very close to those of MAO prepared from liver and brain. The K_m values for lung and liver MAO are compared in Table 1. The two sets of values are very similar, with the non-hydroxylated substrates generally having lower K_m values than the hydroxylated substrates. These results suggested that the lung MAO contained both subtypes of the enzyme, namely MAO-A (deaminating 5-HT and noradrenaline) and MAO-B (with phenylethylamine and benzylamine as typical substrates) (see Fowler et al 1978).

The two subtypes of MAO differ in their inhibitor specificity as well as in their substrates. Clorgyline inhibits MAO-A and deprenyl inhibits MAO-B from the liver (see Fowler et al 1978). We found similar inhibitor specificity in

TABLE 1

Comparison of mitochondrial MAO from rat lung and rat liver

Substrate	*Km (μM)*	
	Lung	*Liver*[a]
Benzylamine	135	245
Phenylethylamine	28	21
Kynuramine	52	71
Tryptamine	27	185
5-Hydroxytryptamine	330	187
Adrenaline	445	400
Noradrenaline	410	416
Dopamine	400	405
Tyramine	305	282

Mitochondria were prepared from rat lungs as described by Youdim (1975) and incubated with a range of concentrations (0.01–3 mM) of substrate. Enzymic activity was assayed fluorimetrically when kynuramine was substrate (Krajl 1963) but otherwise radiochemically using ^{14}C-labelled substrates.

[a]These results are from Houslay & Tipton (1974).

our preparation of lung MAO (Bakhle & Youdim 1979). There seems therefore no reason to doubt that the lung possesses MAO activity almost identical to that in liver and brain. However, there is a difference in monoamine metabolism by lung homogenates and by perfused lung, as indicated by the wide divergence in K_m values for 5-HT between the two systems (Table 2). We have interpreted this difference, in agreement with others (see Alabaster 1977), as showing that 5-HT metabolism in the perfused lung is strictly limited by uptake of substrate.

TABLE 2

Values of K_m for monoamine metabolism by rat lung

Substrate	K_m (μM)	
	Perfused lung	*Mitochondrial MAO*
Phenylethylamine	54	28
5-Hydroxytryptamine	2	330

K_m values for the deamination of two substrates in perfused lung are compared with those already shown in Table 1. ^{14}C-labelled substrate was infused for 3 min into the pulmonary circulation and the metabolite emerging in the lung effluent was determined radiochemically. Concentrations, 0.1–50 μM for 5-HT and 0.1–150 μM for phenylethylamine.

A similar situation almost certainly exists for noradrenaline, which has a K_m of 400 μM for mitochondrial MAO from rat lung (Bakhle & Youdim 1979) but an uptake K_m of about 1 μM in perfused rat lung (see Alabaster 1977). An even greater difference is seen with adrenaline, dopamine and tyramine. These three amines are just as good substrates as 5-HT and noradrenaline for mitochondrial MAO (see Table 1) but they are not inactivated in perfused lung (see Alabaster 1977). Here the restriction of access of substrate to enzyme is absolute.

The selectivity shown by the isolated perfused lung in monoamine inactivation is not shared by the isolated perfused liver. In recent experiments we prepared the livers from rats for perfusion via the portal circulation using the method of Woods et al (1970). A number of monoamines (Table 3) were perfused through the liver over a range of concentrations (0.01–4.0 mM) and samples of the effluent perfusate were analysed for unchanged amine and oxidized metabolite.

With all substrates (Table 3) the formation of deaminated product was a saturable process. We were able to calculate apparent K_m and V_{max} values for each substrate; the K_m values are shown in Table 3 along with the corresponding values for rat liver mitochondrial MAO obtained by Houslay & Tipton (1974). The remarkable feature is the very good correlation between the two

TABLE 3

K_m values for monoamine metabolism in rat liver

Substrate	K_m (μM)	
	Perfused liver	*Mitochondrial MAO*[a]
Benzylamine	200	245
Phenylethylamine	37	21
Kynuramine	75	71
5-Hydroxytryptamine	288	187
Noradrenaline	405	416
Tyramine	270	282
Dopamine	365	405

The amines were infused over a range of concentrations (0.01–4 mM) through isolated rat livers perfused via the portal circulation and the deaminated metabolites emerging from the liver were measured. Kynuramine was measured fluorimetrically and the other substrates were labelled with ^{14}C and determined radiochemically (see Bakhle & Youdim 1979).
[a]Houslay & Tipton (1974).

preparations, perfused liver and mitochondrial MAO. Not only is the full metabolic potential of liver realized for 5-HT and noradrenaline, but dopamine and tyramine are also inactivated in perfused liver as efficiently as they are metabolized by liver mitochondrial MAO. Clearly, in the liver, the cell membrane does not exert a selectivity comparable to that observed in lung.

A similar situation holds for another biogenic amine, histamine, which is extensively metabolized by perfused liver but passes through the pulmonary circulation unchanged in spite of the presence, in lung homogenates, of *two* histamine-inactivating enzymes, diamine oxidase and *N*-methyltransferase (see Alabaster 1977 for references).

METABOLISM OF β-PHENYLETHYLAMINE

Another naturally occurring substrate for lung MAO is β-phenylethylamine, a monoamine with predominantly central actions (see Sabelli et al 1978). An intriguing result of the work so far presented is that although metabolism of 5-HT and noradrenaline in the perfused lung is limited by uptake, that of β-phenylethylamine (PEA) was not so clearly affected by changing from studies *in vitro* to the perfused lung (see Table 2). This result and other evidence (see Bakhle & Youdim 1979) suggested very strongly that the uptake of PEA in rat lung is different from that of 5-HT and noradrenaline. Our recent experiments (Ben-Harari & Bakhle 1980) measured uptake of [^{14}C]PEA as the total radioactivity in lung after a 3-min infusion through rat isolated lungs. Metabolism during this time was derived from the sum of metabolites in lung and metabolites in the effluent. These two variables (uptake and metabolism) are shown in Fig. 1 over a range of concentrations. It is clear that although the deamination of PEA is a saturable process, the uptake is not saturable up to 200 μM. This is immediately different from 5-HT and noradrenaline, where uptake is saturable and at a much lower concentration, approximately 10 μM (see Alabaster 1977). A closer analogy for PEA uptake is the uptake of amphetamine (α-methylphenylethylamine) in rabbit lung (Anderson et al 1974), which has been resolved into two components, a saturable (perhaps facilitated diffusion) process, rate-determining at low concentrations, and a diffusion process which is the limiting step at high concentrations. We have analysed our data for PEA uptake in this way and find that, above 50 μM, the limiting uptake process is linearly related to the perfusate concentration but below 50 μM uptake of PEA seems to be in excess of the simple diffusion component. This analysis of PEA uptake is shown in Fig. 2. An estimate of K_m for the saturable process is 25 μM, a value remarkably close to the K_m of PEA for MAO *in vitro* (Table 1).

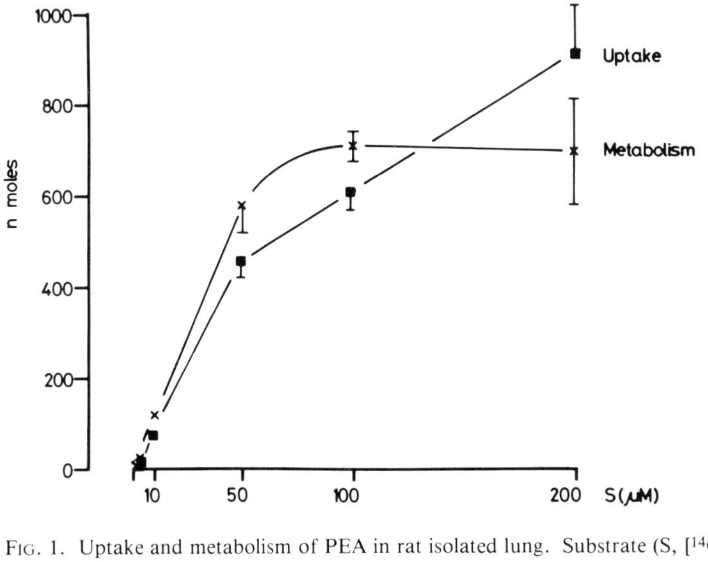

FIG. 1. Uptake and metabolism of PEA in rat isolated lung. Substrate (S, [^{14}C]PEA; 0.15–200 μM) was infused for 3 min through the pulmonary circulation of the rat lung. The perfusion was stopped and radioactivity in lung was measured. Total radioactivity in lung is shown as 'uptake'. The values for 'metabolism' are the sum of radioactive metabolites retained in lung together with the metabolite in lung effluent collected during the 3-min infusion. The values shown are the means (± SEM) of 4–8 lungs at each concentration.

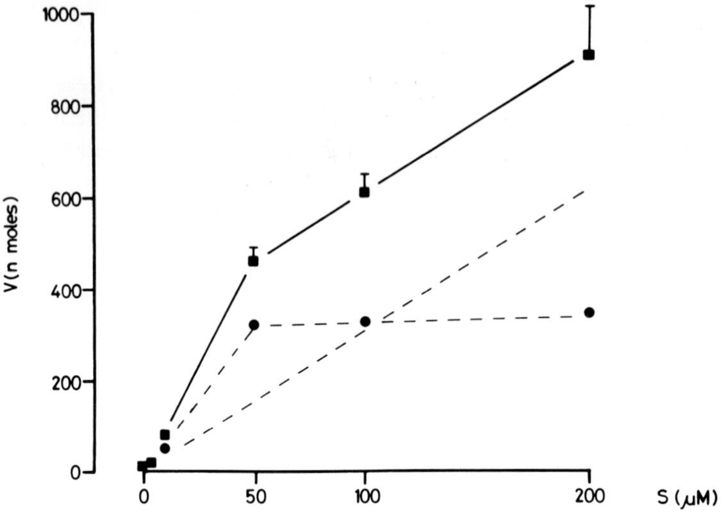

FIG. 2. Analysis of uptake of PEA (substrate, S) by rat isolated lung. The solid line is drawn through points representing the observed uptake (nmol/g lung) of PEA. The broken lines are two possible components of the observed values. The straight line is a diffusion component calculated from a straight line drawn through the three highest observed uptake values. Subtraction of the diffusion component from the observed values yields the values shown as filled circles; the broken line joining these points represents the saturable component of PEA uptake.

Another difference between the inactivation of PEA on one hand and 5-HT and noradrenaline on the other was found in the effect of MAO inhibitors. For 5-HT and noradrenaline, MAO inhibitors did not change the uptake of amine (see Alabaster 1977). However, with PEA, uptake was drastically reduced at every concentration of PEA when the lungs were treated with deprenyl, a selective inhibitor of MAO-B (Fig. 3). This is the clearest evidence that the inactivation of PEA is not uptake limited but enzyme limited, quite unlike 5-HT or noradrenaline.

Further analysis of the inactivation of PEA showed it to be sensitive to a variety of conditions (Table 4) and the uptake in particular to be inhibited by a number of basic amines (Fig. 4). All the drugs used reduced the total ^{14}C retained in the lung after a 3-min infusion of [^{14}C]PEA, but it is significant that normetanephrine and dexamethasone did not decrease the proportion of metabolite in lung (Fig. 4). Thus the inhibitory effect of amphetamine, propranolol and benzylamine on uptake may be ascribed at least in part to the ability to inhibit the intracellular MAO, a deprenyl-like effect. However, normetanephrine and dexamethasone showed no ability to depress the metabolism of the PEA taken up and these drugs are thus capable of blocking

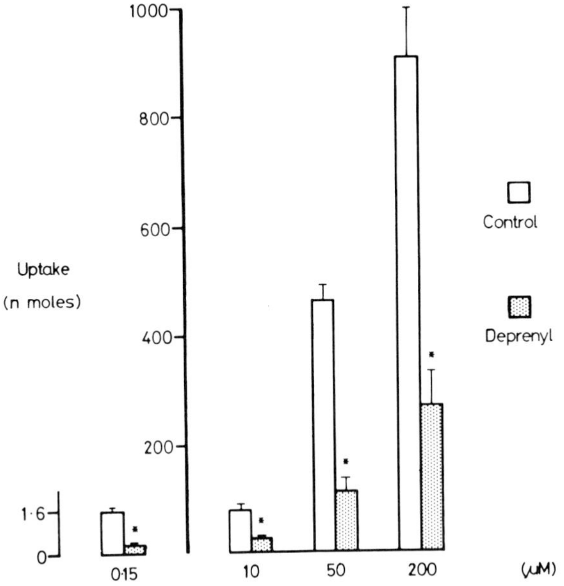

FIG. 3. Inhibition by deprenyl of PEA uptake (μM) by rat isolated lung. The open bars show the mean uptake (± SEM; n = 4–8) of PEA in untreated lungs and the stippled bars the uptake in lungs treated with deprenyl. Deprenyl (5 μM) was infused before and during the infusion of PEA.

TABLE 4

Inhibition of metabolism of phenylethylamine in rat lung under different conditions

Condition	*% Inhibition*
Na^+ lack	33 ± 4
Cold (4°C)	83 ± 3
Amphetamine	70 ± 2
Propranolol	40 ± 2
Benzylamine	41 ± 5
Normetanephrine	49 ± 10
Dexamethasone	64 ± 11

The metabolism of PEA was measured by collecting lung effluent for 30 min, during and after a 3-min infusion of [^{14}C]PEA (50 μM) through the pulmonary circulation of the isolated rat lung and analysing the whole effluent for ^{14}C-deaminated metabolite (Ben-Harari & Bakhle 1980). Values are mean (± SEM) % inhibition of metabolism brought about by each treatment (n = 4–8 lungs per treatment). Metabolism of PEA under control conditions was 708 ± 24 nmoles (n = 42).

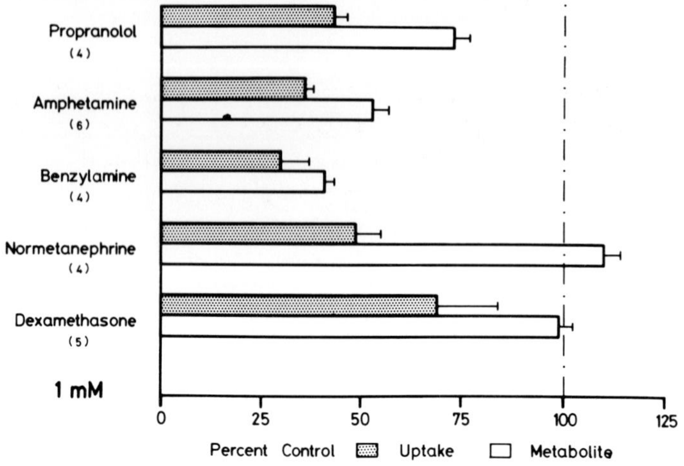

FIG. 4. Effect of various drugs on uptake and metabolism of PEA by rat isolated lung. The uptake of ^{14}C (stippled bars) and the metabolite (open bars) derived from a 3-min infusion of [^{14}C]PEA (50 μM) after treatment of the isolated lung with the different drugs is expressed as % of control values (100%, broken line). All five drugs (1 mM final concentration) decreased uptake. Three drugs (propranolol, amphetamine and benzylamine) also decreased the proportion of metabolite present in lung; normetanephrine and dexamethasone did not. The values shown are the means ($\pm$ SEM) from the number of experiments shown in brackets.

the uptake process alone. From this and the high K_m of PEA uptake we are tempted to classify a part of the PEA uptake as resembling the $Uptake_2$ of catecholamines (Iversen 1971).

In other ways the uptake of PEA by lung seems closer to that described for basic drugs like amphetamine (Anderson et al 1974) and propranolol (Dollery & Junod 1976). It may be that PEA is the endogenous substrate for a system capable of handling basic exogenous drug molecules in lung, rather as the steroids are the natural substrates for oxidative enzymes also capable of oxidizing drug molecules.

PATHOLOGICAL AND PHYSIOLOGICAL FACTORS AFFECTING MONOAMINE INACTIVATION

In parallel with investigations into the mechanisms of monoamine inactivation in normal lung we have been interested in the way monoamine inactivation might respond to changes brought about either pathologically or physiologically.

Pathological factors

Two pathological changes in the environment of the lung have been studied, both concerned with its external environment: exposure *in vivo* to cigarette smoke or to high concentrations (> 95%) of oxygen. The experiments with cigarette smoke were not extensive but they did show that exposure to smoke for up to 10 days did not affect 5-HT metabolism in perfused lung, whereas the metabolism of both angiotensin I and prostaglandin E_2 was changed (Bakhle et al 1979a). We need more experiments on the effects of tobacco smoke in order to assess the effects of this common insult to the lung on its pharmacokinetic potential.

The effects of hyperoxic atmospheres on monoamine inactivation were studied because of the report by Kistler et al (1967) that during the development of oxygen toxicity in rats, damage was first seen in pulmonary endothelial cells, known to be a major site of monoamine inactivation (see Alabaster 1977). Block & Fisher (1977) found a significant decrease in 5-HT metabolism in perfused lung taken from rats after only 18 hours of exposure to high oxygen tensions (97% O_2); after the longest exposure (48 hours) 5-HT metabolism had fallen to about 60% of the control level. In our study (Bakhle et al 1979b), in which we used a slightly lower oxygen concentration (90–95%), we saw no change in 5-HT metabolism in perfused lung until after 60 hours of exposure. At this time mortality was high (40% of the rats died) and only a 20% decrease in metabolism resulted. It is particularly noticeable that we could not reproduce the early change in 5-HT metabolism and, even allowing for differences in experimental methods, it seems that 5-HT metabolism may not provide a *reliable* early warning of pulmonary oxygen toxicity. A better test of oxygen toxicity may prove to be prostaglandin inactivation, which was found to decrease relatively early by both groups (Klein et al 1978, Bakhle et al 1979b). The mechanism by which oxygen might diminish 5-HT and prostaglandin metabolism could involve the inactivation of enzymic SH groups. There are eight moles of SH per mole of MAO (Youdim 1975) and the SH content is important for full catalytic activity, as the oxidation of SH to disulphide (S—S) bonds leads to a reduction in enzymic activity (Youdim & Sourkes 1965). Less direct evidence, obtained from the effects of SH inhibitors and the effect of thiols, shows that prostaglandin dehydrogenase, the rate-limiting enzyme in the pulmonary inactivation of prostaglandins, also contains SH groups essential for activity (Hansen 1976). We do not know enough about the nature of the transport systems for these substrates to be able to assess the effect of oxygen on this component of the inactivation process.

A more common, iatrogenic, insult to the lung is provided by inhalation anaesthetics. Animal lungs, isolated or *in vivo,* responded to nitrous oxide and halothane with a reduced inactivation of 5-HT and noradrenaline (Naito & Gillis 1973, Bakhle & Block 1976). Recently, pulmonary 5-HT clearance in patients was measured during and after surgical operations (that is, in anaesthetized and unanaesthetized subjects), and no significant difference could be found (Gillis et al 1979). The discrepancy between the results from animals and man may be due to the different measurement techniques used but the need for more assays in man is obvious. Nevertheless, it seems clear that changes in the ventilating gas can affect the ability of lung to metabolize substrates in the pulmonary circulation.

Physiological factors

The physiologically induced changes in the lung's environment that we have investigated are the oestrous cycle and postnatal development in rats. There are many reports that MAO activity changes with the sexual cycle in animals and man and after treatment with sex hormones (Youdim & Holzbauer 1976a). These changes are confined to the central nervous system and to other sex hormone 'target' organs such as uterus, ovary and adrenal gland. Organs not considered to be target organs, such as liver, heart and kidney, are unaffected (Holzbauer & Youdim 1973). The lung is not considered a target organ for ovarian steroids and we expected that monoamine inactivation in this tissue, like that in heart, would remain unaltered over the oestrous cycle. Our results proved otherwise (Bakhle & Ben-Harari 1979a, b). Using both 5-HT and PEA, as substrates of MAO types A and B respectively, we first studied MAO activity in homogenates, since this was the experimental system used in previous studies (Holzbauer & Youdim 1973). For both substrates there was a clear change in MAO activity during the four-day oestrous cycle. At a single concentration, activity towards 5-HT was highest at met-oestrus and, for PEA, the increased activity persisted until the following stage, di-oestrus (Fig. 5). With a range of concentrations, estimates of K_m and V_{max} were obtained for both substrates at each stage of the cycle and a further difference between the substrates appeared. As illustrated in Fig. 6, the major effect on 5-HT metabolism was on the K_m whereas for PEA V_{max} changes were more obvious. We think this might reflect a change in affinity for 5-HT and a change in the synthesis of MAO catalytic protein for PEA.

Changes in MAO activity can also be produced by treating female rats with oestradiol or progesterone, using the regime of Holzbauer & Youdim (1973). This treatment decreased (with oestradiol) or increased (with progesterone)

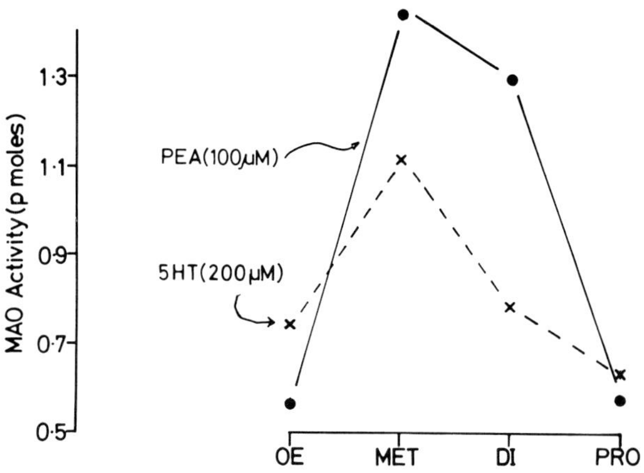

FIG. 5. MAO activity in rat lung homogenates during the oestrous cycle. The activity (pmol metabolite min^{-1} μg protein^{-1}) of lung homogenates from rats at different stages of the 4-day oestrous cycle (OE, oestrus; MET, met-oestrus; DL, di-oestrus; PRO, pro-oestrus) was measured at a single concentration of 5-HT (×-----×; 200 μM) and of PEA (•——•; 100 μM).

enzyme activity in uterus and ovary towards kynuramine but, again, heart, liver and kidney had proved resistant. Our results (Table 5) using lung homogenates showed that the metabolism of both substrates was never decreased and that oestradiol treatment was more effective in increasing PEA metabolism whereas, for 5-HT, progesterone was more effective. There is no simple correlation between the results of treatment with exogenous steroids and those during the natural cycle, but these experiments emphasize the susceptibility of lung MAO to changes in levels of ovarian steroids. These results also underline the point made by Youdim & Holzbauer (1976a) that the effects of steroids on monoamine oxidation depend on the substrates chosen to estimate enzyme activity.

Having established the *potential* for changes in monoamine inactivation during the oestrous cycle, we then studied 5-HT and PEA inactivation in perfused lungs to see how this potential was expressed. We chose met-oestrus and pro-oestrus as the stages showing the largest differences in MAO activity and studied the metabolism over a range of concentrations of each substrate in perfused lungs from rats at these stages. The results were again unexpected.

For 5-HT there was a difference only at low concentrations (0.15–5 μM) and metabolism was greater during pro-oestrus, the converse of the results with the homogenates. This we believe to be another illustration of the strict control of 5-HT metabolism by the uptake step. Because for 5-HT there is

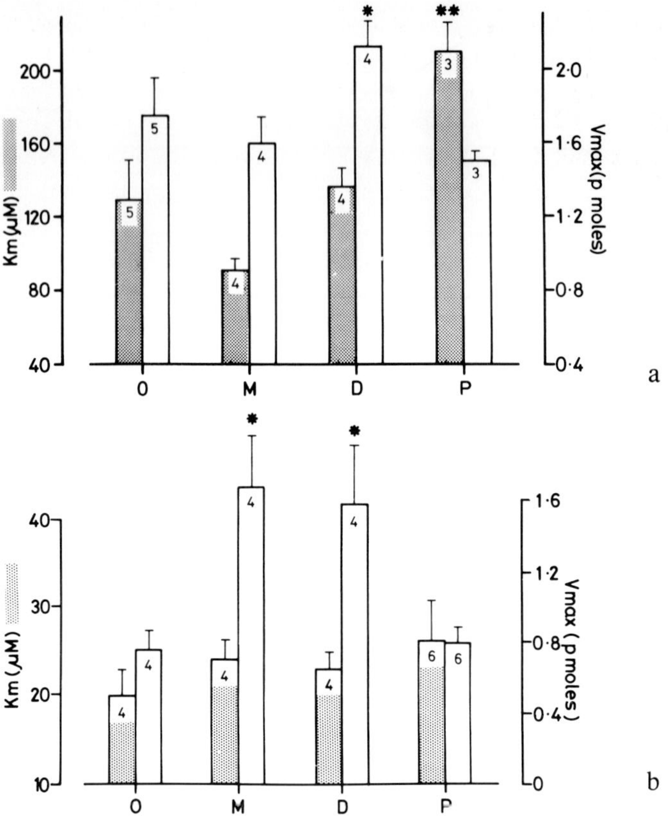

FIG. 6. Values of K_m and V_{max} of MAO activity in rat lung homogenates during the oestrous cycle. In (a) for 5-HT, the K_m is highest at pro-oestrus and lowest at met-oestrus. In (b), for PEA, there is no change in K_m but V_{max} at met- and di-oestrus is higher than at the other two stages. The height of the bars represents the mean (± SEM) values from 4–8 lungs at each stage for either substrate.

TABLE 5

Effect of steroid treatment *in vivo* on metabolism of monoamines by rat lung homogenates

Treatment	*5-HT*		*PEA*	
	K_m	V_{max}	K_m	V_{max}
Control (saline)	114 ± 4	1.1 ± 0.1	30 ± 5	1.4 ± 0.2
Oestradiol (0.5 mg/kg)	92 ± 1*	1.2 ± 0.1	58 ± 8*	2.2 ± 0.2*
Progesterone (1.0 mg/kg)	85 ± 8*	1.9 ± 0.2*	16 ± 1	1.2 ± 0.1

The values shown are the means (± SEM) of 4–7 experiments. K_m is expressed as μM and V_{max} as pmole product μg protein^{-1} min^{-1}. Steroids were injected intraperitoneally as a saline suspension, daily for 8 days at the dose shown.
*Significantly different from control values ($P < 0.05$; Student's t-test).

always a large excess of MAO activity, changes in intracellular activity can be entirely irrelevant to metabolism in the whole lung, which will respond more strikingly to comparatively small changes in uptake. To test this hypothesis we measured uptake of 5-HT at a single concentration (0.5 μM) at all four stages of the cycle. Uptake was highest at pro-oestrus (Fig. 7a) and lowest at oestrus and di-oestrus. Fig. 7a also shows the metabolism expected in

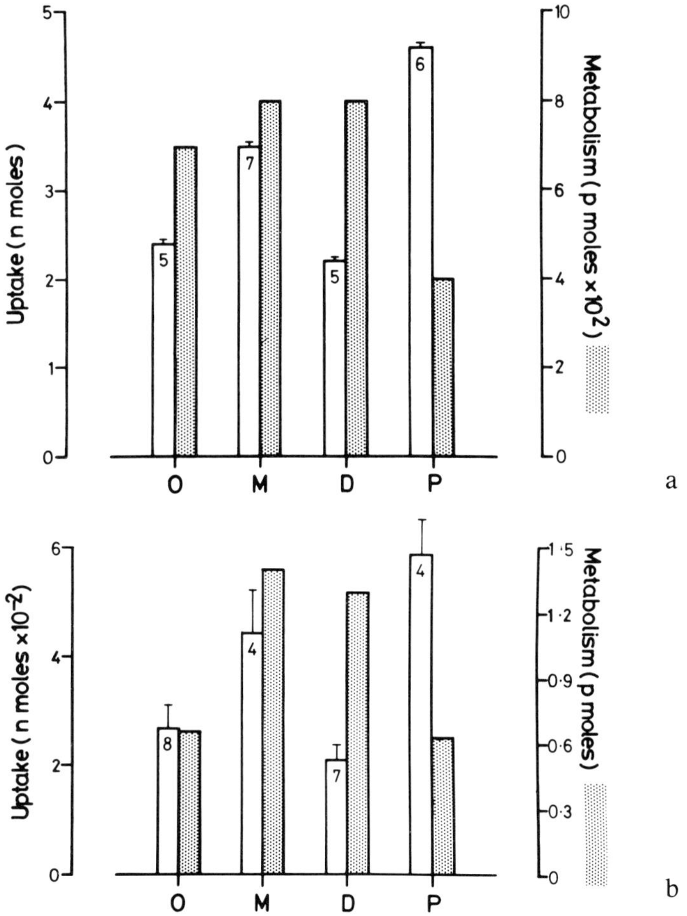

FIG. 7. Comparison of uptake in perfused lung and metabolism in lung homogenate for (a) 5-HT and (b) PEA. In (a), with a low concentration of substrate (0.5 μM), uptake was greatest during pro-oestrus, whereas metabolism in homogenates was the lowest. Metabolism in perfused lung was more closely correlated with uptake than with metabolism *in vitro*. In (b), with PEA, note the 100 times increase in the uptake scale. Here again there is little correlation between uptake and metabolism *in vitro*.

homogenates at this concentration and it is clear that there is little correlation between the two variables for 5-HT. Furthermore, the inactivation of 5-HT in whole perfused lung followed the changes in uptake more closely than changes in MAO activity.

For PEA, metabolism in perfused lung from rats during met- and pro-oestrus was identical over the whole concentration range (0.15–150 μM) in spite of large differences shown in homogenates. Direct measurement of the uptake of PEA (100 μM) showed no difference at met- and pro-oestrus. Here also there was no clear correlation between results in homogenates and in perfused lung (Fig. 7b), and the uptake values were a better guide to metabolism in perfused lung.

The conclusions from these experiments are quite clear. First, the enzymic activity towards monoamines does change with the oestrous cycle and from the susceptibility of this activity to exogenous oestradiol and progesterone it seems reasonable to assume that it is the changing steroid levels in the cycle that are responsible for the effects seen. For this reason alone, lung should now be considered a target organ for ovarian steroids as it is for corticosteroids. Second, another distinct effect of the oestrous cycle is to change the movement of substrate into the cell (which we have rather loosely referred to as 'uptake'). Since steroids are known to affect monoamine uptake in other systems (Iversen 1971) it seems reasonable to assume that the change in ovarian steroids causes the change in monoamine uptake in lung. Third, the crucial importance of this uptake step in determining metabolism and hence inactivation in whole perfused lung is re-emphasized.

The other physiological factor studied was the age of the animal. Age-dependent changes in MAO activity in various tissues of the rat and other species including man have often been reported (see Youdim & Holzbauer 1976b for review). We have examined the postnatal development of MAO activity in rat lung using 5-HT, dopamine and PEA as substrates. Our results (Fig. 8) showed that MAO activity increased with age, and thus lung MAO responds like that from other tissues (see Blatchford et al 1976). An interesting feature of our results is the difference between the development of MAO activity toward 5-HT and PEA. Whereas enzyme activity for 5-HT deamination is well developed by the 10th day and reaches its maximum on the 40th day, the enzyme activity for PEA lags behind up to the 20th day and then develops rapidly but does not reach a maximum by the 80th day. This observation may help to explain the higher V_{max} of MAO toward PEA than 5-HT, observed by us using mitochondrial or isolated perfused lung preparations. Lung MAO activity increases with age in parallel with the development of other tissue components, which reach their adult composition and function

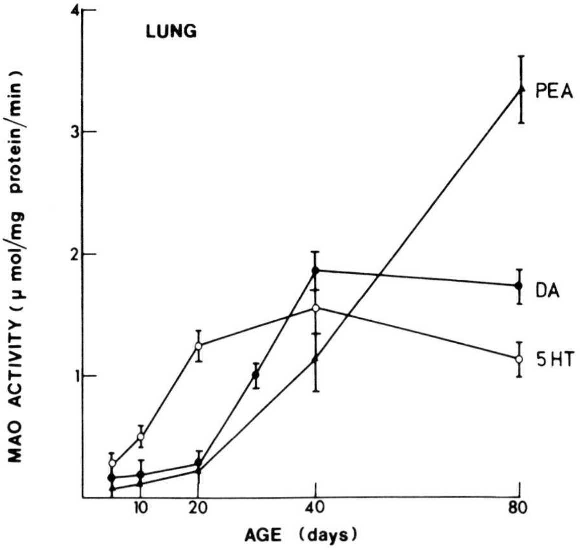

FIG. 8. Postnatal development of MAO activity in homogenates of lung from male rats between 5 and 80 days old. The activity towards three substrates (5-HT, PEA and dopamine, DA) was measured in litter-mates.

after several weeks or months. For example, covalently bound flavin, as FAD, is an essential co-factor of MAO (Youdim 1976). The enzyme that synthesizes flavin is known to increase with age and is thought to be regulated by thyroid hormones (Rivlin et al 1976). The low tissue content of flavin in the newborn and its development with age (Youdim 1979) may be the consequence of the lack of either its synthesizing enzyme or the enzyme which attaches it to its apoenzyme. Developmental changes in other factors – for example, phospholipids in the immediate environment of the enzyme in the outer mitochondrial membrane, which are required for its full activity – will certainly contribute to the progressive rise in MAO activity in the young rat lung. Lipid concentrations are low at birth and increase gradually during the first three months (Crawford & Sinclair 1972). Furthermore, it may be that in newborn rats relatively less apoenzyme protein is present. Whatever the mechanism of these changes may be, further studies are needed to elucidate the biochemical basis and the physiological importance of these findings. We also need to know if changes occur in the uptake system for 5-HT and PEA as the animal develops.

CONCLUSIONS

From this discussion of recent work on factors affecting monoamine inactivation in lung we should like to draw two conclusions.

First, the fact that physiological changes such as those occurring during the oestrous cycle and in the developing animal can affect monoamine inactivation strengthens our belief that this inactivation has a physiological role. Although inactivation is ultimately dependent on enzymic deamination by MAO, uptake of substrate may be the crucial step. It is the selectivity of this process that gives the lung three distinct systems for handling monoamines in the pulmonary vasculature: a high affinity, low capacity system for 5-HT and noradrenaline; a lower affinity, high capacity system for PEA and perhaps amphetamine and propranolol; and a total exclusion system for substrates like adrenaline and dopamine.

Furthermore, it is this selectivity of uptake that differentiates pulmonary monoamine inactivation from hepatic inactivation in spite of identical enzymic content. The physiological significance of the contrast between the 'open door' policy of liver and the selectivity of lung is not immediately apparent but it does suggest that the purpose of this function in the two organs is different – in liver to protect against ingested exogenous amines, but in lung to control levels of endogenous monoamines.

The crucial importance of uptake under normal conditions and during the oestrous cycle emphasizes that, for lung, prediction of inactivation in perfused tissues based solely on a knowledge of metabolism in homogenates is likely to be misleading (Bakhle & Vane 1974, Youdim & Woods 1975).

Our second conclusion is that this function of lung can be affected by external factors acting through the gas phase in lung. Although the effect of inhaled anaesthetics may turn out to be negligible, long-term exposure to atmospheric pollutants could be more effective in altering monoamine metabolism. If so, this would suggest one way in which changes in inspired air could lead to changes in blood levels of endogenous vasoactive substances.

It would be unjustified at present to attempt to relate the observed changes in monoamine inactivation by lung to observed changes in the whole body brought about by the stimulus in question, be it the oestrous cycle or 20 years of cigarette smoking, if only because changes in metabolism of other relevant hormones have not yet been studied. Nevertheless, the results so far obtained are clear encouragement to pursue the investigation of physiological and pathological factors affecting the metabolism of monoamines and other substrates in lung.

ACKNOWLEDGEMENT

The Medical Research Council and the Royal Society supported much of the work reported here by Y.S.B. and R.R.B.-H.

References

Alabaster VA 1977 Inactivation of endogenous amines in the lungs. In: Bakhle YS, Vane JR (eds) Metabolic functions of the lung (Lung biology in health and disease, vol 4) Dekker, New York, p 3-31

Anderson MW, Orton TC, Pickett RD, Eling TE 1974 Accumulation of amines in the isolated perfused rabbit lung. J Pharmacol Exp Ther 186:456-466

Bakhle YS, Ben-Harari RR 1979a Effects of oestrous cycle and exogenous ovarian steroids on 5-hydroxytryptamine metabolism in rat lung. J Physiol (Lond) 291:11-18

Bakhle YS, Ben-Harari RR 1979b Effects of the oestrous cycle and exogenous ovarian steroids on metabolism of β-phenylethylamine in rat lung. Br J Pharmacol 67:109-114

Bakhle YS, Block AJ 1976 Effects of halothane on pulmonary inactivation of noradrenaline and prostaglandin E_2 in anaesthetized dogs. Clin Sci Mol Med 50:87-90

Bakhle YS, Vane JR 1974 Pharmacokinetic function of the pulmonary circulation. Physiol Rev 54:1007-1045

Bakhle YS, Youdim MBH 1979 The metabolism of 5-hydroxytryptamine and β-phenylethylamine in perfused rat lung and *in vitro*. Br J Pharmacol 65:147-154

Bakhle YS, Hartiala J, Toivonen H, Uotila P 1979a Effects of cigarette smoke on the metabolism of vasoactive hormones in rat isolated lungs. Br J Pharmacol 65:495-500

Bakhle YS, Hartiala J, Toivonen H 1979b Exposure to oxygen inhibits metabolism of vasoactive hormones in rat isolated lungs. J Physiol (Lond) 293:27P

Ben-Harari RR, Bakhle YS 1980 Uptake of β-phenylethylamine in rat isolated lung. Biochem Pharmacol 29:489-494

Blatchford D, Holzbauer M, Grahame-Smith DG, Youdim MBH 1976 Ontogenesis of enzyme systems deaminating different monoamines. Br J Pharmacol 57:279-294

Block ER, Fisher AB 1977 Depression of serotonin clearance by rat lungs during oxygen exposure. J Appl Physiol 42:33-38

Crawford MA, Sinclair AJ 1972 Nutritional influences in the evolution of the mammalian brain. Lipids, malnutrition and the developing brain. Excerpta Medica, Amsterdam (Ciba Found Symp 3), p 267-292

Dollery CT, Junod AF 1976 Concentration of ($\pm$) propranolol in isolated perfused lungs of rat. Br J Pharmacol 57:67-71

Fowler CJ, Callingham BA, Mantle TJ, Tipton KF 1978 Monoamine oxidase A and B; a useful concept? Biochem Pharmacol 27:97-101

Gaddum JH, Hebb CO, Silver A, Swan AAB 1953 5-Hydroxytryptamine. Pharmacological action and destruction in perfused lungs. Q J Exp Physiol Cogn Med Sci 38:255-262

Gillis CN, Cronau LH, Mandel S, Hammond GL 1979 Indicator dilution measurement of 5-hydroxytryptamine clearance by human lung. J Appl Physiol 46:1178-1183

Hansen HS 1976 15-Hydroxyprostaglandin dehydrogenase – a review. Prostaglandins 12:647-679

Holzbauer M, Youdim MBH 1973 The oestrous cycle and monoamine oxidase activity. Br J Pharmacol 48:600-608

Houslay MD, Tipton MF 1974 A kinetic evaluation of monoamine oxidase activity in rat liver mitochondrial outer membranes. Biochem J 139:645-652

Iversen LL 1971 The role of transmitter uptake mechanisms in synaptic neurotransmission. Br J Pharmacol 41:571-591

Klein LS, Fisher AB, Soltoff S, Colburn RF 1978 Effect of oxygen exposure on pulmonary metabolism of prostaglandin E_2. Am Rev Respir Dis 118:622-625

Kistler GS, Caldwell PRB, Weibel ER 1967 Development of fine structural damage to alveolar and capillary lining cells in oxygen poisoned rat lungs. J Cell Biol 33:605-628

Krajl M 1963 A rapid fluorimetric determination of monoamine oxidase. Biochem Pharmacol 14:1684-1686

Naito H, Gillis CN 1973 Effects of halothane and nitrous oxide on removal of noradrenaline from the pulmonary circulation. Anesthesiology 39:575-580

Rivlin RS, Fazekas AG, Hung YP, Chaudhuri R 1976 Flavin metabolism and its control by thyroid hormones. In: Singer TP (ed) Flavins and flavoproteins. Elsevier, Amsterdam, p 747-753

Sabelli HC, Borison RL, Diamond BI, Havdala HS, Narasimhachari N 1978 Phenylethylamine and brain function. Biochem Pharmacol 27:1707-1712

Starling EH, Verney EB 1925 The secretion of urine as studied on the isolated kidney. Proc R Soc London B Biol Sci 97:321-363

Woods HF, Eggleston LV, Krebs HA 1970 The cause of hepatic accumulation of fructose-1-phosphate on fructose loading. Biochem J 119:501-510

Youdim MBH 1975 Monoamine deaminating system in mammalian tissue. In: Blaschko H (ed) International review of science. Butterworth, London, p 169-211

Youdim MBH 1976 Rat liver mitochondrial monoamine oxidase: an iron requiring flavoprotein. In: Singer TP (ed) Flavins and flavoproteins. Elsevier, Amsterdam, p 651-661

Youdim MBH 1979 Development of monoamine deaminating systems. Animal and human correlates. In: Mesami E, Brazier MAB (eds) Neural growth and differentiation. Raven Press, New York, p 71-90

Youdim MBH, Holzbauer M 1976a Physiological aspects of the oxidative deamination of monoamines. In: Monoamine oxidase and its inhibition. Excerpta Medica, Amsterdam (Ciba Found Symp 39), p 105-131

Youdim MBH, Holzbauer M 1976b Physiological and pathological changes in tissue monoamine oxidase activity. J Neural Transm 38:193-230

Youdim MBH, Sourkes TL 1965 The effect of heat, inhibitors and riboflavin deficiency on monoamine oxidase. Can J Biochem 43:1305-1323

Youdim MBH, Woods HF 1975 The influence of tissue environment on the rate of metabolic processes and properties of enzymes. Biochem Pharmacol 24:317-323

Youdim MBH, Holzbauer M, Woods HF 1974 Physicochemical properties, development and regulation of central and peripheral monoamine oxidase. Adv Biochem Psychopharmacol 12:11-28

Discussion

Morishige: Have you tested the effect on phenylethylamine uptake of doses of dexamethasone lower than 1 mmol/l?

Bakhle: Yes, but you need this high concentration of steroid to see any effect on the uptake of phenylethylamine.

Morishige: At that concentration it would seem that the steroid might be exerting a steric hindrance effect on the transport mechanism of the membrane. That is, by insertion into the membrane, this high concentration of steroid may be altering the fluidity of the membrane in a non-physiological manner.

Vane: You suggested that phenylethylamine (PEA) is taken up by a process resembling the Uptake$_2$ of catecholamines (p 112). However, PEA has no polar groups, unlike the catechols with their two hydroxyl groups, so it could pass straight through the cell membrane without needing an uptake process. Isn't that a simpler explanation?

Bakhle: It is reputed to go through the blood–brain barrier without any hindrance (Nakajima et al 1964), but when we measured uptake of 5-HT and PEA, whereas 5-HT gives a saturable curve, the curve of PEA uptake did not show saturation (see Fig. 1, p 109) but neither did it show a simple linear relationship. This is exactly what was reported for amphetamine (Anderson et al 1974). One possibility is that this curve represents a saturable system with a diffusional component.

Youdim:* I agree with Professor Vane's simpler explanation, that non-polar amines pass through the cell membrane. This is what actually happens, in the brain with PEA (Oldendorf 1971) and tryptamine (Martin et al 1976). The similarity of uptake of PEA and amphetamine can be explained by their structural and pharmacological resemblance (Wyatt et al 1977). For comparison we should look at the uptake and deamination of benzylamine and tryptamine in the isolated lung since both amines, like PEA, are substrates for MAO type B (Tipton et al 1976).

Junod: In radioautographic studies we have obtained evidence for heterogeneity of the function of the pulmonary endothelium, depending on the nature of the substrate. For example, 5-HT is taken up by endothelial cells in the lung evenly along the vascular bed, whereas there is a preferential uptake of noradrenaline (norepinephrine) in certain segments of the pulmonary vasculature, namely in the pre- and postcapillary vessels and in veins (Strum & Junod 1972, Nicholas et al 1974). So even though the uptake mechanism looks similar, the distribution of labelling is not the same for 5-HT and noradrenaline – hence the concept of heterogeneity of function of the endothelial cells.

You mentioned that propranolol inhibited the uptake of PEA as part of your evidence that PEA uptake corresponds to Uptake$_2$. However, I do not think the characteristics of propranolol uptake by the lung correspond to those of PEA.

Bakhle: Our evidence for an Uptake$_2$ type of mechanism for PEA does not rest on inhibition by propranolol but on inhibition by normetanephrine and dexamethasone and on its high K_m, of about 50 μM (see p 111). On the second

*Comments added in writing after the symposium.

point, didn't you show that uptake of propranolol appeared to have two components in rat lung (Dollery & Junod 1976)?

Junod: Yes, but the kinetics were different. Propranolol accumulation is not related to metabolism, because propranolol is not metabolized by the lung, and the apparent V_{max} for propranolol accumulation is one order of magnitude higher than the value you found for PEA (Dollery & Junod 1976). The uptake of a drug is probably completely different from the uptake of naturally occurring substances and one can't really compare the two types of substrates.

Bakhle: The combination of saturation and diffusion is not seen with 5-HT or noradrenaline and it is seen with amphetamine. There is a suggestion of it with propranolol and also with PEA. There are other points of interest: propranolol doesn't interfere with 5-HT uptake, nor does amphetamine. PEA, amphetamine and propranolol all interfere with each other and they seem to have kinetically the same sort of uptake. One can speculate therefore that the same system is moving these three substrates.

Junod: Have you shown that propranolol uptake is inhibited by various concentrations of PEA?

Bakhle: We haven't done that experiment. However, 5-HT and noradrenaline don't inhibit each other's uptake but they have very similar uptake systems. Do you think that propranolol inhibits PEA uptake without sharing its uptake mechanism?

Junod: In a completely different way, yes, just as imipramine blocks 5-HT or noradrenaline uptake but without being taken up by the same system (Junod 1972).

Moncada: How do the various MAO substrates interact? Do they compete for the same uptake mechanism? For example, will noradrenaline facilitate or create the possibility for adrenaline uptake?

Bakhle: Nobody has looked at the interaction of noradrenaline and adrenaline uptake, but we found no interaction between 5-HT and PEA uptake (Bakhle & Youdim 1976). 5-HT and noradrenaline do not compete for the carrier; in fact Iwasawa & Gillis (1974) have separated the two carrier sites pharmacologically. So although 5-HT and noradrenaline behave as if they use the same uptake system, the systems must be different. It may be, as Dr Junod suggested, that these substrates go to different cells, but I don't think that is an adequate explanation.

Morishige: Have you studied the effects of giving oestrogens or progesterone on the uptake of monoamines by the lung in animals?

Bakhle: No. We have studied only variations in uptake of amines over the oestrous cycle, so far.

Youdim: If the results that have been reported for the *in vitro* and *in vivo* actions of oestrogens and progesterone on 5-HT and noradrenaline uptake by the brain are any guide, I suspect that they will have a similar effect on the lung amine uptake system (Endersby & Wilson 1974, Kendall & Tonge 1977, Wirz-Justice et al 1974).

Morishige: We have measured sex steroid receptors in the rat lung and your evidence that uptake of 5-HT is greatest in pro-oestrus coincides somewhat with an elevated level of oestrogen receptors in lung at oestrus. The curious point is that in the rat the circulating blood level of oestradiol is high in late di-oestrus and lowest in oestrus, so there doesn't seem to be a direct relation to oestrogens as such.

Bakhle: No. I think the low level of MAO activity that we find at pro-oestrus in the rat may be related to oestradiol, because oestradiol is inhibitory to MAO, according to Collins & Southgate (1970), although the doses they used were large. That would be the only correlation we would suggest. For the rest, I am just saying that we find that, in lung, amine metabolism *is* affected by the cycle; we can't say what the significance is. We want to go on to look at amine inactivation in pregnancy.

Youdim: It is already known that MAO activity and 5-HT, dopamine and noradrenaline metabolism change during pregnancy (Parvez et al 1975, Greengrass & Tonge 1974). If the lung is a target organ for the steroids, as we suspect it to be, we should expect similar changes in monoamine metabolism in this tissue during pregnancy.

Soffer: You find a change in K_m of monoamine oxidase in a homogenate using 5-HT as substrate, during oestrus. How do you think that happens? Do you think this is due to a change in the physicochemical characteristics of the enzyme itself or to the presence of regulatory molecules which modify its kinetic properties?

Bakhle: I don't know enough about how ovarian steroids affect enzyme behaviour to know exactly why there is a change in K_m for 5-HT. One possibility could be a natural inhibitor of MAO. With phenylethylamine the K_m is unchanged but V_{max} alters. This suggests that there is an increase in the synthesis of the enzyme catabolizing phenylethylamine (MAO type B) during met-oestrus and di-oestrus, but the catalytic properties are the same, whereas for 5-HT, which is catabolized by the A form of MAO, perhaps an inhibitor is present, whose production varies over the oestrous cycle.

Youdim: On previous occasions we have suggested that the observed changes in MAO activity during the oestrous cycle can be explained by simultaneous changes in the blood concentrations of progesterone (stimulator) and oestrogens (inhibitor), because there is a parallel between the tissue concentrations of these steroids in adrenal gland and ovaries and MAO activity (Youdim et al 1974, Youdim & Holzbauer 1976). It has already been established that in steroid-synthesizing glands the tissue content is a valid indicator for the rates at which steroids are secreted (Fajer et al 1971, Holzbauer 1971, Youdim et al 1974).

The mechanism by which steroids alter MAO activity is not fully understood, but there are a number of ways in which these effects could be achieved. Steroids could act as allosteric effectors, by changing the lipid environment of the enzyme in the mitochondrial outer membrane (Singer et al 1979); or they could act by inducing new enzyme formation at the transcriptional or post-transcriptional level, by decreasing or increasing enzyme degradation, by changing the permeability of the outer mitochondrial membrane (the site of MAO), or by modulating the covalent incorporation of FAD (the MAO cofactor) into the apoenzyme (Youdim et al 1974, Youdim & Holzbauer 1976, Youdim 1979). We are now in a position to answer some of these questions using a technique of MAO A or MAO B protein titration. Recently it has been shown that radiolabelled selective inhibitors of the A and B enzyme, namely clorgyline and deprenyl, bind covalently and stoichiometrically to the active site of the enzyme. The amount of MAO protein can therefore be titrated (Youdim et al 1976, Youdim 1976, Salach et al 1979).

I am not happy about Dr Bakhle's suggestion of an MAO inhibitor. It must be remembered that the ovary secretes several active progesterone derivatives at varying rates during the cycle (Holzbauer 1971) and the possible effects of these compounds should be considered. Furthermore, corticosteroids have been reported to decrease MAO activity (Parvez & Parvez 1973a,b) and cyclic variations in their secretion are possible.

Vane: Dr Flower, does prostaglandin dehydrogenase also change in activity during the oestrous cycle?

Flower: You can certainly produce changes in enzyme activity by injecting oestradiol or progesterone, and there are also marked increases during pregnancy (Sun & Armour 1974, Bedwani & Marley 1975, Blackwell & Flower 1976). I don't know of any work in which changes in prostaglandin dehydrogenase activity during the oestrous cycle have been carefully studied.

References

Anderson MW, Orton TC, Pickett RD, Eling TE 1974 Accumulation of amines in the isolated perfused rabbit lung. J Pharmacol Exp Ther 186:456-466

Bakhle YS, Youdim MBH 1976 Metabolism of phenylethylamine in rat isolated perfused lung; evidence for monoamine oxidase 'Type B' in lung. Br J Pharmacol 56:125-127

Bedwani JR, Marley PB 1975 Enhanced inactivation of prostaglandin E_2 by the rabbit lung during pregnancy or progesterone treatment. Br J Pharmacol 53:547-554
Blackwell GJ, Flower RJ 1976 Effects of steroid hormones on tissue levels of prostaglandin 15-hydroxydehydrogenase in the rat. Br J Pharmacol 56:343-344P
Collins GGS, Southgate J 1970 The effect of progesterone and oestradiol on rat uterine monoamine oxidase activity. Biochem J 117:38P
Dollery CT, Junod AF 1976 Concentration of (±)propranolol in isolated, perfused lungs of rat. Br J Pharmacol 57:67-71
Endersby CA, Wilson C 1974 The effect of ovarian steroids on the accumulation of ^{3}H-labelled monoamines by hypothalamic tissue *in vitro*. Brain Res 73:321-331
Fajer AB, Holzbauer M, Newport HM 1971 The contribution of the adrenal gland to the total amount of progesterone produced in the female rat. J Physiol (Lond) 214:115-126
Greengrass PM, Tonge SR 1974 The concentrations of the monoamines and their precursor amino acids in three areas of mouse brain during pregnancy. Arch Int Pharmacodyn Ther 210:75-84
Holzbauer M 1971 *In vivo* production of steroids with central depressant actions by the ovary of the rat. Br J Pharmacol 43:560-569
Iwasawa Y, Gillis CN 1974 Pharmacological analysis of norepinephrine and 5-hydroxytryptamine removal from the pulmonary circulation; differentiation of uptake sites for each amine. J Pharmacol Exp Ther 188:386-393
Junod AF 1972 Accumulation of ^{14}C-imipramine in isolated perfused rat lungs. J Pharmacol Exp Ther 183:182-187
Kendall DA, Tonge SR 1977 Effects of testosterone and ethinyloestradiol on the synthesis and uptake of noradrenaline and 5-hydroxytryptamine in rat hindbrain: evidence for a presynaptic regulation of monoamine synthesis. Br J Pharmacol 60:310-311P
Martin WR, Sloan JW, Vaupel DB, Bell JA, Nozaki M 1976 Tryptamine in the brain and the spinal cord: its role in the LSD response. In: Usdin E, Sandler M (eds) Trace amines and the brain. Dekker, New York, p 83-102
Nakajima T, Kakimoto Y, Sano I 1964 Formation of β-phenylethylamine in mammalian tissue and its effect on motor activity in the mouse. J Pharmacol Exp Ther 143:319-325
Nicholas TE, Strum JM, Angelo LS, Junod AF 1974 Site and mechanism of uptake of ^{3}H-L-norepinephrine by isolated perfused rat lungs. Circ Res 35:670-680
Oldendorf WH 1971 Brain uptake of radiolabelled amino acids, amines and hexoses after arterial injection. Am J Physiol 221:1629-1639
Parvez H, Parvez S 1973a The effect of metopirone and adrenalectomy on the regulation of the enzymes monoamine oxidase and catechol-*O*-methyltransferase in different brain regions. J Neurochem 20:1011-1020
Parvez H, Parvez S 1973b The regulation of monoamine oxidase activity by adrenal corticoid steroids. Acta Endocrinol 73:509-517
Parvez S, Parvez SH, Youdim MBH 1975 Variation in activity of monoamine metabolizing enzymes in rat liver during pregnancy. Br J Pharmacol 53:241-246
Salach JI, Detmer K, Youdim MBH 1979 The reaction of bovine and rat liver monoamine oxidase with (^{14}C)-clorgyline and (^{14}C)-deprenyl. Mol Pharmacol 16:234-241
Singer TP, Von Korff RW, Murphy DL 1979 Monoamine oxidase structure, function and altered function. Academic Press, New York
Strum JM, Junod AF 1972 Radioautographic demonstration of 5-hydroxytryptamine-^{3}H uptake by pulmonary endothelial cells. J Cell Biol 54:456-467
Sun FF, Armour SB 1974 Prostaglandin 15-hydroxydehydrogenase and Δ^{13}-reductase levels in the lungs of maternal, fetal and neonatal rabbits. Prostaglandins 7:327-338
Tipton KF, Houslay MD, Mantle TJ 1976 The nature and location of the multiple forms of monoamine oxidase. In: Monoamine oxidase and its inhibition. Excerpta Medica, Amsterdam (Ciba Found Symp 39), p 5-32
Wyatt JR, Gillin JC, Stoff DM, Moha EA, Tinklenberg JR 1977 β-Phenylethylamine and

the neuropsychiatric disturbances. In: Usdin E et al (eds) Neuroregulators and psychiatric disorders. Oxford University Press, New York, p 31-45

Wirz-Justice A, Hackman E, Lichtsteiner M 1974 The effect of oestradiol dipropionate and progesterone on monoamine uptake in rat brain. J Neurochem 22:187-189

Youdim MBH 1976 Monoamine oxidase – an iron requiring flavoprotein. In: Singer TP (ed) Flavins and flavoproteins. Elsevier, Amsterdam, p 590-599

Youdim MBH 1979 Development of monoamine deaminating systems: animal and human correlates. In: Mesami E, Brazier MAB (eds) Neural growth and differentiation. Raven Press, New York, p 71-90

Youdim MBH, Holzbauer M 1976 Physiological aspects of the oxidative deamination of monoamines. In: Monoamine oxidase and its inhibition. Excerpta Medica, Amsterdam (Ciba Found Symp 39), p 105-134

Youdim MBH, Holzbauer M, Woods HF 1974 Physicochemical properties, development and regulation of central and peripheral monoamine oxidase activity. In: Usdin E (ed) Neuropharmacology of monoamines and their regulatory enzymes. Raven Press, New York, p 11-28

Youdim MBH, Grahame-Smith DG, Woods HF 1976 Some properties of human platelet monoamine oxidase in iron-deficiency anaemia. Clin Sci Mol Med 50:479-585

The fate of circulating biologically active peptides in the lungs

SERGIO H. FERREIRA, LEWIS J. GREENE, MARIA CRISTINA O. SALGADO and E.M. KRIEGER

Departments of Pharmacology, Biochemistry and Physiology, School of Medicine of Ribeirão Preto, São Paulo, Brazil

Abstract The factors which regulate the disappearance of endogenous active substances during pulmonary transit are discussed. The presence of hydrolytic enzymes in the cytosol is not the only factor regulating pulmonary metabolism. An uptake–transport process is required to permit access to intracellular enzymes. No endothelial cell transport mechanism has yet been described for peptides. However, bradykinin and angiotensin I are metabolized by the pulmonary circulation because the enzyme is localized on the luminal surface of the endothelial cells.

The pulmonary and extrapulmonary conversion of angiotensin in rat is still a matter of debate. Evidence is presented which supports the idea that when low doses of angiotensin I (< 10 ng) are given intravenously, most of the conversion is pulmonary. With higher doses, extrapulmonary conversion also contributes to the final pressor effect of angiotensin I.

The fate of several biologically active peptides in the pulmonary circulation is quite different from that in other vascular beds. While peptides are generally extensively removed from the circulation by other vascular beds, most peptides pass through the lungs untouched. Two physiologically important peptides, bradykinin and angiotensin I, are exceptions. Bradykinin is inactivated and angiotensin I is converted to the biologically active peptide angiotensin II by enzyme-mediated hydrolytic processes.

LUNG METABOLISM OF PEPTIDES

Lung homogenates contain a great variety of hydrolytic enzymes with the capacity to inactivate all known biologically active peptides and most endogenous mediators. However, as previously pointed out (Ferreira & Bakhle 1977), the presence of inactivating enzymes in intracellular compartments or in tissue homogenates does not necessarily mean that the biologically active

Metabolic activities of the lung
(Ciba Foundation symposium 78) p 129-145

substance will be removed and inactivated during passage through the pulmonary circulation. As shown in Fig. 1, an uptake–transport mechanism is a limiting step necessary to permit the access of any biologically active material to intracellular inactivating enzymes. The absence of an uptake–transport mechanism explains why adrenaline and histamine are not removed and metabolized during passage through the lungs (Alabaster 1977). The same seems to be true for prostacyclin (Moncada & Vane 1979) and prostaglandins of the A series (McGiff et al 1967). An active transport mechanism has been suggested to be present in the lung for prostaglandins of the E series (Bito & Baroody 1975). The behaviour of most peptides in the pulmonary circulation does not differ substantially from that of other biologically active substances. *In vivo* experiments support the idea that the pulmonary endothelial cell membrane seems to be impermeable to peptides for which there is no uptake mechanism. Although angiotensin II, substance P, oxytocin, vasopressin, eledoisin and other peptide hormones are hydrolysed by lung homogenates, they are not removed during passage through the lungs. As we shall discuss here, the limited number of peptides that are hydrolysed *in vivo* during transit through the lungs are substrates for the enzymes present on the luminal surface of the endothelial cells (for references see reviews: Bakhle 1974, Bakhle & Vane 1974, Ferreira & Bakhle 1977, Longenecker & Huggins 1977, Erdös 1979).

Thus it is either the presence of membrane-bound enzymes in direct contact with blood or the existence of an uptake–transport mechanism coupled with intracellular inactivating enzymes which allows the lung to control circulating levels of biologically active substances. If uptake–transport occurs, but the substance is not inactivated, it will eventually return to the circulation (Bakhle 1979).

Bradykinin was the first peptide shown to be removed by passage through the lung. Using the blood-bathed organ technique, Ferreira & Vane (1967a) compared the concentration of bradykinin in femoral arterial blood after its infusion into the right ventricle or into the ascending aorta, and found that about 80% of the infused bradykinin disappeared during a single passage through the lungs and heart chambers. This degree of disappearance greatly exceeded that seen in the other vascular beds and that expected on the basis of bradykinin inactivation by blood kininases during pulmonary transit (~30%). A six-fold increase in the amount of bradykinin surviving pulmonary circulation (dog and cat) was observed after treatment with bradykinin-potentiating factor (BPF) derived from *Bothrops jararaca* venom (Ferreira & Vane 1976b). Since it was known that BPF inhibits the enzymic inactivation of bradykinin (Ferreira 1965), it was suggested that the disappearance

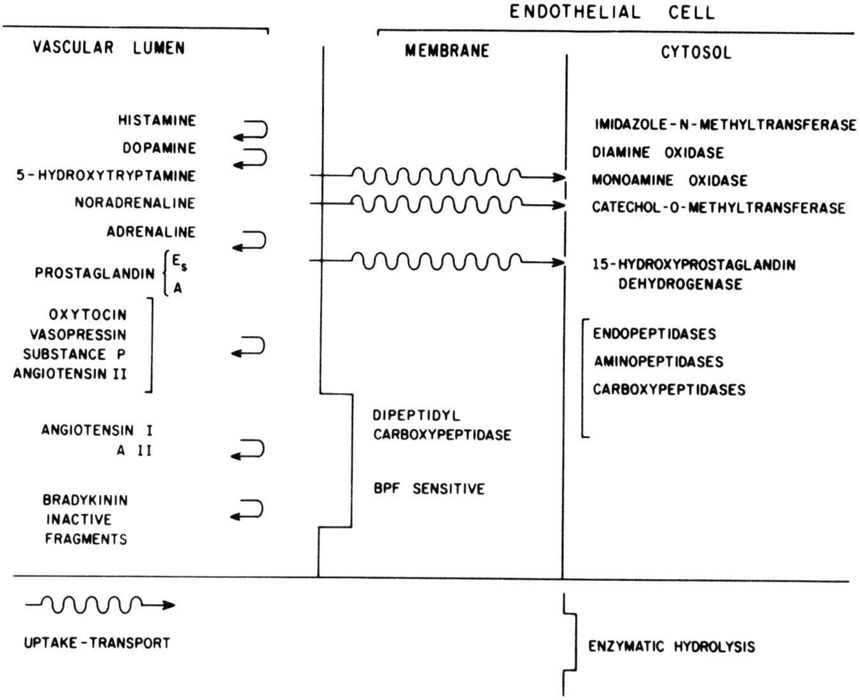

FIG. 1. Mechanism controlling the disappearance of biological substances during a single passage through the pulmonary circulation. If the substance is not a substrate for the enzymes present on the luminal surface of endothelial cells it may pass untouched or be removed by an uptake–transport mechanism. This mechanism makes the substance accessible to hydrolytic enzymes within the cell.

of bradykinin in the lungs was due to its inactivation by lung kininases. Shortly after these observations, Ng & Vane (1967, 1968, 1970) found that, in dogs, the lungs were able to convert angiotensin I. Conversion in the lung circulation (50% in 10 seconds) was quicker than that observed in blood (17% in 30 seconds). It was already known that *in vivo* angiotensin II is not removed during its passage through the pulmonary vascular beds (Goffinet & Mulrow 1965).

Bakhle (1968) first demonstrated the enzymic nature of the conversion by lung using a particulate preparation. Bradykinin was also inactivated by this fraction and both activities were inhibited by BPF peptides. The ability to discriminate between activity for angiotensin conversion and bradykinin inactivation with mercaptoethanol, 8-hydroxyquinoline and by chloride activation suggested that different enzymes were responsible for the activity. Later it was found that the enzyme purified from either lung or plasma can hydrolyse both substrates and is strongly inhibited by BPF-derived peptides (see Soffer 1976, Erdös 1979 for recent reviews).

The demonstration that lung kininase and angiotensin conversion were markedly inhibited *in vitro* and *in vivo* by BPF strongly stimulated research in this area. At least three main lines evolved. One was related to the purification, sequence determination and synthesis of the peptides responsible for the biological activity of BPF. The second line was concerned with purification of the lung angiotensin-converting enzyme, and the third was oriented towards locating the activity and determining the specificity of the BPF-sensitive peptidase(s).

PEPTIDES FROM BOTHROPS JARARACA VENOM

We have been involved in the first line of this research. We purified the nine peptides responsible for the biological activity of BPF (Ferreira et al 1970a). All of them potentiate bradykinin and inhibit angiotensin conversion and a general parallelism existed for the potency of these natural peptides in the two systems (Ferreira et al 1970b). The smallest of the peptides, the pentapeptide BPP_{5a}, was sequenced (Ferreira et al 1970a). Activity *in vitro* and *in vivo* was demonstrated for synthetic BPP_{5a} (Stewart et al 1971). Using this peptide we showed for the first time that it is possible to control overactivity of the renin–angiotensin system in some models of hypertension (Krieger et al 1971; see Greene et al 1972 for a review).

Our studies stimulated others to determine the structures of most of the other peptides (Ondetti et al 1971) and to confirm their biochemical (Cheung & Cushman 1973) and pharmacological properties (Engel et al 1972, 1973). Developments in this area were crowned by the design and synthesis of captopril by Cushman et al (1977). This is an orally active peptidylpeptide hydrolase inhibitor. For many years it had been known that sulphydryl compounds are potent inhibitors of kininase activity *in vitro* and *in vivo* (Ferreira & Rocha e Silva 1962, Erdös & Wöhler 1963). Captopril (D-3-mercapto-2-methylpropanoyl-L-proline) is an *N*-acyl derivative of proline (carboxyl terminus of all BPF peptides) correctly spaced from a sulphydryl group. Captopril is now under intense experimental investigation and is undergoing clinical trial. It is still uncertain whether its hypotensive effect is due only to inhibition of the angiotensin-converting activity. Part of the antihypertensive effect of the synthetic nonapeptide from *Bothrops jararaca*, BPP_{9a} (Thurston & Swales 1978), and of captopril (Gavras et al 1978) in man may also be due to potentiation of endogenous bradykinin.

CONVERTING ENZYME OR KININASE

The availability of homogeneous preparations of lung angiotensin-converting enzyme permitted the demonstration that the enzyme was identical to kininase II. Since the enzyme releases the carboxyl terminal dipeptide from bradykinin and angiotensin I it is appropriate to use its biochemical name dipeptidyl carboxypeptidase (EC 3.4.15.1) rather than either of its trivial names, kininase II or angiotensin-converting enzyme. On the basis of K_m, bradykinin is a better substrate for this enzyme than angiotensin I. The Cl^- ion dependence is more pronounced for converting enzyme activity than for kininase. The peptides from *B. jararaca* as well as captopril are extremely effective inhibitors. Specific antibodies prepared against the pure enzyme have been shown to inhibit bradykinin inactivation and angiotensin conversion in the lung, and to reverse renovascular hypertension. As we shall discuss later, antibodies provided the final proof for the localization of this enzyme on the luminal surface of the endothelial cells of the lung (Igic et al 1972, Dorer et al 1972, 1974, Cheung & Cushman 1973, Soffer 1976, Soffer & Sonnenblick 1978, Markle et al 1978, Erdös 1979).

LOCALIZATION OF DIPEPTIDYL CARBOXYPEPTIDASE

Over the years, several different approaches have been used to support the idea that angiotensin I conversion and bradykinin inactivation are mediated by the same enzyme(s) located in the cell membranes in direct contact with the blood. When infused through the isolated perfused lungs bradykinin was extensively removed (Ryan et al 1968, 1970a, Alabaster & Bakhle 1972a,b), angiotensin II passed through untouched and angiotensin I was converted to angiotensin II (Bakhle et al 1969). The speed of angiotensin I conversion indicated that converting enzyme activity was easily accessible. Furthermore, kininase and angiotensin-converting activity could be blocked by BPF or by the synthetic peptides (BPP_{5a}, BPP_{9a}).

Ryan et al (1970a,b), using radioactively labelled bradykinin or angiotensin I, showed that the radioactivity had the same transit time as blue dextran (mol.wt. 2 000 000), suggesting that bradykinin inactivation or angiotensin conversion probably occurs in the vascular space, at the endothelial cell level. The kinetics of metabolism of these peptides by perfused lung were identical to those of adenine nucleotides, known to be metabolized on the luminal surface of endothelial cells in the pulmonary circulation (Ryan & Ryan 1977). These results were confirmed by Fanburg & Glazier (1973), who also demonstrated that the conversion was a function of vascular surface and transit time.

Another line of evidence supporting the idea that bradykinin and angiotensin I are metabolized on the luminal surface of pulmonary endothelial cells came from the location in the various cell fractions of the kininase and converting activity sensitive to inhibition by BPF or derived synthetic peptides. As already pointed out, Bakhle (1968) demonstrated that angiotensin-converting activity in dog lung was associated with a particulate fraction, later shown by Sander & Huggins (1971) (in the rabbit) to be associated with plasma membranes. The location of the enzyme was demonstrated by Ryan et al (1972) with a highly effective separation process that allowed a clean separation of plasma membranes from intracellular components. This membrane fraction inactivated bradykinin, rapidly converted angiotensin I and did not inactivate angiotensin II. The location of the enzyme on the surface of the endothelial cell membrane of the lung arterioles and venules was definitively demonstrated by Ryan et al (1976) (in tissue and cell culture) using a microperoxidase-antibody reagent and by Caldwell et al (1976) using fluorescein-labelled antibody.

IS DIPEPTIDYL CARBOXYPEPTIDASE THE PHYSIOLOGICALLY IMPORTANT ENZYME FOR KININ INACTIVATION AND ANGIOTENSIN CONVERSION?

The fact that this membrane-bound enzyme is inhibited by BPF links it to the important physiological events demonstrated in the pulmonary vascular bed *in vivo*. BPF and related peptides are very effective *in vivo*. For example, in the rat, BPP_{9a} completely inhibits bradykinin inactivation and angiotensin conversion by the lungs (Engel et al 1972, 1973). However, the inability to reproduce this intense inhibition in the rat perfused lung, where BPP_{9a} reduced bradykinin inactivation only from 97 to 91% (Bakhle 1976), clearly indicates that rat perfused lung has an abnormal kininase activity. Furthermore, 7-homo-Pro-bradykinin is inactivated by the perfused rat lung by a mechanism not affected by BPP_{9a}. These observations may result from increased membrane permeability of perfused lung to peptides, which facilitates access to intracellular peptidases. The inactivation of angiotensin II by perfused preparations also supports this interpretation. *In vivo*, angiotensin II is known to pass freely through the pulmonary circulation (Goffinet & Mulrow 1965, Hodge et al 1967, Biron et al 1967). In perfused lungs, however, this probably depends on the state of the preparation, for there have been reports of no inactivation (Bakhle et al 1969) and of inactivation (Turker 1973). Inactivation of angiotensin II by perfused lung seems to be a function of the tissue damage, as it occurred only when the lung was oedematous (Bakhle 1976). This abnormal permeability to peptides may explain the low recovery of angiotensin II after administration of angiotensin I (Ryan et al 1970b) and the large number of small peptides obtained by injecting bradykinin into the isolated perfused lung (Ryan et al 1970a).

The absence of an uptake mechanism for bradykinin and angiotensin can be inferred from the experiments of Ryan et al (1970a,b), for there was no delay in the release of metabolites, in contrast to other substrates such as adrenaline for which an uptake mechanism has been described (Alabaster 1977).

All of these observations suggest that during a single passage through the lung *in vivo*, because of the absence of an uptake–transport mechanism for biologically active peptides, only those peptides that are substrates for peptidases present on the luminal surface of endothelial cells are metabolized.

PULMONARY OR NON-PULMONARY CONVERSION

The relative contribution of non-pulmonary vascular beds to the overall conversion of angiotensin I is still a matter of dispute. The bulk of the evidence points to the lungs as the major site of angiotensin I conversion in most species (Ng & Vane 1967, 1968, 1970, Aiken & Vane 1970). However, Oparil et al (1979), using the synthetic peptide BPP_{9a}, recently showed that angiotensin I in the dog had a pressor effect which was independent of pulmonary conversion. They demonstrated that when conversion of angiotensin I in the lung was inhibited, intra-arterial administration of angiotensin I was able to cause a hypertensive effect. Pulmonary conversion in the rat has been suggested to be unimportant (Stewart & Freer 1973, Freer & Stewart 1975, Kraye & Gross 1971). Moreover, Freer & Stewart (1975) questioned whether a single enzyme is responsible for kinin inactivation and angiotensin I conversion in the rat.

Recently, Krieger et al (1980) re-evaluated this problem in conscious rats. In these animals, low doses (1–10 ng) of angiotensin I injected intravenously induced much larger responses than when injected intra-arterially (Fig. 2). These results clearly show that rat lung converts angiotensin I *in vivo*. As the dose is increased the percentage of conversion diminishes. At doses higher than 30 ng of angiotensin I, providing 40–50 mmHg pressure rise, there is no longer any difference in the magnitude of the observed effect between the two routes of injection. The times of onset of the effect of intravenous administration of angiotensin I and II were similar; however, the time of onset and the time to reach maximum effect were shorter when angiotensin I was administered intravenously rather than intra-arterially (Table 1), indicating that the lungs played a part in the conversion of high as well as low doses of angiotensin I. As shown in Table 1, the time of onset of the effect of intra-arterial administration was greater for angiotensin I than angiotensin II but

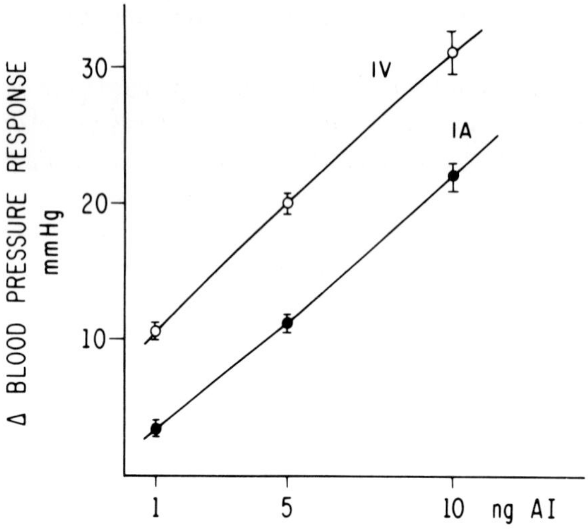

FIG. 2. Increase in blood pressure induced by low doses of angiotensin I injected intravenously (IV) or intra-arterially (IA) into conscious rats. The participation of the lung in angiotensin I conversion is indicated by the higher blood pressure response after intravenous injection.

TABLE 1

Comparison between intravenous (IV) and intra-arterial (IA) administration of large doses of angiotensin I (>30 ng) and II to give a rise in blood pressure of 0–50 mm Hg in conscious rats

Angiotensin	*Onset time of effect (seconds)*		*Maximum effect (seconds)*	
	IV	*IA*	*IV*	*IA*
I	2.9 ± 0.3	3.4 ± 0.3	6.1 ± 0.6	9.9 ± 0.9
II	3.1 ± 0.3	1.0 ± 0.2	7.3 ± 0.3	5.4 ± 0.4

this period of time, 3–4 seconds, is too short to allow one complete recirculation, since the circulation time is of the order of 6–7 seconds in the conscious rat. This result suggests an extrapulmonary conversion of high doses of angiotensin I. In summary, it seems that for very low doses of angiotensin I injected intravenously most of the conversion occurs in the pulmonary circulation. At high doses of angiotensin I, conversion in peripheral vascular beds becomes important.

The blockade of conversion of angiotensin I by BPP_{5a} and BPP_{9a} clearly illustrates these points. With low, intravenously injected doses of angiotensin I these peptides totally inhibited the blood pressure increase (inhibition of pulmonary conversion). However, the effect of increasing doses of BPP_{9a} on high doses of angiotensin I (i.v.) is observed first on the time of onset, suggesting an effect on pulmonary conversion. With increasing amounts of BPP_{9a}, the hypertensive effect of high doses of angiotensin I (i.v.) can be totally blocked, suggesting an inhibition of pulmonary and peripheral conversion. In this context it is interesting that Oparil et al (1979) showed that extrapulmonary conversion is less sensitive to BPP_{9a}. Using antibody to angiotensin II, Oates & Stokes (1974) concluded that, in addition to pulmonary conversion, peripheral conversion also occurs in the anaesthetized rat. It is interesting to note that peripheral conversion was demonstrable in the presence of antibody to angiotensin II, which required using much higher doses of angiotensin I (10–50 ng).

Freer & Stewart (1975), using BPP_{5a} and high doses of angiotensin I, concluded that lung kininase and angiotensin-converting activity were due to different enzymes. Our results do not support this view since threshold doses of BPP_{5a} for bradykinin potentiation also inhibited pulmonary conversion of low doses of angiotensin I (Krieger et al 1980).

In summary, we have discussed the concept that the disappearance or activation of a biologically active peptide during its transit through the pulmonary circulation is the result of the presence of a hydrolytic enzyme (dipeptidyl carboxypeptidase) on the luminal surface of endothelial cells, since there is no active uptake–transport mechanism in lung endothelial cells to permit the access of such peptides to other intracellular peptidases. Conversion of intravenously administered low doses of angiotensin I in the conscious rat seems to occur mainly in the pulmonary circulation. At high doses, extrapulmonary conversion seems to operate as well. The extrapulmonary enzyme responsible for angiotensin I conversion is less susceptible to inhibition by BPP_{9a} (Oparil et al 1979). Thus, because bradykinin is a better substrate than angiotensin I for the rat lung enzyme (bradykinin is inactivated 90–97%, whereas angiotensin I conversion is ~30%), the peripheral metabolism of intravenously injected bradykinin is less important than that of high intravenous doses of angiotensin I. This may explain why BPP peptides apparently affect bradykinin more than angiotensin I.

References

Aiken JW, Vane JR 1970 The renin-angiotensin system: inhibition of converting enzyme in isolated tissues. Nature (Lond) 228:30-34

Alabaster VA 1977 Inactivation of endogenous amines in the lungs In: Bakhle YS, Vane JR (eds)

Metabolic functions of the lung (Lung biology in health and disease, vol 4) Dekker, New York, p 3-25

Alabaster VA, Bakhle YS 1972a The inactivation of bradykinin in the pulmonary circulation of isolated lungs. Br J Pharmacol 45:299-309

Alabaster VA, Bakhle YS 1972b Converting enzyme and bradykininase in the lung. Circ Res 30 & 31 (Suppl 2):72-81

Bakhle YS 1968 Conversion of angiotensin I to angiotensin II by cell-free extracts of dog lung. Nature (Lond) 220:919-921

Bakhle YS 1974 Converting enzyme *in vitro*: measurement and properties. In: Page IH, Bumpus FM (eds) Angiotensin. Springer-Verlag, Berlin (Handbook of experimental pharmacology vol 50) p 41-80

Bakhle YS 1976 The nature of the bradykinin inactivating system in isolated lungs. Br J Pharmacol 56:349-350P

Bakhle YS 1979 Action of prostaglandin dehydrogenase inhibitors on prostaglandin uptake in rat isolated lung. Br J Pharmacol 65:635:639

Bakhle YS, Reynard AM, Vane JR 1969 Metabolism of the angiotensins in isolated perfused tissues. Nature (Lond) 222:956-959

Bakhle YS, Vane JR 1974 Pharmacokinetic function of the pulmonary circulation. Physiol Rev 54:1007-1045

Biron P, Meyer P, Panisset JC 1967 Removal of angiotensins from the systemic circulation. Can J Physiol Pharmacol 46:175-178

Bito LZ, Baroody, RA 1975 Inhibition of pulmonary prostaglandin metabolism by inhibitors of prostaglandin bio-transport (probenecid and bromocresol green). Prostaglandins 10:633-639

Caldwell PR, Seegal BC, Hsu KC, Das M, Soffer RL 1976 Angiotensin converting enzyme: vascular endothelial localization. Science (Wash DC) 191:1050-1051

Cheung HS, Cushman DW 1973 Inhibition of homogeneous angiotensin converting enzyme of rabbit lung by synthetic venom peptide of *Bothrops jararaca*. Biochim Biophys Acta 293:451-463

Cushman DW, Cheung HS, Sabo EF, Ondetti MA 1977 Design of potent competitive inhibitors of angiotensin-converting enzyme. Carboxyalkanoyl and mercaptoalkanoyl amino acids. Biochemistry 16:5484 5491

Dorer FE, Kahn JR, Lentz KE, Levine M, Skeggs LT 1972 Purification and properties of angiotensin-converting enzyme from hog lung. Circ Res 31:356-366

Dorer FE, Kahn JR, Lentz KE, Levine M, Skeggs LT 1974 Hydrolysis of bradykinin by angiotensin-converting enzyme. Circ Res 34:824-827

Engel SL, Schaeffer TR, Gold BI, Rubin B 1972 Inhibition of pressor effects of angiotensin I and augmentation of depressor effects of bradykinin by synthetic peptides. Proc Soc Exp Biol Med 140:240-244

Engel SL, Schaeffer TR, Waugh MH, Rubin B 1973 Effects of the nonapeptide SQ 20881 on blood pressure of rats with experimental renovascular hypertension. Proc Soc Exp Biol Med 143:483-487

Erdös EG 1979 Kininases. In: Erdös EG (ed) Bradykinin, kallidin and kallikrein: supplement. Springer-Verlag, Berlin (Handbook of experimental pharmacology 25, Suppl) p 427-487

Erdös EG, Wöhler JR 1963 Inhibition in vivo of the enzymatic inactivation of bradykinin and kallidin. Biochem Pharmacol 12:1193-1199

Fanburg BL, Glazier JB 1973 Conversion of angiotensin I to angiotensin II in the isolated perfused dog lung. J Appl Physiol 35:325-331

Ferreira SH 1965 A bradykinin potentiating factor (BPF) in the venom of *Bothrops jararaca*. Br J Pharmacol Chemother 24:163-169

Ferreira SH Bakhle YS 1977 Inactivation of bradykinin and related peptides in the lung. In: Bakhle YS, Vane JR (eds) Metabolic functions of the lung (Lung biology in health and disease, vol 4) Dekker, New York, p 33-53

Ferreira SH, Bartelt DC, Greene LJ 1970a Isolation of bradykinin potentiating peptides from *Bothrops jararaca* venom. Biochemistry 9:2583-2593

Ferreira SH, Greene LJ, Alabaster VA, Bakhle YS, Vane JR 1970b Activity of various fractions of bradykinin potentiating factor against angiotensin I converting enzyme. Nature (Lond) 225:379-380

Ferreira SH, Rocha e Silva M 1962 Potentiation of bradykinin by dimercaptopropanol (BAL) and other inhibitors of its destroying enzyme in plasma. Biochem Pharmacol 11:1123-1128

Ferreira SH, Vane JR 1967a The disappearance of bradykinin and eledoisin in the circulation and vascular beds of the cat. Br J Pharmacol Chemother 30:417-424

Ferreira SH, Vane JR 1967b The detection and estimation of bradykinin in the circulating blood. Br J Pharmacol Chemother 29:367-377

Freer RJ, Stewart JM 1975 *In vivo* pulmonary metabolism of bradykinin, angiotensin I, and 5-hydroxytryptamine in the rat. Arch Int Pharmacodyn Ther 217:97-109

Gavras H, Brunner HR, Turini GA, Kershaw GR, Tifft CP, Cuttelod S, Gavras I, Vukovich RA, McKinsky DN 1978 Antihypertensive effect of the oral angiotensin converting enzyme inhibitor SQ 14255 in man. N Engl J Med 298:991-995

Goffinet JA, Mulrow PJ 1965 Estimation of angiotensin clearance by an *in vivo* assay. Clin Res 11:408

Greene LJ, Camargo ACM, Krieger EM, Stewart JM, Ferreira SH 1972 Inhibition of the conversion of angiotensin I to II and potentiation of bradykinin by small peptides present in *Bothrops jararaca* venom. Circ Res 30 & 31 (Suppl 2): 62-71

Hodge RL, Ng KKF, Vane JR 1967 Disappearance of angiotensin from the circulation of the dog. Nature (Lond) 215:138-141

Igic R, Erdös EG, Yeh HSJ, Sorrells K, Nakajima T 1972 Angiotensin I converting enzyme of the lung. Circ Res 30 & 31 (Suppl 2):51-61

Kraye VAW, Gross F 1971 Conversion of angiotensin I to angiotensin II in peripheral vascular beds of the rat. Am J Physiol 220:1294-1296

Krieger EM, Salgado HC, Assan CJ, Greene LJ, Ferreira SH 1971 Potential screening test for detection of overactivity of renin-angiotensin system. Lancet 1:269-271

Krieger EM, Salgado MC, Trindade IEK, Ferreira SH, Greene LJ 1980 Inactivation of bradykinin and conversion of angiotensin I in conscious rats with experimental renal hypertension. Proceedings of the IIIrd Simposio Interamericano sobre Hipertensión Arterial, Mexico City, February 11–15, 1979

Longenecker GL, Huggins CG 1977 Biochemistry of the pulmonary angiotensin-converting enzyme. In: Bakhle YS, Vane JR (eds) Metabolic functions of the lung (Lung biology in health and disease, vol 4) Dekker, New York, p 55-83

Markle R, Sonnenblick EH, Conroy JM, Soffer RL 1978 Reversal of renovascular hypertension by antibodies specific for angiotensin-converting enzyme. Proc Natl Acad Sci USA 75:5702-5705

Moncada S, Vane JR 1979 Pharmacology and endogenous roles of prostaglandin endoperoxides, thromboxane A_2 and prostacyclin. Pharmacol Rev 30: 293-331

McGiff JC, Terragno NA, Strand JC, Lee JB, Lonigro AJ, Ng KKF 1967 Selective passage of prostaglandins across the lung. Nature (Lond) 223:742-745

Ng KKF, Vane JR 1967 Conversion of angiotensin I to angiotensin II. Nature (Lond) 216:762-776

Ng KKF, Vane JR 1968 Fate of angiotensin I in the circulation. Nature (Lond) 218:144-150

Ng KKF, Vane JR 1970 Some properties of the angiotensin converting enzyme in the lung *in vivo*. Nature (Lond) 225:1142-1144

Oates HF, Stokes GS 1974 Role of extrapulmonary conversion in mediating the systemic pressor activity in angiotensin I. J Exp Med 140:79-86

Ondetti MA, Williams NJ, Sabo EF, Pluscec J, Weaver ER, Kocy O 1971 Angiotensin converting enzyme inhibitors from the venom of *Bothrops jararaca*. Isolation, elucidation of structure and synthesis. Biochemistry 10:4033-4039

Oparil S, Koerner TBS, O'Donoghue JK 1979 Mechanism of angiotensin I converting enzyme inhibition by SQ 20,881 (Glu-Trp-Pro-Arg-Pro-Gln-Ile-Pro-Pro) *in vivo*. Hypertension 1:13-22

Ryan US, Ryan JW 1977 Correlation between the fine structure of the alveolar-capillary unit and its metabolic activities. In: Bakhle YS, Vane JR (eds) Metabolic functions of the lung (Lung biology in health and disease, vol 4) Dekker, New York, p 197-232
Ryan JW, Roblero J, Stewart JM 1968 Inactivation of bradykinin in the pulmonary circulation. Biochem J 110:795-797
Ryan JW, Roblero J, Stewart JM 1970a Inactivation of bradykinin in rat lung. Adv Exp Med Biol 8:263-271
Ryan JW, Stewart JM, Leary WP, Ledingham JG 1970b Metabolism of angiotensin I in the pulmonary circulation. Biochem J 120:221-223
Ryan JW, Smith U, Niemeyer RS 1972 Angiotensin I: metabolism by plasma membrane of lung. Science (Wash DC) 176:64-66
Ryan JW, Ryan US, Schultz DR, Day AR, Dorer FE 1976 Further evidence on the subcellular sites of kininase II (angiotensin converting enzyme). Adv Exp Med Biol 70:235-243
Sander GE, Huggins CG 1971 Subcellular localization of angiotensin I converting enzyme in rabbit lung. Nat New Biol 230:27-29
Soffer RL 1976 Angiotensin-converting enzyme and the regulation of vasoactive peptides. Annu Rev Biochem 45:73-94
Soffer RL, Sonnenblick EH 1978 Physiologic, biochemical and immunologic aspects of angiotensin-converting enzyme. Prog Cardiovasc Dis 21:167-175
Stewart JM, Freer RJ 1973 Inhibitors of the pulmonary destruction of bradykinin in the rat. In: Peeters H (ed) Protides of the biological fluids (20th Colloquium) Pergamon Press, Oxford & New York, p 331-333
Stewart JM, Ferreira SH, Greene LJ 1971 Bradykinin potentiating peptide PCA-Lys-Trp-Ala--Pro. An inhibitor of the pulmonary inactivation of bradykinin and conversion of angiotensin I to II. Biochem Pharmacol 20: 1557-1567
Thurston H, Swales JD 1978 Converting enzyme inhibitor and saralasin infusion in rats. Evidence for an additional vasodepressor property of converting enzyme inhibitor. Circ Res 42:588-592
Turker RK 1973 Change of activity of angiotensins I and II in the isolated perfused guinea pig lung. Arch Int Physiol Biochim 81:523-536

Discussion

Junod: Is there any possibility of competition between bradykinin and angiotensin, at physiological concentrations, for converting enzyme?

Bakhle: This seems unlikely, because at physiological concentrations of these peptides one is far below the K_m of both substrates. Such concentrations are never achieved *in vivo* (K_m for bradykinin, 4 μM; for angiotensin I, 30 μM; Dorer et al 1974).

Junod: Dr Ferreira showed a result suggesting that circulating bradykinin could be affected by the inhibitor, because there was a fall in blood pressure.

Ferreira: Yes. When we started inhibiting lung kininase with peptides from *Bothrops jararaca* venom, giving small amounts of angiotensin I, there was a parallel effect on bradykinin and on angiotensin I conversion. There is an assay dependency. If the assay is sensitive to angiotensin I conversion, destruction of bradykinin and conversion of low doses of AI are similarly inhibited.

Bakhle: The problem is that with the inhibitory peptides, and with captopril also, there is potentiation of bradykinin at receptor level, plus inhibition of its destruction, so that you observe the sum of two effects.

Ferreira: Potentiation, through an allosteric change of the receptor, may occur in an isolated preparation but has not been proved to occur *in vivo*. When bradykinin is injected intra-arterially in the rat and the animal is treated with a bradykinin potentiator like BPP_{9a} there is no apparent potentiation. If BPF acted on the bradykinin receptor one would see potentiation.

Aiken: In anaesthetized dogs Dr Vane and I (Aiken & Vane 1972) showed that the effects of a close intra-arterial injection of bradykinin to the hind leg could be potentiated by the pentapeptide, BPP_{5a}. But that doesn't necessarily mean a change in receptor sensitivity because the potentiation could still have been prevention of inactivation by an enzymic route, but in this case the enzyme would have had to have been in blood or the hindlimb vascular bed.

Reid: Where are the receptors for, say, AI or AII? We know about the surface caveolae of the endothelial cells, but is there any evidence of the fate of the molecule or its metabolite? Does it remain in the endothelial cell or does it move to cells external to it, in either the lung or any other organ?

Vane: I don't know any evidence that angiotensin II gets through the endothelial cells, but it certainly causes contraction of the smooth muscle cells behind them.

Alberti: We have heard about the peptidases on the cell surface. Is it known yet how they bind peptides, where they are in the membrane, and whether there is a change in membrane properties once they bind their substrate? In other words, is this something rather like a receptor that has peptidase properties? Has anyone isolated these peptidases from the membrane?

Soffer: Let me first summarize the current information on receptors for the vasoactive peptides. As far as I know, a specific receptor for bradykinin has yet to be characterized. Two kinds of experimental approach have been used to identify specific receptors for angiotensin II. In the first, various antagonists of angiotensin II have been injected into animals and their effects on the vasopressor or aldosteronogenic responses to this octapeptide have been examined. In the second, the binding of radioactive angiotensin II by isolated cells or by membrane fractions from various tissue homogenates has been studied. A substantial body of information has emerged from these approaches which indicates that most tissues contain specific angiotensin II receptors associated with their plasma membrane fraction (see for example Lin & Goodfriend 1970, Needleman et al 1976, Bennett & Snyder 1976, Douglas et al 1978, Capponi & Catt 1979). These angiotensin II receptors have not yet been purified from any source, so specific anti-receptor antibodies are unavailable. It has not, therefore, generally been possible to establish with certainty the cellular and subcellular localization of the receptor in different organs. It is interesting, however, that there is evidence suggesting that cultured vascular endothelial cells contain receptors for the octapeptide (Buonassisi & Venter 1976).

In contrast to the angiotensin II receptor, angiotensin-converting enzyme (EC 3.4.15.1) has been obtained in pure form and its physicochemical and immunological properties (reviewed by Soffer & Sonnenblick 1978) and its mechanism of action (reviewed by Cushman et al 1978) have been characterized. An interesting aspect that has not yet been investigated is the structural relationship of the enzyme to the vascular endothelial membrane of which it is a part. It may be, for example, that its participation in an organized membranous structure results in different catalytic properties from those documented with isolated, solubilized enzyme preparations. Converting enzyme may be a good model for exploring the structural basis and functional significance of membrane–protein interaction since it can be isolated as a pure, water-soluble molecule and since antibodies to it are available.

Incidentally, it is my impression that there is as yet no certainty whether bradykinin is normally present in the circulation. If it is, the concentration is presumably vanishingly low, while that of angiotensin I may be of the order of 10^{-10}M.

Reid: Does that include the fetus and newborn?

Soffer: I don't know. As Dr Bakhle said, the K_m for angiotensin I is high, perhaps 40-80 μM, whereas that for bradykinin is much lower (~ 1 μM). But compared with the circulating levels, these are high concentrations of either substrate.

Vane: The fact that endothelial cells in culture have angiotensin receptors could be interpreted in at least two ways. One is that these cells act as a transducer for the effects of angiotensin II on the smooth muscle behind them. The other is that the angiotensin receptor in the endothelial cell is doing something quite different, like releasing prostacyclin.

One point that came clearly out of the paper by Dr Youdim and Dr Bakhle is that the endothelial cells of the lungs have a selective uptake mechanism for catecholamines or 5-HT which is missing from endothelial cells of the portal vessels in the liver. Is there any morphological difference between the endothelium of the portal vessels and the lungs?

Simionescu: Yes. The capillaries of the lung, like those of muscle, are provided with continuous endothelium and a continuous basal lamina. The pulmonary endothelium contains, characteristically, a large population of plasmalemmal vesicles, 60–70 nm in diameter. The liver has discontinuous capillaries (sinusoids) characterized by a very thin endothelium which displays large gaps (up to hundreds of nanometres in diameter); its basal lamina is either discontinuous or absent. A third type of capillary is present in viscera, namely the fenestrated capillary, the endothelium of which is also highly attenuated and characteristically has numerous transcellular circular openings, the fenestrae (60–80 nm in diameter). The fenestra is usually closed by a thin, single-layered diaphragm with a central knob (10–15 nm diameter). These capillaries have a continuous basal lamina.

Meyrick: We have compared the endothelial cell of the hilar pulmonary artery and that of the normally non-muscular peripheral pulmonary artery, and find differences between these two regions of lung (Meyrick & Reid 1979a,b, 1980). The endothelial cell in the hilar pulmonary artery is larger in diameter and thicker than that in the peripheral arteries. The hilar cell has more Weibel–Palade bodies and its basement membrane is more complete than in the peripheral cells. The labelling index of the hilar endothelial cell is less, about 30% of that found at the periphery.

With exposure to hypoxia further differences emerge. The organelles of the hilar endothelial cells hypertrophy, particularly those organelles associated with protein synthesis (Meyrick & Reid 1980); the organelles in the peripheral cells also hypertrophy but here it is mainly an increase in pinocytic vesicles and in intracellular matrix (B. Meyrick, unpublished observations 1980). After just 24 hours of hypoxia the labelling index of the hilar endothelial cells increases threefold. At the periphery an increase in labelling index also occurs but here it is a fourfold increase and only after Day 7. At the hilum the areal density of Weibel–Palade bodies decreases, while at the periphery it increases (Meyrick & Reid 1978, 1980).

Ferreira: If the enzyme is more effective as a kininase, acting on bradykinin, than as a converting enzyme acting on angiotensin I, perhaps we should call it a kininase, and the inhibitors such as captopril should be called kininase inhibitors!

Vane: They should in fact be called dipeptidyl carboxypeptidase inhibitors.

Soffer: That is right. After all, the inhibitors happened to be discovered in the context of blood pressure, but almost certainly there are other reactions contributing to other processes where this enzyme is involved.

Said: You stressed the minute circulating concentrations of bradykinin, but this is a local hormone and it might occur in much higher concentrations in a local or regional circulation, while at the same time being at a very low concentration in the general circulation.

Soffer: That is certainly possible. I am curious whether anyone has definitely established that it is present in the general circulation.

Ferreira: One can detect bradykinin in the circulation by radioimmunoassay but the question is whether it is important for the normal control of blood pressure. It seems that it is not, because you can give BPF or captopril in large amounts without changing the blood pressure, in a normal or non-hypertensive animal.

Soffer: There is a tribe of Amazonian Indians, the Yanomamos, who eat almost no salt (Oliver et al 1975). They have a very high renin level and their renin–angiotensin system presumably contributes enormously to the maintenance of their blood pressure. Nobody has ever given them a converting enzyme inhibitor, but in these Indians such an agent would be likely to elicit a profoundly hypotensive response unrelated to its bradykinin-potentiating action.

Stalcup: Niarchos et al (1979) have shown that normal individuals on a normal salt intake show a fall in blood pressure if treated acutely with SQ 20 881, a specific inhibitor of converting-enzyme activity.

Ferreira: If there were circulating angiotensin or bradykinin, captopril should cause hypotension.

Bakhle: That isn't necessarily true; it's a matter of controlling mechanisms. If the production of angiotensin II in normal individuals is not a part of the mechanism maintaining blood pressure, you can give as much inhibitor as you like and there won't be any change in blood pressure.

References

Aiken JW, Vane JR 1972 Inhibition of converting enzyme of the renin–angiotensin system in the kidneys and hindlegs of dogs. Circ Res 30:203-273

Bennett JP, Snyder SH 1976 Angiotensin II binding to mammalian brain membranes. J Biol Chem 251:7423-7430

Buonassisi V, Venter JC 1976 Hormone and neurotransmitter receptors in an established vascular endothelial cell line. Proc Natl Acad Sci USA 73:1612-1616

Capponi AM, Catt KJ 1979 Angiotensin II receptors in adrenal cortex and uterus. Binding and activation properties of angiotensin analogues. J Biol Chem 254:5120-5127

Cushman DW, Cheung HS, Sabo EF, Ondetti MA 1978 Design of new antihypertensive drugs: potent and specific inhibitors of angiotensin-converting enzyme. Prog Cardiovasc Dis 21:176-182

Dorer FE, Kahn JR, Lentz KE, Levine M, Skeggs LT 1974 Hydrolysis of bradykinin by angiotensin converting enzyme. Circ Res 34:824-827

Douglas J, Aguilera G. Kondo T, Catt K 1978 Angiotensin II receptors and aldosterone production in rat glomerulosa cells. Endocrinology 102:685-696

Lin SY, Goodfriend TL 1970 Angiotensin receptors. Am J Physiol 218:1319-1328

Meyrick B, Reid L 1978 The effect of continued hypoxia on rat arterial circulation: an ultrastructural study. Lab Invest 38:188-200

Meyrick B, Reid L 1979a Ultrastructural features of the distended pulmonary arteries of the normal rat. Anat Rec 193:71-97

Meyrick B, Reid L 1979b Hypoxia and incorporation of ^{3}H-thymidine by cells of the rat pulmonary arteries and alveolar wall. Am J Pathol 96:51-70

Meyrick B, Reid L 1980 Endothelial and subintimal changes in rat hilar pulmonary artery during recovery from hypoxia. A quantitative ultrastructural study. Lab Invest 42:603-615

Needleman P, Douglas JR, Jakschik BA, Blumberg AL, Isakson PC, Marshall GR 1976 Angiotensin antagonists as pharmacological tools. Fed Proc 35:2488-2493

Niarchos AP, Pickering TG, Case DB, Sullivan P, Laragh JH 1979 Role of the renin–angiotensin system in blood pressure regulation. The cardiovascular effects of converting enzyme inhibition in normotensive subjects. Circ Res 45:829-837

Oliver WJ, Cohen EL, Neel JV 1975 Blood pressure, sodium intake, and sodium related hormones in the Yanomamo Indians, a 'no-salt' culture. Circulation 52:146-151

Soffer RL, Sonnenblick EH 1978 Physiologic, biochemical and immunologic aspects of angiotensin-converting enzyme. Prog Cardiovasc Dis 21:167-175

The lung as a generator of prostacyclin

R.J. GRYGLEWSKI

Department of Pharmacology, N. Copernicus Academy of Medicine, Grzegórzecka 16, 31-531 Kraków, Poland

Abstract Under physiological conditions prostacyclin is the main metabolite of arachidonic acid that is generated and released by the lungs. In man and in cat prostacyclin seems to be a circulating hormone whose concentration is 100–200 pg ml^{-1} higher in arterial blood than in mixed venous blood. Generation of prostacyclin by lungs can be increased by angiotensin II, bradykinin and arachidonic acid provided that low concentrations of these substances are infused into the pulmonary artery. Air pulmonary emboli and mechanical hyperventilation stimulate the lungs to generate more prostacyclin. Respiratory stimulants such as lobeline or almitrine are also effective prostacyclin releasers from the lung. It is proposed that this para-endocrine function of the lung protects coronary and cerebral arteries against thrombosis and atherosclerosis while pharmacological amplification of the pulmonary release of prostacyclin may constitute a new means of treating thromboembolic diseases.

METABOLIC FUNCTION OF THE LUNG

Vane (1969) has developed the concept that the selective removal or activation of certain biogenic amines, peptides and lipids in the pulmonary circulation either protects the organism against endogenous intoxication by vasoactive substances or reveals biological activity of relatively inactive prohormones (e.g. angiotensin). This is the so-called metabolic function of the lung and it consists in the uptake and/or biochemical transformation of a number of substrates that are brought to the lungs in mixed venous blood. In some instances the uptake of a substrate seems to be more important than its subsequent enzymic inactivation by the lung, as in the case of catecholamines and prostaglandins.

Approximately 20 to 35% of noradrenaline (norepinephrine) is removed on passage through the pulmonary circulation while the pulmonary removal of

Metabolic activities of the lung
(Ciba Foundation symposium 78) p 147-164

adrenaline (epinephrine) is negligible. The lung treats adrenaline—a circulating hormone—in a different way from noradrenaline—a neuromediator, or 5-hydroxytryptamine (serotonin)—a local hormone (Vane 1969, Bakhle & Vane 1977).

Inactivation of prostaglandins (PGs) during their passage through the pulmonary circulation also requires their active transportation into the lung cells. This transport mechanism exists for PGE_2 and $PGF_{2\alpha}$, but not for PGA_2 (Eling et al 1977) or prostacyclin (Dusting et al 1978). The catabolism of PGs by 15-hydroxyprostaglandin dehydrogenase is secondary to their uptake into the lung cells.

Ferreira & Vane (1967) have found that the biological activity of bradykinin is largely lost during passage through the pulmonary circulation. Ryan & Ryan (1977a,b) have shown that bradykinin is hydrolysed at 5 of its 8 peptide bonds by enzymes situated near the luminal surface of pulmonary endothelial cells. The same lung peptidase, namely kininase II (converting enzyme, dipeptidyl carboxypeptidase, EC 3.4.15.1), activates angiotensin I to angiotensin II (Ng & Vane 1968).

Unlike catecholamines or prostaglandins, kinins and angiotensin I are not taken up by pulmonary endothelial cells from the bloodstream. The molecules of these peptides are enzymically split on the surface of the pulmonary endothelium as they pass (Ryan & Ryan 1977a,b).

Adenosine triphosphate (ATP), diphosphate (ADP) and monophosphate (AMP) are eliminated across the pulmonary circulation by phosphate esterases which are situated on the surface of the pulmonary endothelial cells (Ryan & Ryan 1977b). In this respect the pulmonary metabolism of nucleotides resembles that of peptides.

The lungs receive the entire cardiac output. The bloodstream brings to the pulmonary endothelium both circulating hormones (e.g. adrenaline), prohormones (e.g. angiotensin I) and 'local hormones', or chemical mediators which have escaped peripheral tissue inactivation (e.g. bradykinin, serotonin, prostaglandins and nucleotides). The specificity of the intracellular uptake mechanism and the availability of the appropriate enzymes enable the lung to deal with these substances in a highly selective manner.

RELEASE OF PROSTANOIDS BY THE LUNG

Prostanoids are not only metabolized by the lungs; they are also generated in this organ. Indeed, the lungs contain an entire set of enzymes for the oxidation and cyclization of arachidonic acid to a variety of metabolites. When isolated perfused lungs from sensitized guinea-pigs are challenged with an antigen, PGE_2, $PGF_{2\alpha}$, PGD_2, prostacyclin (PGI_2) and thromboxane A_2 (TXA_2) are released into the lung effluent (Hamberg & Samuelsson 1974) along with a number of their metabolites (Boot et al 1978, Pace-Asciak & Rangaraj 1977). Several of those prostanoids are released by the lungs after mechanical stimulation (Piper & Vane 1971), hyperventilation and hypoxia as well as after chemical stimulation with large doses of histamine, serotonin, bradykinin, arachidonic acid, slow-reacting substance C (SRS-C) and a rabbit aorta contracting substance releasing factor (RCS-RF) (Piper & Vane 1971).

$PGF_{2\alpha}$, PGE_2, PGD_2, TXA_2 and prostacyclin (Pace-Asciak & Rangaraj 1977) have all been claimed to be the major products of the enzymic transformation of arachidonic acid in lung tissue. We have proposed (Gryglewski et al 1976b, 1978b) the following pulmonary compartmentalization for the generation of prostanoids: prostaglandins—smooth muscle of large airways; thromboxane—interstitial cells of lung parenchyma; and prostacyclin—pulmonary endothelium. We also suggest that the generation of PGs and TXA_2 by the lung is associated neither with its metabolic nor with its hormonal functions. These prostanoids are 'local hormones' which modulate inflammatory and anaphylactic responses in the lung as they do in other tissues. The only 'true' hormonal function of the lungs is to release prostacyclin.

HORMONAL FUNCTION OF THE LUNG

We have discovered that cat lungs *in vivo* continuously generate prostacyclin (Gryglewski et al 1978a,b,c, Gryglewski 1979a,b). Vane's group (Moncada et al 1978) has confirmed our finding in rabbits. In the light of these results it has been postulated that prostacyclin is a circulating hormone and that the endocrine function of the lung represents an important mechanism for the control of platelet aggregation in the arterial circulation and, perhaps, for preventing atherogenesis, since prostacyclin has two main biological properties: it relaxes arteries and it prevents blood platelets from aggregating (Gryglewski et al 1976a, Moncada et al 1976). This last property of prostacyclin is closely related to its capacity to stimulate adenylate cyclase in platelets. In addition to its anti-aggregatory action, prostacyclin also disperses preformed platelet clumps, both in animals and in man (Szczeklik & Gryglewski 1979). This last property of prostacyclin enabled us to develop an *in vivo* technique for its bioassay (Gryglewski et al 1978b), which is as follows.

Strips of tendinous collagen when superfused with heparinized blood of anaesthetized cats (Gryglewski et al 1978b), rabbits (Moncada et al 1978) or man (Szczeklik & Gryglewski 1979) gain in weight because of deposition of platelets aggregates on the surface of the strips. The maximum gain in weight

(200–400 mg) occurs usually after 30–45 min of superfusion. Prostacyclin infused directly into the superfusing bloodstream (0.2–5.0 ng ml^{-1}), or infused intravenously either into anaesthetized animals (100–2000 ng $kg^{-1}min^{-1}$) or into humans (2–20 ng $kg^{-1}min^{-1}$) causes a dose-dependent disaggregation of the platelet clumps. The degree of disaggregation is higher in arterial blood than in mixed venous blood. This difference in disaggregatory potency of prostacyclin does not depend on the difference in Po_2, Pco_2 and pH between arterial and venous blood. On the other hand, the higher disaggregatory potency of prostacyclin in arterial blood disappears after pretreating animals with a large dose of aspirin (200 mg kg^{-1}) or after arterial blood is allowed to circulate in a silicone delay coil for 10 min before it reaches the collagen detector. We came to the conclusion that the disaggregatory action of exogenous prostacyclin is supplemented by endogenous prostacyclin released from the lung into arterial blood.

The dog lung generates prostacyclin that partially disappears on passage through the peripheral circulation but is not removed by the lung itself (Dusting et al 1978). Also, perfused guinea-pig and rat lungs generate prostacyclin (Gryglewski et al 1978b). Moncada et al (1978) have presented evidence that the lung of anaesthetized rabbits generates prostacyclin. This hormone in arterial blood can be neutralized by an antiserum to PGI_1 which cross-reacts with prostacyclin (PGI_2) (Moncada et al 1978). Recently, Hensby et al (1979) demonstrated in five human volunteers a difference in concentration of 6-oxo-$PGF_{1\alpha}$ between blood taken from the pulmonary artery and from the left ventricle. Mass spectrometric determinations were used. This last finding extends our concept of the hormonal functioning of the lungs from animals to humans.

STIMULATION OF PROSTACYCLIN RELEASE BY THE LUNG

Isolated perfused guinea-pig and cat lungs spontaneously release prostacyclin (Gryglewski et al 1978b,c). Half an hour after preparation of the lungs prostacyclin is found in the effluent at concentrations as high as 2–5 ng ml^{-1} (Gryglewski et al 1978c, Gryglewski 1979b). Gentle massage or intra-arterial infusions of arachidonic acid (0.1–0.5 μg ml^{-1}) (Gryglewski 1979a), bradykinin (0.5–5 ng ml^{-1}) or angiotensin II (5–50 ng ml^{-1}) (Gryglewski et al 1979, Gryglewski 1979b) stimulate the release of an additional amount of prostacyclin from the lungs. On the other hand, several other biologically active peptides, amines and nucleotides do not release prostacyclin from perfused guinea-pig lungs (Gryglewski 1979a,b).

In anaesthetized cats angiotensin (0.3–1.5 μg kg^{-1}, i.v.) and bradykinin

(1–5 μg kg^{-1}, i.v.) induce the release of prostacyclin into circulation; however, the lung is not the only organ responsible for the secretion of prostacyclin (Gryglewski et al 1979). Angiotensin II seems to stimulate the release of prostacyclin from any cell that has angiotensin receptors on its surface and prostacyclin synthetase in the cell body. The selective generation of prostacyclin by the lungs *in vivo* is stimulated by pulmonary air emboli, by choking or by hyperventilation.

These procedures lead to an increase in concentration of prostacyclin in arterial blood while an increase in prostacyclin level in venous blood is much lower or not detectable. This indicates that prostacyclin having been released from the lungs is then inactivated in the peripheral circulation. Mechanical hyperventilation can be replaced by giving a respiratory stimulant such as lobeline (Fig.1). Lobeline is a potent releaser of prostacyclin from the lungs. A disaggregatory prostacyclin-like substance released by lobeline into arterial blood is biologically inactivated during a 10-min period of extracorporeal recirculation at 37 °C (Fig.1).

Another respiratory stimulant that releases prostacyclin from the lung is almitrine bis(methane) sulphonate (i.e. bis-(allylamine)-4,6[{bis(fluoro-4-phenyl)methyl}-4-piperazinyl]-2-triazine bis(methane) sulphonate; Research

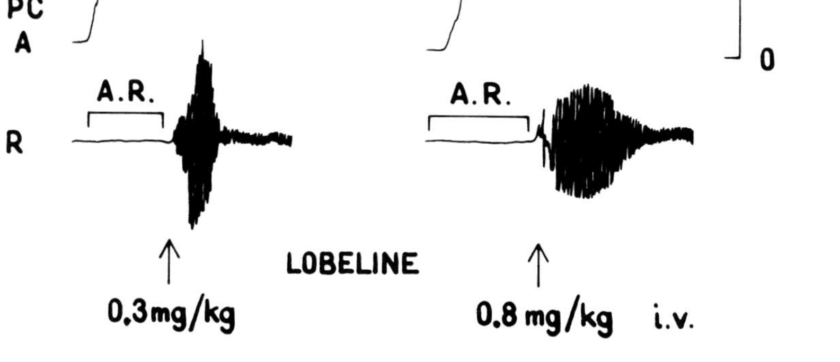

FIG.1. Lobeline-induced release of prostacyclin-like substance into aortic blood as evidenced by disaggregation of platelet clumps on collagen strips (PCA) and lack of this effect after a 10 min extracorporeal recirculation of blood (delay). R, respiratory tidal volume, A.R., artificial respiration, 25 min^{-1}.

Institute Servier, Paris). Almitrine (up to 30 μg ml^{-1}) does not stimulate the release of prostacyclin from perfused guinea-pig and cat lungs; however, when injected intravenously almitrine stimulates the lungs of anaesthetized cats to generate a disaggregatory prostacyclin-like substance (Fig.2). This effect is dose-dependent (Fig.3). The stimulatory effect of almitrine on the release of prostacyclin into arterial blood is abolished by pretreating the cats with a high dose of indomethacin (20 mg kg^{-1}). In these animals almitrine still stimulates the rate of respiration and it increases tidal volume. The release of prostacyclin by almitrine is greatly diminished when almitrine cannot stimulate respiratory movements, for example after bilateral vagotomy or in curare-treated cats (Fig.4).

In summary, there are two distinct methods for stimulating the generation

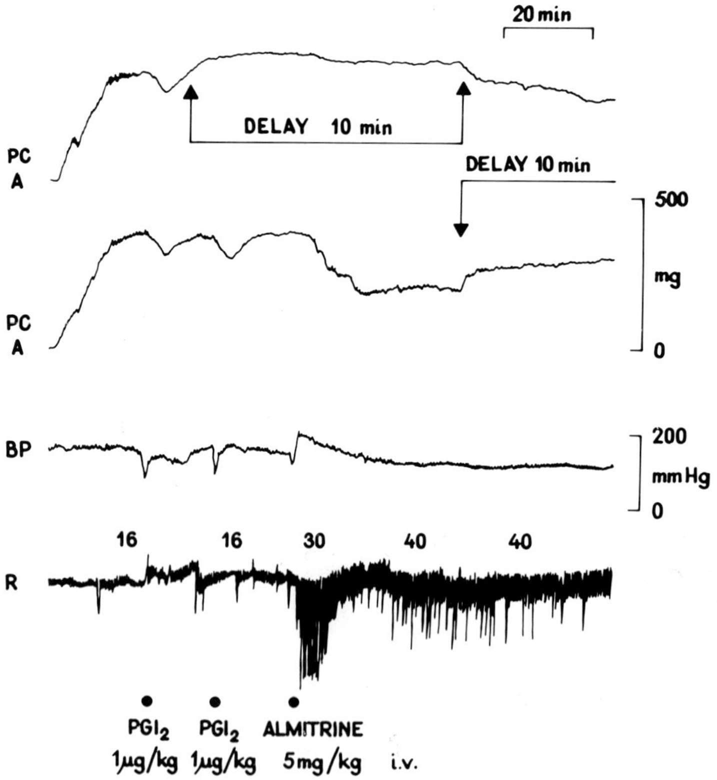

FIG.2. Almitrine-induced release of a prostacyclin-like substance into aortic blood (PCA) of anaesthetized cat. The position of a 10-min delay silicone coil is shown by arrows. BP, arterial blood pressure. R, respiratory tidal volume and frequency of respiratory movements.

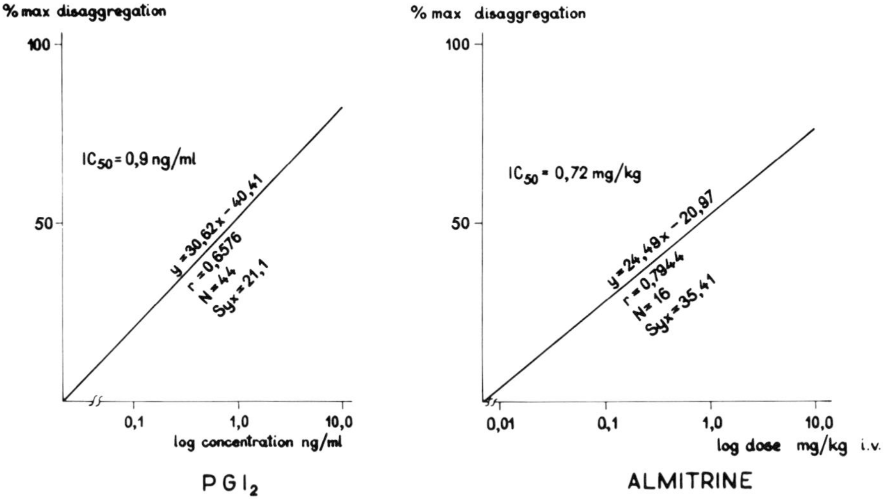

FIG.3. The disaggregatory effect of a prostacyclin-like substance released by almitrine into aortic blood compared with the disaggregatory action of synthetic prostacyclin instilled into the blood superfusing collagen strips.

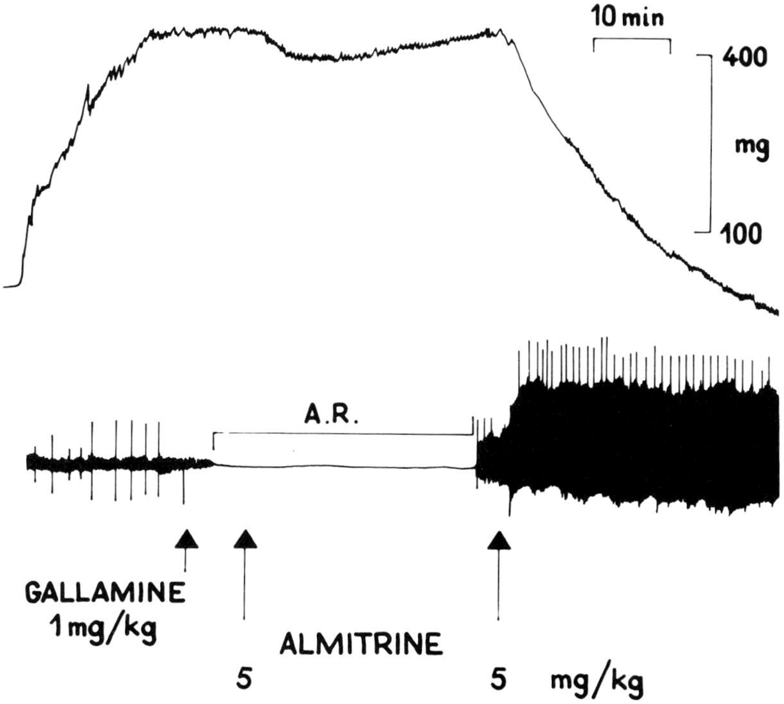

FIG.4. A diminution of the prostacyclin-releasing activity of almitrine in a curarized cat (gallamine + artificial respiration, A.R.) as shown by a difference in the disaggregatory effects of the first and second i.v. injections of almitrine.

of prostacyclin by the lung *in vivo*. Biologically active peptides (such as angiotensin II) can do it; however, other organs apart from the lung are also the target organs for the prostacyclin-releasing action of angiotensin II or bradykinin. A change in the respiratory rate or in respiratory tidal volume is also associated with the release of prostacyclin-like substance from the lung. A respiratory stimulant, almitrine, can induce the protracted generation of prostacyclin by the lungs. Alkalosis following an intravenous infusion of sodium bicarbonate (2–5 ml of 5% solution) is not associated with the generation of prostacyclin by the lungs. Therefore, it might be that a simple stretching of the pulmonary tissue is responsible for the release of prostacyclin from the lungs. It would be of a great practical importance to learn about the effect of almitrine on the difference in blood levels of 6-oxo-$PGF_{1\alpha}$ between the pulmonary artery and the left ventricle in man (Hensby et al 1979).

HYPOTHESIS

In the lung, the classical prostaglandins and TXA_2 play a role as 'local hormones' which influence airway resistance, mainly in pathological circumstances. Although these prostanoids may appear in arterial blood, in principle they are not supposed to be released into the circulation since they fulfil their functions at the site of their generation and should be destroyed there. When there is a leakage of PGs into blood they are efficiently removed from the circulation through the metabolic function of the lung. The endocrine function of the lung is to secrete prostacyclin. Prostacyclin has little or no effect on the respiratory function of the lung; however, when administered by inhalation to asthmatic patients, prostacyclin evokes vasodilatation and it suppresses platelet aggregability (Szczeklik & Gryglewski 1979).

The site of generation of prostacyclin in the lung remains unknown. Although there is no direct evidence we assume that prostacyclin is secreted by pulmonary endothelial cells, the same cells that metabolize angiotensin I, bradykinin and nucleotides (Ryan & Ryan 1977a,b). The basis of this assumption is the fact that arterial endothelium is a rich source of prostacyclin synthetase. This assumption fits our concept of the anatomical compartmentalization of arachidonic acid metabolism in the lung (Gryglewski et al 1976b), according to which classical prostaglandins are generated by smooth muscle of large airways, TXA_2 is likely to be formed by interstitial cells of lung parenchyma and now prostacyclin may be secreted by pulmonary endothelium directly into the bloodstream (Gryglewski et al 1978a,b, Moncada et al 1978).

To summarize, we put forward the hypothesis that the pulmonary endothelium may be considered a huge 'endocrine' gland which generates prostacyclin. It is suggested that the 'hormonal' prostacyclin supplements the local anti-aggregatory and vasodilatory actions of 'vascular' prostacyclin. If so, this phenomenon would be of utmost importance for the coronary and cerebral circulation. The amount of prostacyclin released by the lungs is too small (100–200 pg ml^{-1}, according to Hensby et al 1979 and Gryglewski et al 1978a) to influence blood pressure or platelet aggregability by itself; however, the lungs can be stimulated to secrete more prostacyclin.

Respiratory stimulants with a particular mode of action, such as lobeline or almitrine, increase the pulmonary production of prostacyclin and their action is related to the hyperventilation caused by these drugs. On the other hand, low doses of angiotensin II and bradykinin stimulate several organs (the lungs among them) to generate prostacyclin. The treatment of atherosclerotic patients with their own 'endogenous prostacyclin' is the final goal of the experimental trials aiming to increase the hormonal function of the lungs.

The strategic position of the lungs in the circulation and a high degree of 'saturation' of this organ with blood exposed to endothelial cells make pulmonary endothelium the best candidate for the site of the metabolic and hormonal functions of the lungs. We believe that generation of prostacyclin by the lungs increases the natural resistance of the organism to thrombosis and atherosclerosis, predominantly in the cerebral and cardiac arteries.

References

Bakhle YS, Vane JR (eds) 1977 Metabolic functions of the lung (Lung biology in health and disease, vol 4) Dekker, New York

Boot JR, Cockerill AF, Dawson W, Mallen DNB, Osborne DJ 1978 Modification of prostaglandin and thromboxane release by immunological sensitization and successive immunological challenges from guinea-pig lungs. Int Arch Allergy Appl Immunol 57:159-164

Dusting GJ, Moncada S, Vane JR 1978 Disappearance of prostacyclin (PGI_2) in the circulation of the dog. Br J Pharmacol 62:414P

Eling TE, Hawkins HJ, Anderson MW 1977 Structural requirements for and the effects of chemicals on the rat pulmonary inactivation of prostaglandins. Prostaglandins 14:51-60

Ferreira SH, Vane JR 1967 Half-lives of peptides and amines in the circulation. Nature (Lond) 215:1237–1240

Gryglewski RJ 1979a Is the lung an endocrine organ that secretes prostacyclin? In: Vane JR, Bergström S (eds) Prostacyclin. Raven Press, New York, p 275-288

Gryglewski RJ 1979b Prostacyclin as a circulating hormone. Biochem Pharmacol 28:3161-3166

Gryglewski RJ, Bunting S, Moncada S, Flower RJ, Vane JR 1976a Arterial walls are protected against deposition of platelet thrombi by a substance (prostaglandin X) which they make from prostaglandin endoperoxides. Prostaglandins 12:685-713

Gryglewski RJ, Dembińska-Kieć A, Grodzińska L, Panczenko B 1976b Differential generation of substances with prostaglandin-like and thromboxane-like activities by guinea pig trachea and lung strips. In: Bouhuys A (ed) Lung cells in disease. North-Holland, Amsterdam, p 289-307

Gryglewski RJ, Korbut R, Ocetkiewicz A 1978a Generation of prostacyclin by lungs *in vivo* and its release into the arterial circulation. Nature (Lond) 273:765-767

Gryglewski RJ, Korbut R, Ocetkiewicz A, Spławiński J, Wojtaszek B, Świes J 1978b Lungs as a generator of prostacyclin—hypothesis on physiological significance. Naunyn-Schmiedebergs Arch Pharmacol 304:45-50

Gryglewski RJ, Korbut R, Spławiński J 1978c A new endocrine-like function of the lungs: generation of prostacyclin. Mater Med Pol 10:247-253

Gryglewski RJ, Korbut R, Spławiński J 1979 Endogenous mechanisms which regulate prostacyclin release. Haemostasis 8/3-5:294-299

Hamberg M, Samuelsson B 1974 Prostaglandin endoperoxides. VII. Novel transformations of arachidonic acid in guinea pig lung. Biochem Biophys Res Commun 61:942-949

Henbsy CN, Barnes PY, Dollery CT, Dragie H 1979 Production of 6-oxo-$PGF_{1\alpha}$ by human lung *in vivo*. Lancet 2:1162-1163

Moncada S, Gryglewski RJ, Bunting S, Vane JR 1976 An enzyme isolated from arteries transforms prostaglandin endoperoxides to an unstable substance that inhibits platelet aggregation. Nature (Lond) 263:663-665

Moncada S. Korbut R, Bunting S, Vane JR 1978 Prostacyclin is a circulating hormone. Nature (Lond) 273:767-768

Ng KKF, Vane JR 1968 Fate of angiotensin I in the circulation. Nature (Lond) 218:144-150

Pace-Asciak C, Rangaraj G 1977 Distribution of prostaglandin biosynthetic pathways in several rat tissues. Formation of 6-keto-prostaglandin $F_{1\alpha}$. Biochim Biophys Acta 486:579-582

Piper PJ, Vane JR 1971 The release of prostaglandins from the lung and other tissues. Ann N Y Acad Sci 180:363-385

Ryan JW, Ryan US 1977a Is the lung a para-endocrine organ? Am J Med 63:595-603

Ryan JW, Ryan US 1977b Pulmonary endothelial cells. Fed Proc 36:2683-2691

Szczeklik A, Gryglewski RJ 1979 Actions of prostacyclin in man. In: Vane JR, Bergström S (eds) Prostacyclin. Raven Press, New York, p 393-407

Vane JR 1969 The release and fate of vasoactive hormone in the circulation. Br J Pharmacol 35:209-242

Discussion

Stubbs: I frequently see diabetic patients with macroangiopathy or atherosclerosis and microangiopathy. We know that lung metabolism is sensitive to insulin; is there any evidence that the generation or release of prostacyclin is sensitive to insulin, or that it is altered in the diabetic?

Gryglewski: Yes. Silberbauer et al (1980) have shown that in miniature swine with streptozotocin-induced diabetes the generation of prostacyclin in arteries is reduced. (It is also decreased in omental arteries from patients with atherosclerosis.) On the other hand, we find that during the infusion of prostacyclin in man a short-lasting hyperglycaemia develops. This effect of prostacyclin is not necessarily involved in the suppression of insulin secretion.

Moncada: There is increasing evidence that in diabetic patients and in animals with induced diabetes, prostacyclin production by the vascular wall is decreased. This is accompanied by an increase in *ex vivo* platelet reactivity and the formation of thromboxane B_2 (Harrison et al 1978, Johnson et al 1979). We have some unpublished results in streptozotocin-induced diabetic rats which confirm those observations. After pancreas transplantation in these rats there seems to be a recovery not only of the diabetes but also of the ability of the vessel wall to produce prostacyclin.

Stubbs: Have you tried to block this with aspirin or indomethacin?

Moncada: No.

Alberti: Did you investigate whether these diabetic rats had more platelet aggregates than normal, and whether they had cardiovascular problems later on?

Moncada: We didn't measure micro-aggregates in the circulation; we measured *ex vivo* platelet aggregation and TXB_2 formation and both parameters were increased, as has been described before. We are now trying to induce atherosclerosis in our diabetic rats. We want to see whether these diabetic rats are more susceptible to an atherosclerotic diet than normal rats and to correlate the induction of atherosclerosis with deficient prostacyclin formation.

Collier: You propose that the lung is an endocrine organ producing prostacyclin, Professor Gryglewski, and you suggest that atherosclerosis may be a prostacyclin deficiency disease. May I support the alternative possibility that you also raised: that prostacyclin is a local hormone and that what emerges from the lungs is simply an overflow of excessive production. Since there are about 1500 miles of capillaries in the human lung there must be an enormous possibility of platelets adhering to the capillary wall, and therefore teleologically it would seem necessary for the lungs to produce prostacyclin locally, more or less continuously, to avoid that danger. Hence it seems unnecessary to postulate any other function for the lung prostacyclin. If prostacyclin does prevent atherosclerosis, however, would you not expect atherosclerosis rather commonly in patients with rheumatoid arthritis, since they are treated with large doses of prostaglandin synthesis inhibitors?

Gryglewski: On your first point, I don't know whether prostacyclin is released from the lungs as a true hormone or just as an overflow of its endothelial production. According to our findings, prostacyclin is continuously released from lungs into arterial blood. From the practical point of view, it is important that we can stimulate the release of prostacyclin from lungs *in vivo*.

Secondly, so far as I know, people suffering from rheumatoid arthritis and taking large doses of aspirin are supposed to be *less* prone to a second myocardial infarction than others, although the results of the recent AMIS study cast doubt on this statement (Aspirin Myocardial Infarction Study Research Group 1980). Nonetheless I agree that the lack of atherogenic properties of aspirin appears to be against the concept that I am proposing. May I add, however, that the lungs *in vivo* are extremely resistant to the aspirin-induced blockade of cyclo-oxygenase (Gryglewski et al 1978a).

Vane: We all have circulating platelet aggregates in our venous bloodstream and they do get stuck in the lungs. It is a nice concept that the formation of PGI_2 by the lungs serves the function of dispersing those platelet aggregates.

Aiken: We are studying platelet aggregation by monitoring continuously the formation of these aggregates in the circumflex coronary artery of the dog. We place a plastic cylinder around the artery, which produces about 90–95% reduction in lumen size (Aiken et al 1979). The platelets stick in the narrowed lumen and reduce blood flow from its normally constant rate of 20–30 ml/min to zero in 3–4 minutes. At the point when flow is near zero we grab the obstructor with forceps and shake loose the platelet aggregate to restore flow. If we infuse prostacyclin intravenously (50 ng/kg per minute) we see a spontaneous shedding of the aggregates from the obstructed site and no further aggregation (flow reduction) until we stop the infusion. A bolus injection of prostacyclin (0.3 to 1 μg/kg) inhibits aggregation for 8–10 minutes. If we now inject a fairly large dose (100 μg/kg) of ADP intravenously we see a fall in blood pressure and an inhibition of platelet aggregation lasting several minutes. This amount of ADP is enough to aggregate platelets, causing a transient drop in the platelet count. We wanted to see whether part of the response to ADP was due to release of prostacyclin. We therefore bioassayed prostacyclin, using a superfused bovine coronary artery, which is relaxed by the injection of 0.5 ng of prostacyclin. ADP applied directly to the artery produces a contraction, but if ADP is injected intravenously there is a dramatic relaxation of the artery which coincides with the fall in blood pressure. The release of this prostacyclin-like activity is blocked by indomethacin, as is a large part of the ADP-induced fall in blood pressure. We therefore feel that ADP given intravenously releases a prostacyclin-like substance.

We have proposed that, when we inject ADP, platelets in the venous circulation aggregate and plug small vessels in the pulmonary vascular bed (Hemker et al 1980). It is possible that this platelet plug is the stimulus for prostacyclin release, the precursor coming perhaps from the platelets themselves or from arachidonic acid in the vessel wall. We think that prostacyclin, generated locally at the point where aggregates plug the artery, causes platelet disaggregation and that both the free platelets and some of the prostacyclin wash off into the arterial blood.

Vane: We have two concepts, therefore—firstly that in normal circumstances there is a continuous release of small amounts of prostacyclin from the lungs and, secondly, that this release can be stimulated in various ways, by platelet aggregates or by stimulating respiration. Perhaps when you go jogging, one effect is to make you breathe harder and faster and this releases prostacyclin, which is good for your cardiovascular system!

Gryglewski: How much prostacyclin appears in the blood, as assayed on the bovine coronary artery preparation, when you give 100 μg/kg ADP?

Aiken: It is equivalent in effect to 0.1–1.0 μg/kg injected intravenously, which is a rather large amount of prostacyclin, but this level of release is not maintained for long and is not easily repeated in the same animal. There seems to be a kind of tachyphylaxis (rapid adaptation) to it.

Herbaczyńska-Cedro: Professor Gryglewski has shown that adrenaline does not stimulate the release of prostacyclin from isolated lung. In our recent unpublished experiments we infused adrenaline (1 $\mu g\ kg^{-1} min^{-1}$) into rabbits for 20–30 minutes and observed that the weight of the isolated collagen tissue (rabbit tendon) superfused with arterial blood decreases slowly during the infusion. This could also be seen in the cat. It looked as if an anti-aggregatory substance was generated, most likely from peripheral sources. Intravenous injection of angiotensin caused a more rapid disaggregation of platelets, as shown by the decrease in the tendon weight, suggesting that a disaggregatory substance was now being released from lungs. Is it possible that infusion of adrenaline provokes a widespread release of prostacyclin, generated from peripheral vessels and not from the lungs?

Gryglewski: Our results on cats are different. In our experiments adrenaline does not release prostacyclin from lungs or from any other organ. On the contrary, adrenaline prevents the release of prostacyclin into the circulation when this release is stimulated by cholinergic drugs.

Stalcup: When we examined the effect of infusing catecholamines on the kallikrein–kinin system in the dog we found a dose-dependent increase of bradykinin in the circulation, with infusion of catecholamines in fairly good pressor doses. Identical findings have been published by Constania & Rothschild (1974). Perhaps there is an intermediate generation of kinin that could lead to prostacyclin generation.

Said: When your cats breathed mechanically, Dr Gryglewski, and you increased the breathing rate from 30 to 80/min, what was the effect of this rapid and shallow breathing on the arterial P_{CO_2}?

Secondly, if you postulate that prostacyclin originates mainly from endothelium, what is it about the movement of the lung which brings about greatly increased prostacyclin synthesis? Presumably the hypernoea or the increased rate of breathing mainly influences the airways and alveoli. Is that consistent with prostacyclin coming mainly from the endothelium?

Gryglewski: We haven't studied P_{CO_2}, so I can't answer your first question. However, we have found recently that stimulation of chemoreceptors in cats with mixed hypoxia and hypercapnia (breathing a mixture of 8% O_2, 5% CO_2 and 87% N_2) is a much better means of stimulating prostacyclin release than mechanical hyperventilation.

Vane: On Dr Said's second point, each time an alveolus expands it presumably causes some distortion of the endothelial cells around it. We know that any distortion of a cell is likely to generate prostaglandin, so that could be the basis for prostacyclin release. The lungs are actively distorted several times a minute, which could account for continuous generation of PGI_2. The other tissue which is actively distorted several times each minute is the heart, and we know that heart tissue can also produce prostacyclin (see Moncada & Vane 1978).

Alberti: Can you elaborate on the effects of infusing prostacyclin in patients with thromboembolic disease?

Gryglewski: The experimental basis for our clinical studies has been the finding that in experimental atherosclerosis in rabbits the capacity of arteries and the heart to generate prostacyclin is suppressed earlier than any detectable anatomical damage to the arteries (Gryglewski et al 1978b). We think that prostacyclin deficiency is due to intoxication with lipid peroxides and that atherosclerosis is a hormonal disease resulting from deficiency of prostacyclin. We therefore decided to treat this deficiency with infusions of the synthetic hormone (Szczeklik et al 1979). So far we have treated over 50 patients suffering from advanced arteriosclerosis obliterans (rest pain, ischaemic ulcers). Prostacyclin is infused intra-arterially or intravenously (2–10 ng kg^{-1} min^{-1} for 72 hours). Speaking broadly, about 40% of patients showed a good response during the observation period of 4–17 months. The criteria for improvement were increase in muscle blood flow, alleviation of rest pain and healing of ischaemic ulcerations. We believe that this therapeutic success is related to the action of prostacyclin on platelets rather than to its action on blood vessels. Because of its disaggregatory properties (Gryglewski et al 1978c), prostacyclin may prevent the development of atheromatous plaques in the collateral arterial circulation.

Vane: The general experience now, in the clinic, is that about half the patients with major occlusions of the arteries of the legs benefit for a considerable period from a three-day infusion of prostacyclin. There are also indications of benefit in Raynaud's disease. We are starting double-blind clinical trials in both conditions.

Alberti: Can you separate out yet the potential long-term effects on the arterial lipid deposits from the effects on vessel circumference?

Gryglewski: No. There is no evidence of a direct effect of prostacyclin on the atherosclerotic plaques in major arteries, at least judging from angiographic studies. Plethysmographic and xenon-clearance techniques have shown a persistent increase in muscular blood flow after prostacyclin treatment.

Slater: What is the intracellular distribution of prostacyclin synthetase within the lung endothelial cells?

Moncada: In general prostaglandin synthetases are located in the endoplasmic reticulum of cells.

Slater: If the enzyme is inside the cell, in the endoplasmic reticulum, it may be less susceptible to the damaging action of lipid peroxidation, which you have shown to inhibit prostacyclin synthetase (Moncada et al 1976). There are, of course, several mechanisms for controlling and regulating lipid peroxidation in the membranes of the endoplasmic reticulum (see Dianzani & Ugazio 1978). Professor Gryglewski mentioned lipid peroxidation. Has he tried the effects of increased lipid peroxidation in the perfused lung on the release of prostacyclin?

Gryglewski: We infused 15-hydroperoxy arachidonic acid into isolated lung to see whether this lipid peroxide would stop the spontaneous generation of prostacyclin. We failed to find this effect in cat, rabbit and guinea-pig lungs. In the rat lung this blockade occurs occasionally.

Professor Szczeklik has measured plasma levels of malondialdehyde in humans. Increased plasma malondialdehyde levels are found in patients with inborn hyperlipidaemia or hypercholesterolaemia (Szczeklik & Gryglewski 1980). I believe that the lipid peroxide content should be measured in low density lipoproteins rather than in plasma. After all, low density lipoproteins and not plasma triglycerides, cholesterol or fatty acids were found to be of predictive value for the development of atherosclerosis (Vergani et al 1978).

Moncada: We have been trying, unsuccessfully so far, to induce lipid peroxidation in the lung *in vivo* to see whether as a result of this there is a change in the metabolism of arachidonic acid. One problem of course is to measure how much peroxidation we can induce. The other relates to the rapid metabolism of lipid peroxides *in vivo* or in isolated perfused organs.

Slater: The intravenous infusion of lipid peroxides is associated with a variety of toxic effects (see Cortesi & Privett 1973, Olcott & Dolev 1963), even though the lipid peroxides are relatively rapidly metabolized by glutathione peroxidase (Christopherson 1968) and by non-enzymic pathways. Since the prostaglandin and prostacyclin biosynthetic enzymes are intracellular, it would seem better to generate the lipid peroxides within the cell rather than to infuse them parenterally if inhibitory actions on the biosynthetic pathways are desired. It may be possible, for example, to stimulate lipid peroxidation in lung tissue by exposure to ozone (Goldstein et al 1969), especially if this treatment is combined with an associated depletion of glutathione, for example with methyl phenylazoformate (Kosower et al 1965).

Moncada: We have used ozone. What about paraquat?

Slater: Paraquat is a widely used herbicide and may produce lung injury under certain conditions of exposure or administration. It undergoes a ready oxidation–reduction interaction with nicotinamide-adenine dinucleotides and oxygen, and may stimulate lipid peroxidation in lung endoplasmic reticulum (Shu et al 1979). Another substance reported to stimulate lipid peroxidation in the lungs is nitrogen dioxide (Thomas et al 1968).

Datta: The effect of toxic but non-lethal oxygen tension and other oxidants on the lung leads to a phenomenon termed 'tolerance'. Stimulation of the pentose phosphate pathway may contribute to producing tolerance to lung injury and to reducing oxidants inhaled by the lung (Tierney et al 1973). It has been suggested that oxygen tolerance may be linked to the increased glucose-6-phosphate dehydrogenase activity observed after exposure to 85% oxygen or after injection of α-naphthylthiourea (Finder et al 1972).

Reid: Has anyone looked at the effect on prostacyclin release of either hypoxia or hyperoxia? The production of superoxides might be important in shock lung (adult respiratory distress syndrome). Superoxide dismutase might be used to prevent damage due to superoxides.

Herbaczyńska-Cedro: We looked at the effect of hypoxia, induced by inhalation of a hypoxic gas mixture, on the release of prostacyclin from the lungs in dogs. We bioassayed prostacyclin-like activity in arterial blood using isolated strips of bovine coronary artery. Hypoxic ventilation did not cause any detectable release of prostacyclin into the arterial blood.

In another series of experiments in which an isolated collagen preparation (rabbit tendon) was superfused with cat arterial blood, hypoxic ventilation did not evoke any detectable disaggregation of platelets aggregated on the tendon. We concluded that in these experiments hypoxia did not stimulate prostacyclin generation (Truskolaski et al 1979).

Bakhle: Professor Weibel studied hyperoxia in rat lungs (Kistler et al 1967). Were there more platelet aggregates than usual in these lungs? The hyperoxia might have caused more peroxidation of unsaturated fatty acids and thus a depression of prostacyclin production.

Burri: The endothelial cells were heavily damaged and capillaries obliterated and destroyed. There would have been platelet aggregation in any case, due to the desquamation of the endothelial cells (Kistler et al 1967).

Stalcup: Crapo et al (1978) found that an early sign of oxygen toxicity is aggregation of platelets in the pulmonary microcirculation.

References

Aspirin Myocardial Infarction Study Research Group 1980 A randomized, controlled trial of aspirin in persons recovered from myocardial infarction. J Am Med Assoc 243: 661-669
Aiken JW, Gorman RR, Shebuski RJ 1979 Prevention of blockage of partially obstructed coronary arteries with prostacyclin correlates with inhibition of platelet aggregation. Prostaglandins 17:483-494
Christopherson BO 1968 Formation of monohydroxy-polyenic fatty acids from lipid peroxides by a glutathione peroxidase. Biochim Biophys Acta 164:35-46
Constania A, Rothschild AM 1974 Lowering of kininogen in rat blood by adrenaline and its inhibition by sympatholytic agents, heparin and aspirin. Br J Pharmacol Chemother 50:375-381
Cortesi R, Privett OS 1973 Toxicity of fatty ozonides and peroxides. Lipids 7:715-721
Crapo JD, Peters-Golden M, Marsh-Salin J, Shelburne JS 1978 Pathologic changes in the lungs of oxygen-adapted rats. A morphometric analysis. Lab Invest 39:649-653
Dianzani MU, Ugazio G 1978 In: Slater TF (ed) Biochemical mechanism of liver injury. Academic Press, London, p 669-707
Finder E, LaForce M, Huber G 1972 Prevention of pulmonary oxygen toxicity. Clin Res 20:577
Goldstein BD, Collinson C, Balchum OJ 1969 Arch Environ Health 18:631-635
Gryglewski RJ, Korbut R, Ocetkiewicz A, Spławiński J, Wojtaszek B, Świes J 1978a Lungs as a generator of prostacyclin—hypothesis on physiological significance. Naunyn-Schmiedeberg's Arch Pharmacol 304:45-50
Gryglewski RJ, Dembińska-Kieć A, Żmuda A, Gryglewska T 1978b Prostacyclin and thromboxane A_2 biosynthesis capacities of heart, arteries and platelets at various stages of experimental atherosclerosis in rabbits. Atherosclerosis 31:385-394
Gryglewski RJ, Korbut R, Ocetkiewicz A 1978c Reversal of platelet aggregation by prostacyclin. Pharmacol Res Commun 10:185-189
Harrison HE, Reece AH, Johnson M 1978 Decreased vascular prostacyclin in experimental diabetes. Life Sci 23:351-356
Hemker DP, Shebuski RJ, Aiken JW 1980 Release of a prostacyclin-like substance into the circulation of dogs by intravenous adenosine 5'-diphosphate. J Pharmacol Exp Ther 212:246-252
Johnson M, Reece AH, Harrison HE 1979 Decreased vascular prostacyclin in experimental diabetes. Adv Pharmacol Ther 4:865p
Kistler GS, Caldwell PRB, Weibel ER 1967 Development of fine structural damage to alveolar and capillary lining cells in oxygen-poisoned rat lungs. J Cell Biol 32:605
Kosower NS, Vanderhoff GA, Kosower EM, Huang PC 1965 Decreased glutathione content of human erythrocytes produced by methyl phenylazoformate. Biochem Biophys Res Commun 20:469-474
Moncada S, Vane JR 1978 Pharmacology and endogenous roles of prostaglandin endoperoxides, thromboxane A_2 and prostacyclin. Pharmacol Rev 30:293-331
Moncada S, Gryglewski RJ, Bunting S, Vane JR 1976 A lipid peroxide inhibits the enzyme in blood vessel microsomes that generates from prostaglandin endoperoxides the substance (prostaglandin X) which prevents platelet aggregation. Prostaglandins 12:715-737
Olcott HS, Dolev A 1963 Toxicity of fatty acid ester hydroperoxides. Proc Soc Exp Biol Med 114:820-822
Shu H, Talcott RE, Rice SA, Wei ET 1979 Lipid peroxidation and paraquat toxicity. Biochem Pharmacol 28:327-331
Silberbauer K, Clopath P, Sinzinger H, Schernthaner G 1980 Effect of experimentally induced diabetes on swine vascular prostacyclin (PGI_2) synthesis. Atherogenesis 4: Suppl 3:150 (abstr)
Szczeklik A, Niżankowski R, Skawiński S, Głuszko P, Gryglewski RJ 1979 Successful therapy of advanced arteriosclerosis obliterans with prostacyclin. Lancet 1:1111-1114
Szczeklik A, Gryglewski RJ 1980 Low density lipoproteins (LDL) are carriers for lipid peroxides and invalidate prostacyclin biosynthesis in arteries. Artery, in press

Thomas HV, Mueller PK, Lyman RL 1968 Lipoperoxidation of lung lipids in rats exposed to nitrogen dioxide. Science (Wash DC) 159:532-534

Tierney D, Ayer L, Herzog S, Yang J 1973 Pentose pathway and production of reduced nicotinamide adenine dinucleotide phosphate. Am Rev Respir Dis 108:1348-1351

Truskolaski P, Herbaczyńska-Cedro K, Huszczuk A 1979 Blood from hypoperfused lungs contains biological activity which resembles PGI_2 and is not susceptible to prostaglandin synthetase inhibitors. Eur J Clin Invest 9:36 (abstr)

Vergani C, Trovato G, Dioguardi N 1978 Serum total lipids, lipoproteins A and B in cardiovascular disease. Clin Chim Acta 87:127-133

Interrelationships between prostacyclin and thromboxane A_2

S. MONCADA and J.R. VANE

Wellcome Research Laboratories, Langley Court, Beckenham, Kent, BR3 3BS, UK

Abstract Prostacyclin is a product of arachidonic acid metabolism generated by the vessel wall of all mammalian species studied including man. Prostacyclin is a potent vasodilator and the most potent inhibitor of platelet aggregation so far described. It inhibits platelet aggregation through stimulation of adenylate cyclase leading to an increase in cyclic AMP in the platelets. The enzyme which synthesizes prostacyclin is mainly localized in the endothelial layer of the vascular wall. Prostacyclin can also be a circulating hormone constantly released by the pulmonary circulation. On the basis of these observations we proposed that platelet aggregability *in vivo* is controlled via a prostacyclin mechanism.

In contrast to the vessel wall, in blood platelets arachidonic acid is converted by the enzyme thromboxane synthetase to a potent vasoconstrictor and proaggregating substance, thromboxane A_2. Therefore arachidonic acid is metabolized in the vessel wall and the platelets to potent substances with opposing biological activities. The balance between the activities of these substances is important in the homeostatic interaction of the platelets and the vessel wall. The different ways of interfering with this balance and its impact in the development of thrombosis and atherosclerosis are discussed.

The balance between thromboxane A_2 and prostacyclin might be important in the control of the pulmonary circulation. This possibility is discussed in the light of the present evidence.

Recent discoveries in the field of prostaglandins (PGs) have substantially added to our knowledge of platelet–vessel wall interactions and opened up exciting new therapeutic possibilities. In this brief review we deal mainly with the way in which the balance between metabolites of arachidonic acid which either induce or prevent platelet aggregation affects the physiology and pathophysiology of haemostasis and thrombosis. In addition we shall discuss the way in which the lungs may play a role in these control mechanisms. We have previously reviewed in more detail the biosynthesis, metabolism and

Metabolic activities of the lung
(Ciba Foundation symposium 78) p 165-183

general pharmacology of prostaglandins and the unstable products of arachidonic acid (see Moncada & Vane 1978).

REGULATION OF PLATELET BEHAVIOUR IN VIVO BY THROMBOXANE A_2 AND PROSTACYCLIN

In 1970, Smith and Willis demonstrated that during aggregation, platelets release among other products prostaglandins of the E and F type. Shortly afterwards it was demonstrated that aspirin-like drugs inhibited prostaglandin biosynthesis and as a result the general theory was proposed (Vane 1971) that this enzyme inhibition accounts for the anti-inflammatory effects (and perhaps the side-effects) of aspirin-like drugs. Since then, substantial evidence to support this theory has been generated and it is now widely accepted that the analgesic, antipyretic and anti-inflammatory effects of aspirin-like drugs are mediated via inhibition of prostaglandin biosynthesis (see Moncada & Vane 1979).

It has been known for several years that aspirin inhibits the platelet release reaction induced by ADP and collagen *in vitro*. Additionally, aspirin prolongs the bleeding time and this effect occurs at low concentrations that are achieved in plasma after an oral therapeutic dose. Aspirin also inhibits prostaglandin production in platelets after oral administration. Because of this, it was suggested that inhibition of prostaglandin biosynthesis could account for the inhibitory effect of aspirin on platelet aggregation. At that time, however, it was difficult to support that proposition since the known prostaglandins did not induce platelet aggregation. A further step in the knowledge of arachidonic acid metabolism was achieved with the isolation of the unstable prostaglandin endoperoxides and thromboxane A_2 (TXA_2) (Hamberg & Samuelsson 1973, Hamberg et al 1975, Nugteren & Hazelhof 1973).

Prostaglandin endoperoxides (PGG_2 and PGH_2) are unstable in aqueous solution (half-life approximately five minutes at 37 °C) and isomerize to stable prostaglandins. In platelets, the prostaglandin endoperoxides are further metabolized into an even more unstable compound, thromboxane A_2 (half-life of 30 seconds) (Hamberg et al 1975) by an enzyme that has been designated thromboxane synthetase (Needleman et al 1976). Thromboxane A_2 is more potent than the parent endoperoxides as an inducer of platelet aggregation, and as a constrictor of arterial smooth muscle *in vitro* (see Moncada & Vane 1978) and *in vivo* in the hind limb and mesenteric vascular beds of the dog (see Moncada & Vane 1978). Thromboxane A_2 is, in fact, responsible for most if not all of the activity of a substance discovered by Piper &

Vane (1969) to be released during anaphylactic shock in guinea-pig isolated lungs. Because of the activity by which they detected it, they called it 'rabbit aorta contracting substance' or 'RCS'. They showed that its release was inhibited by aspirin-like drugs. In platelets the prostaglandin endoperoxides generated during aggregation most probably exert their aggregating effect through conversion to thromboxane A_2.

In contrast to cyclo-oxygenase, thromboxane synthetase is poorly inhibited by indomethacin. Selective inhibition of thromboxane synthetase has been demonstrated using different types of compounds, including some endoperoxide analogues (see Moncada & Vane 1978). The involvement of endogenous cyclic endoperoxides (and thromboxane A_2) in platelet aggregation and the prevention of their formation by inhibition of cyclo-oxygenase by aspirin provides a satisfactory explanation for the inhibitory effects of aspirin-like drugs on platelet aggregation and the release reaction.

In 1976, while studying the conversion of cyclic endoperoxides by different tissues, we found that a microsomal fraction of vascular tissue converted prostaglandin endoperoxides into an unstable product which, in contrast to thromboxane A_2, was a potent inhibitor of platelet aggregation (Moncada et al 1976). We called it prostaglandin X. The chemical structure of this substance was elucidated (Johnson et al 1976) and PGX was then renamed prostacyclin and given the abbreviation PGI_2 (see Fig. 1).

Prostacyclin is formed by vascular tissue from all species so far tested and is

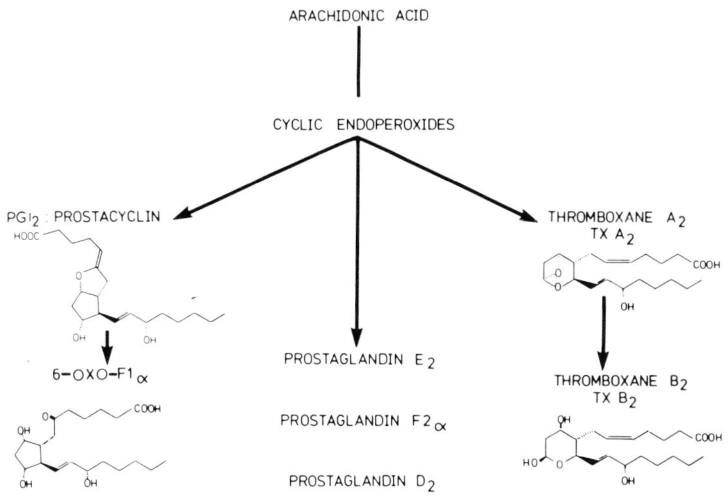

FIG. 1. Production of prostacyclin and thromboxane A_2 from cyclic endoperoxides.

the main metabolic product of arachidonic acid in vascular tissue (see Moncada & Vane 1978). Prostacyclin is the most potent endogenous inhibitor of platelet aggregation yet discovered. It is 30–40 times more potent than PGE, and more than 1000 times more active than adenosine. *In vivo*, prostacyclin applied locally in low concentrations or given systemically inhibits thrombus formation in different animal models and increases cutaneous bleeding time. The duration of these effects *in vivo* is short, disappearing within 30 min of stopping intravenous administration. Prostacyclin disaggregates platelets *in vitro*, *in vivo*, in extracorporeal circulation models, and in the circulation of man (see Moncada & Vane 1978).

Prostacyclin is unstable and its activity disappears within 15 s on boiling or within 10 min at 22 °C at neutral pH. In blood at 37 °C, prostacyclin has a half-life of 2–3 min (see Moncada & Vane 1978). Basic pH increases the stability of prostacyclin, so that at pH 10.5, at 25 °C, it has a half-life of 100 h.

In the vasculature the enzyme which metabolizes prostaglandin endoperoxides to prostacyclin (prostacyclin synthetase) is most highly concentrated in the intima and progressively decreases in activity towards the adventitia. The production of prostacyclin by cultured cells from vessel walls also shows that endothelial cells are the most active producers of prostacyclin (see Moncada & Vane 1978).

Clearly, the generation of prostacyclin is an active means by which the vessel wall could protect itself from the deposition of platelet aggregates. Thus, prostacyclin formation provides a comprehensive explanation of the long-recognized fact that contact with healthy vascular endothelium is not a stimulus for platelet clumping. An imbalance between the formation of prostacyclin and of TXA_2 could be of dramatic consequence.

Vascular damage leads to platelet adhesion but not necessarily to thrombus formation. When the injury is minor, platelet thrombi are formed which break away from the vessel wall and are washed away by the circulation. The degree of injury is an important determinant, and there is general agreement that for the development of thrombosis, severe damage or physical detachment of the endothelium must occur. It is not yet clear whether or not prostacyclin is responsible for all the thromboresistant properties of the vascular endothelium. However, recent work by Czervionke et al (1979) with endothelial cell cultures has demonstrated that platelet adherence in the presence of thrombin increases from 4% to 44% after treatment with 1 mM-aspirin. This increase was paralleled by a decrease in 6-oxo-$PGF_{1\alpha}$ formation from 107 nM to <3 nM and could be reversed by adding 25 nM of exogenous PGI_2. This work suggests that prostacyclin, although probably not responsible for all the thromboresistant properties of vascular endothelium, plays a very important role in the control of platelet aggregability.

The fact that prostacyclin inhibits platelet aggregation (platelet–platelet interaction) at much lower concentrations than those needed to inhibit adhesion (platelet–collagen interaction), suggests that, indeed, prostacyclin allows platelets to stick to vascular tissue and to interact with it, while at the same time preventing or limiting thrombus formation. Certainly, platelets adhering to a site where prostacyclin synthetase is present could well feed the enzyme with endoperoxide, thereby producing prostacyclin and preventing other platelets from clumping onto the adhering platelets, limiting the cells to a monolayer.

It is also possible that formed elements of blood such as the white cells, which produce endoperoxides and TXA_2, interact with the vessel wall to allow formation of prostacyclin, as do the platelets (see Moncada & Vane 1978).

PROSTACYCLIN, THROMBOXANE A_2 AND PLATELET BEHAVIOUR

Prostaglandin endoperoxides are at the crossroads of arachidonic acid metabolism, for they are precursors of substances with opposing biological properties. On the one hand, TXA_2 produced by the platelets is a strong contractor of large blood vessels and induces platelet aggregation. On the other hand, prostacyclin produced by the vessel wall is a strong vasodilator and the most potent inhibitor of platelet aggregation known. The two substances have opposing effects on cyclic AMP concentrations (see Moncada & Vane 1978), giving a balanced control mechanism which will, therefore, affect thrombus and haemostatic plug formation. Selective inhibition of the formation of TXA_2 should lead to an increased bleeding time and inhibition of thrombus formation, whereas inhibition of prostacyclin formation should be propitious for a 'pro-thrombotic state'. The amount of control exerted by this system can be tested, for selective inhibitors of each pathway are available (see Moncada & Vane 1978).

The utilization of aspirin as a pharmacological tool to investigate the interaction between these two substances has been fruitful. Aspirin is highly active against platelet cyclo-oxygenase *in vivo* and *in vitro*. Moreover, this effect is long lasting because aspirin acetylates the active site of the enzyme, leading to irreversible inhibition. Platelets are unable to synthesize new protein and cannot replace the cyclo-oxygenase. Therefore, the inhibition will only be overcome by new platelets coming into the circulation after the block of cyclo-oxygenase in megakaryocytes has worn off. Interestingly, the cyclo-oxygenase of vessel walls seems much less sensitive to aspirin than that of platelets. It has also been suggested that endothelial cells *in vitro* and *in vivo* recover from aspirin inhibition by regenerating the cyclo-oxygenase. This has been reinforced by the observation that the recovery of the endothelial cell synthetase in cell cultures can be prevented by treatment with the protein synthesis inhibitor, cycloheximide (for reviews see Majerus, 1976, Moncada & Amezcua 1979, Moncada & Vane 1978).

Studies in rabbits suggest that low doses of aspirin reduce TXA_2 formation to a greater extent than prostacyclin formation. These experiments also showed that inhibition of TXA_2 formation is longer lasting than that of prostacyclin. Indeed, infusions of arachidonic acid into rabbit and cats lead to an anti-thrombotic effect and to an increase in bleeding time which can be potentiated by low doses of aspirin and blocked by larger doses (which would inhibit prostacyclin and TXA_2 formation).

Until the discovery of prostacyclin, the use of aspirin as an anti-thrombotic agent, on the basis of its effects on platelets, looked very clear, although the results of clinical trials were inconclusive. Now, however, the situation needs further clarification, especially with respect to the optimal dose of aspirin. Aspirin in high doses increases thrombus formation in a model of venous thrombosis in the rabbit, and *in vitro* treatment of endothelial cells with aspirin enhances thrombin-induced platelet adherence to them. In addition, there is an inverse correlation between platelet adhesion and aggregation and the amount of prostacyclin produced by the tissue. Moreover, aspirin treatment of arterial tissue *in vitro* increases its thrombogenicity.

In humans, O'Grady & Moncada (1978) showed that a single low dose of aspirin (0.3 g) increased bleeding time 2 h after ingestion, whereas a high dose (3.9 g) had no effect. Some workers have confirmed these results, but others have been unable to do so. The variability might be linked to the differences in methodology or in the age range of the subjects. Indeed, Jorgensen et al (1979) showed that the cutaneous bleeding time in humans decreases with age and that the response to aspirin varies according to the age, being increased in young male volunteers and not in older subjects. An extension of the concept comes from the demonstration that tranylcypromine, an inhibitor of prostacyclin formation, enhances platelet aggregation in an experimental model of thrombosis in the microcirculation of the brain of the mouse. All these results clearly demonstrate that the balance between TXA_2 and PGI_2 is an important mechanism of control of platelet aggregability *in vivo*. Clearly, manipulation of this control mechanism might lead to pro- or anti-thrombotic states of clinical relevance. In this context it is interesting that Blajchman et al (1979) showed that hydrocortisone treatment of normal or thrombocytopenic rats blocks prostacyclin formation in the vessel wall and decreases the bleeding time, a result which would be expected from the interference with arachidonic acid release induced by steroids. The authors mention that for years it has been the clinical impression that steroids decrease the bleeding time in thrombocytopenic patients without increasing the platelet count (for reviews see Majerus 1976, Moncada & Amezcua 1979, Moncada & Vane 1978).

Studies in man attempting to measure TXB_2 and (or) prostacyclin or 6-oxo-$PGF_{1\alpha}$ after different aspirin dose schedules have confirmed the higher sensitivity of platelet cyclo-oxygenase to aspirin. Masotti et al (1979) have reported that aspirin at 3.2–3.4 mg/kg gave a 50% inhibition of *ex vivo* platelet aggregation induced by several agents, while 4.9 mg/kg was needed for 50% inhibition of prostacyclin formation. Also, recently the effectiveness of a single daily dose of aspirin (160 mg) in protecting against thrombosis in patients with arterio-venous shunts has been demonstrated. This dose reduced significantly (40%) the incidence of thrombosis over an observation period of nearly five months (Harter et al 1979).

From all these results it is clear that a selective inhibitor of thromboxane formation should now be tested for anti-thrombotic efficacy, since theoretically this provides an advantage over aspirin in leaving endoperoxides from platelets available for the vessel walls or other cells to synthesize prostacyclin. The demonstration of an increased level of 'active prostacyclin' originating from platelet endoperoxides should be the main criterion for claiming an improved efficacy by comparison with a small dose of aspirin. Studies *in vivo* are not yet available but *in vitro* Needleman et al (1979) showed that when platelets were treated with a TXA_2 synthetase inhibitor, endoperoxides were available for utilization by the vessel wall. Interestingly, in the presence of a thromboxane synthetase inhibitor, arachidonic acid or collagen added to blood *in vitro* lead to the formation of 6-oxo-$PGF_{1\alpha}$ rather than TXB_2, showing that some cell other than platelets has synthesized prostacyclin. These results support our suggestion that thromboxane synthetase inhibitors might have a superior antithrombotic effect to simple cyclo-oxygenase inhibitors (see Moncada & Vane 1978).

Selective inhibition of prostacyclin formation by lipid peroxides could also lead to a condition in which platelet aggregation is increased, and this could play a role in the development of atherosclerosis. Indeed, lipid peroxidation takes place in plasma as a non-enzymic reaction and it is known to occur in certain pathological conditions. Hence, lipid peroxides present in these conditions could shift the balance of the system in favour of TXA_2 and predispose to thrombus formation.

The role of lipid peroxides in the development of atherosclerosis has been debated for the last 25 years, ever since the presence of lipid peroxides in human atherosclerotic aortae was correlated directly to the severity of the atherosclerosis. Subsequent investigations suggested that these findings were artifactual, the presence of lipid peroxides being ascribed to their formation during the preparative procedure. Despite this the presence of hydroperoxides in lipids of human atheroma has again been reported, and lipid peroxides have been found in atherosclerotic rabbit aortae extracted by a procedure that avoids lipid peroxidation *in vitro*. The available evidence, although still incomplete, favours the suggestion that lipid peroxides are present in atherosclerotic plaques, whether or not these peroxides act by inhibiting prostacyclin formation, and as a consequence reduce the wall's defence mechanism. This theory is of interest, especially since other substances related to atherosclerosis, such as the cholesterol carriers low density lipoproteins (LDL), have also been shown to inhibit prostacyclin formation in endothelial cell cultures (for reviews see Moncada & Vane 1978, Vane & Moncada 1979).

PROSTACYCLIN AND THE CARDIOVASCULAR SYSTEM

Unlike other prostaglandins such as PGE_2 and $PGF_{2\alpha}$ prostacyclin is not inactivated on passage through the pulmonary circulation. Indeed, the lungs constantly release small amounts of prostacyclin into the passing blood (Gryglewski et al 1978a, Moncada et al 1978), perhaps because of the huge mass of endothelial cells present. The concentration of prostacyclin is higher in arterial than in venous blood for there is about 50% overall inactivation in one circulation through peripheral tissues (see Moncada & Vane 1978). Recent measurements in humans of 6-oxo-$PGF_{1\alpha}$ in the arterial and venous side of the circulation during cardiac catheterization confirm that arterial blood contains higher concentrations than venous blood (Hensby et al 1979).

Platelets, therefore, may be constantly influenced by prostacyclin and consequently may have higher levels of cyclic AMP and may be less aggregable than has ever been detected *in vitro*, where measurements are made after a 10–30 min delay during which the blood is processed. In this period, prostacyclin and its effects will decay. This possibility would explain the differences in reactivity between platelets *in vitro* and *in vivo* reported by many authors and might throw light on recent controversies about the control of cyclic AMP levels in platelets. Moreover, it has provided a basis for the explanation of the antithrombotic effect of drugs which inhibit the phosphodiesterase, such as dipyridamole (Moncada & Korbut 1978).

The large vascular endothelial mass of the lung circulation (about 50% of the whole vascular endothelial mass) provides an area situated between the venous and arterial circulation in which platelet clumps might be disaggregated during passage. In this sense it is difficult at present to evaluate the importance of the 'prostacyclin levels' in the circulation since this could be a 'spill over' of a system which acts locally when platelets cross the pulmonary circulation. When injected intravenously in the anaesthetized rabbit, rat or dog, prostacyclin causes a fall in blood pressure and is 4–8 times more potent in this respect than PGE_2. Prostacyclin is at least 100 times more active than its degradation product, 6-oxo-$PGF_{1\alpha}$.

In isolated Langendorff-perfused hearts of the guinea-pig and rabbit, not only is prostacyclin a potent vasodilator but it is also the predominant metabolite of arachidonic acid (Dusting et al 1979). We and others have investigated the effects of prostacyclin on the coronary circulation in the intact heart of open-chest dogs. Local injection of prostacyclin (50–500 ng) into the coronary circulation increased coronary blood flow without producing systemic effects; prostacyclin was a more potent coronary dilator than PGE_2. Furthermore, profound and prolonged coronary vasodilation was rapidly elicited by prostacyclin (20–100 μg) absorbed through the myocardium after dripping a solution on to the surface of the left ventricle. Interestingly, the coronary circulation is sensitized to the vasodilator effects of exogenous prostacyclin, but not to those of PGE_2, when endogenous synthesis is inhibited by indomethacin or meclofenamate. These inhibitors of cyclo-oxygenase decrease resting coronary blood flow in anaesthetized, open-chest dogs. Although this is not seen in conscious dogs without acute surgery it does indicate that the generation of a vasodilator metabolite of arachidonic acid increases or maintains coronary blood flow during mildly traumatic conditions. It is clear that this metabolite is prostacyclin.

In the renal circulation of the dog, prostacyclin infused intravenously reduces renal vascular resistance and increases blood flow and urinary excretion of sodium, potassium and chloride ions at doses below those needed for a systemic effect. There is increasing evidence that prostacyclin mediates the release of renin from the renal cortex. Arachidonic acid, prostaglandin endoperoxides or prostacyclin all stimulate renin release from slices of rabbit renal cortex, but PGE_2 has no such effect (Oates et al 1979). Furthermore, indomethacin reduces renin release in animals and man. Prostacyclin-like activity and 6-oxo-$PGF_{1\alpha}$ have been identified when PGG_2 or PGH_2 is incubated with renal cortical microsomes. Thus, prostacyclin may be the obligatory endogenous mediator of renin secretion by the kidney. Indeed, it has been demonstrated that prostacyclin induces renin release when infused intrarenally into dogs, and also that intra-renal infusions of PGI_2 lead to an increased angiotensin II concentration in arterial blood. 6-Oxo-$PGF_{1\alpha}$ is also formed by collecting tubule cells isolated from rabbit papillae. Interestingly, angiotensin II releases prostacyclin from the rat kidney *in vitro* and the dog kidney *in vivo* (for reviews see Moncada & Vane 1978, Dusting et al 1979, Oates et al 1979, Needleman & Kaley 1978).

It has also been demonstrated that bradykinin releases prostacyclin when given intravenously or infused intrarenally in the dog. This has led to the suggestion that the hypotensive effect of angiotensin-converting enzyme inhibitors (which also potentiate bradykinin) might in part be due to an increase in prostacyclin release (Mullane et al 1980).

Prostacyclin is also a strong vasodilator in the mesenteric and hind limb circulations of the dog (where TXA_2 is a vasoconstrictor) and on the precapillary side of the microcirculation of the hamster cheek pouch where it also reverses catecholamine-induced vasoconstriction. In this preparation 6-oxo-$PGF_{1\alpha}$ had 1/20th the vasodilator activity of prostacyclin and was more potent than PGE_2. In the pulmonary circulation of the dog, prostacyclin is the only product of arachidonic acid which produces strong vasodilatation. It also dilates the pulmonary vascular bed of the fetal lamb and of man. Prostacyclin also induces vasodilatation and hypotension in man when given either intravenously or by inhalation (Gryglewski et al 1978a, Moncada & Vane 1978, Dusting et al 1979).

PROSTACYCLIN–TXA_2 INTERACTIONS IN THE LUNG

Although prostaglandins and RCS were identified several years ago in the effluent of normal or sensitized lungs *in vitro* after different stimuli, it has only recently been recognized that the main metabolites of arachidonic acid via the cyclo-oxygenase pathway in the lung are prostacyclin and TXA_2 (Dawson et al 1976). In consequence, the existing hypotheses about the opposing roles played by PGE_2 and $PGF_{1\alpha}$ on bronchial muscle have been losing support. Sensitization followed by immunological challenge increases the amount of TXA_2 (measured as 15-oxo-13, 14-dihydro-TXB_2) and decreases the amount of prostacyclin (measured as 6-oxo-$PGF_{1\alpha}$ or 6,15-dioxo-13,14-dihydro-$PGF_{1\alpha}$) released from endogenous substrate or from exogenously added arachidonic acid. TXA_2 is a bronchoconstrictor and vasoconstrictor whereas prostacyclin, although not a very potent bronchodilator, is effective in antagonizing bronchoconstriction induced by other agents and is a vasodilator. Thus, it is tempting to speculate that the balance between these compounds also plays a role in lung physiology. The release of these compounds appears to be compartmentalized, the parenchyma being the tissue source of TXA_2

and tracheal and vascular tissue being the source of prostaglandin-like material and probably prostacyclin. It is possible that pathological conditions shift the balance away from prostacyclin towards TXA_2, or lead to an increased concentration of prostaglandin endoperoxides, which are bronchoconstrictors (see above) and probably strong stimulants of vagal, lung 'irritant' receptors, like their stable analogues (see Moncada & Vane 1978). It has been postulated that lipid peroxides synthesized by the lungs via the lipoxygenase pathways increase the formation of TXA_2 and other mediators in guinea-pig lungs *'in vitro'* (Adcock et al 1978). In addition, there have been several indications in the past few years that slow-reacting substance in anaphylaxis (SRS-A) could be a product of arachidonic acid. Recently, the structure of a slow-reacting substance (SRS) from mouse mastocytoma cells has been reported as a novel product of the lipoxygenase pathway. It is formed by the addition of glutathione (Hammarström et al 1979, Parker et al 1979) (originally thought to be cysteine; Murphy et al 1979) to an unstable epoxide (at C_5) intermediate in the formation of dihydroxylated arachidonic acid metabolites in leucocytes. 'Leukotriene' has been introduced as a generic name for eicosanoids like SRS which are non-cyclized C_{20} carboxylic acids with one or two oxygen substituents and three conjugated double bonds.

Leukotrienes share certain structural features with some oxygenated products of arachidonic acid in human and rabbit polymorphonuclear leucocytes. It is not known whether this compound is identical to SRS-A released from the lungs, but these findings highlight the importance of the products of the different lipoxygenases in cell migration, inflammation and other conditions such as increased mediator release and airway reactivity during asthma or anaphylaxis.

In conclusion, prostacyclin and thromboxane A_2 seem to be important biological regulators in different systems. Three of the areas in which early developments have led to a better understanding are: (1) the control of platelet aggregability *in vivo*, (2) the interaction between the renin-angiotensin system, bradykinin and prostacyclin, and (3) the interaction between PGI_2 and TXA_2 and the lipoxygenase system in lung physiology. It is interesting that the lung, thought of for so long as a simple respiratory system, is now being considered much more as a metabolic organ exerting biological control or modulation over many systems.

References

Adcock JJ, Garland LG, Moncada S, Salmon JJ 1978 The mechanism of enhancement by fatty acid hydroperoxides of anaphylactic mediator release. Prostaglandins 16:179-187

Blajchman MA, Senyi AF, Hirsh J, Surya Y, Buchanan M, Mustard JF 1979 Shortening of the bleeding time in rabbits by hydrocortisone caused by inhibition of prostacyclin generation by the vessel wall. J Clin Invest 63: 1026-1035

Czervionke RL, Smith JB, Fry GL, Hoak JC 1979 Inhibition of prostacyclin by treatment of endothelium with aspirin. J Clin Invest 63:1089-1092

Dawson W, Boot JR, Cockerill AF, Mallen DNB, Osborne DJ 1976 Release of novel prostaglandins and thromboxanes after immunological challenge of guinea-pig lung. Nature (Lond) 262:699-702

Dusting GJ, Moncada S, Vane JR 1979 Prostaglandins, their intermediates and precursors: cardiovascular actions and regulatory roles in normal and abnormal circulating systems. Prog Cardiovasc Dis 21:405-430

Gryglewski RJ, Korbut R, Ocetkiewicz AC 1978a De-aggregatory action of prostacyclin in vivo and its enhancement by theophylline. Prostaglandins 15:637-644

Gryglewski RJ, Szczeklik A, Nizankowski R 1978b Anti-platelet action of intravenous infusion of prostacyclin in man. Thromb Res 13:153-163

Hamberg M, Samuelsson B 1973 Detection and isolation of an endoperoxide intermediate in prostaglandin biosynthesis. Proc Natl Acad Sci USA 70:899-903

Hamberg M, Svensson J, Samuelsson B 1975 Thromboxanes: A new group of biologically active compounds derived from prostaglandin endoperoxides. Proc Natl Acad Sci USA 72:2994-2998

Hammarström S, Murphy RC, Samuelsson B, Clark DA, Mioskowski C, Corey EJ 1979 Structure of leukotriene C. Identification of the amino acid part. Biochem Biophys Res Commun 91:1266

Harter HR, Burch JW, Majerus PW, Stanford N, Delmez JA, Anderson CB, Weerts CA 1979 Prevention of thromboembolism in patients on hemodialysis by low-dose aspirin. N Engl J Med 301:577-579

Hensby CN, Barnes PJ, Dollery CT, Dargie H 1979 Production of 6-oxo-PGF$_{1\alpha}$ by human lung in vivo. Lancet 2:1162-1163

Jorgensen KA, Olesen AS, Dyerberg J, Stoffersen E 1979 Aspirin and bleeding time: dependency of age. Lancet 2:302

Johnson RA, Morton DR, Kinner JH, Gorman RR, McGuire JR, Sun FF et al 1976 The chemical structure of prostaglandin X (prostacyclin). Prostaglandins 12:915-928

Majerus PW 1976 Why aspirin? Circulation 54:357-359

Masotti G, Galanti G, Poggesi L, Neri Serneri GG 1979 Differential inhibition of prostacyclin production and platelet aggregation by aspirin. Lancet 2:1213-1216

Moncada S, Amezcua JL 1979 Prostacyclin, thromboxane A_2 interactions in haemostasis and thrombosis. Haemostasis 8:252-265

Moncada S, Korbut R 1978 Dipyridamole and other phosphodiesterase inhibitors act as antithrombotic agents through potentiating endogenous prostacyclin. Lancet 1:1286-1289

Moncada S, Vane JR 1978 Pharmacology and endogenous roles of prostaglandin endoperoxides, thromboxane A_2 and prostacyclin. Pharmacol Rev 30:293-331

Moncada S, Vane JR 1979 Mode of action of aspirin-like drugs. In: Stollerman GH (ed) Advances in internal medicine. Year Book Medical Publishers, Chicago, p 1-22

Moncada S, Gryglewski RJ, Bunting S, Vane JR 1976 An enzyme isolated from arteries transforms prostaglandin endoperoxides to an unstable substance that inhibits platelet aggregation. Nature (Lond) 263:663-665

Moncada S, Korbut R, Bunting S, Vane JR 1978 Prostacyclin is a circulating hormone. Nature (Lond) 273:767-768

Mullane K, Moncada S, Vane JR 1980 Prostacyclin release induced by bradykinin may contribute to the antihypertensive action of angiotensin-converting enzyme inhibitors. In: Samuelsson B et al (eds) Advances in prostaglandin and thromboxane research. Raven Press, New York, p 1159-1161 (vol 7)

Murphy RC, Hammarström S, Samuelsson B 1979 Leukotriene C: a slow-reacting substance from murine mastocytoma cells. Proc Natl Acad Sci USA 76:4275

Needleman P, Kaley G 1978 Cardiac and coronary prostaglandin synthesis and function. New Engl J Med 298:1122-1128

Needleman P, Moncada S, Bunting S, Vane JR, Hamberg M, Samuelsson B 1976 Identification of an enzyme in platelet microsomes which generates thromboxane A_2 from prostaglandin endoperoxides. Nature (Lond) 261:558-560

Needleman P, Wyche A, Raz A 1979 Platelet and blood vessel arachidonate metabolism and interactions. J Clin Invest 63:345-349

Nugteren DH, Hazelhof E 1973 Isolation and properties of intermediates in prostaglandin biosynthesis. Biochim Biophys Acta 326:448-461

O'Grady J, Moncada A 1978 Aspirin: A paradoxical effect on bleeding time. Lancet 2:780

Oates JA, Whorton AR, Gerkens JF, Branch RA, Hollifield JW, Frolich JC 1979 The participation of prostaglandins in the control of renin release. Fed Proc 38:72-74

Parker CW, Huber MM, Hoffman MK, Falkenhein SF 1979 Characterization of the two major species of slow reacting substance from rat basophilic leukemia cells as glutathionyl thioethers of eicosatetraenoic acids oxygenated at the 5 position. Evidence that peroxy groups are present and important for spasmogenic activity. Prostaglandins 18:673-686

Piper PJ, Vane JR 1969 Release of additional factors in anaphylaxis and its antagonism by anti-inflammatory drugs. Nature (Lond) 223:29-35

Smith JB, Willis AL 1970 Formation and release of prostaglandins by platelets in response to thrombin. Br J Pharmacol 40:545-546

Vane JR 1971 Inhibition of prostaglandin synthesis as a mechanism of action for aspirin-like drugs. Nature (Lond) 231:232-235

Vane JR, Moncada S 1979 Polyunsaturated fatty acids as precursors of prostaglandins. Acta Cardiol Suppl 23:21-37

Discussion

Soffer: Does bradykinin stimulate the release of prostacyclin by the lung in the presence of captopril?

Moncada: Yes.

Soffer: Since prostacyclin might be a circulating hormone, and you have an antibody that cross-reacts with it (Moncada et al 1978), you might have a probe with which to examine the physiological effects of this putative hormone. Have you studied what happens to an animal after introducing this antibody into its circulation?

Moncada: No. Smith et al (1979) have developed an antibody to 6-oxo-$PGF_{1\alpha}$ in rabbits which cross-reacts with prostacyclin. These animals did not show a shortened bleeding time.

Soffer: The antibody didn't kill the animal, or affect it in any way?

Moncada: Not that we know of. This has not been studied in detail.

Soffer: Do you know where the cross-reacting antibody goes in such animals?

Moncada: No.

Collier: In the isolated guinea-pig trachea prostacyclin does not cause contraction. In the guinea-pig *in vivo*, bradykinin liberates a bronchoconstrictor substance and this liberation is blocked by aspirin, so some other prostaglandin-like substance must be liberated in the guinea-pig, presumably in the lung; possibly it is thromboxane A_2. Have you any evidence of another prostanoid being liberated?

Moncada: No, but there are several possibilities. The 'profile' of products released from the lungs seems to depend on the degree of stimulus and the area that is mainly stimulated (vasculature, bronchial tree or parenchyma). Small infusions of arachidonic acid, for example, release mainly prostacyclin, while larger infusions release thromboxane A_2.

Aiken: You implied that platelet concentrations of cyclic AMP were elevated sufficiently by basal levels of circulating prostacyclin to change platelet reactivity *in vivo*. If so, one would expect a cyclo-oxygenase inhibitor to reduce levels of cyclic AMP in platelets. In dogs we don't see a change in the platelet content of cyclic AMP after treatment with cyclo-oxygenase inhibitors (aspirin, indomethacin and ibuprofen; Aiken et al 1980). Also, studies by Steer et al (1980) showed no increase in the sensitivity of platelets to ADP after removing plasma prostacyclin with antibodies. Finally, as Dr Gryglewski said earlier (p 155) there is probably an arterio-venous difference in prostacyclin concentration of about 100 pg/ml; but is that enough to affect platelet function?

Moncada: There are experimental problems here. Cyclic AMP levels are measured in platelets after several stages of separation from the blood. This takes time and also stimulates the platelets. Prostacyclin being unstable will disappear, together with its effects, during the preparative procedure. Second, if you add less than 100 pg/ml prostacyclin to platelet-rich plasma, platelet aggregation is not inhibited after one minute's incubation; probably far less than this amount of prostacyclin circulating in the blood continuously will have some effect, but we don't know this. In addition, the cyclic AMP in platelets will probably disappear at different rates, depending on the conditions. For example, the rate of disappearance will be different in unstirred platelet-rich plasma and in the circulation, where platelets are subjected to different rheological conditions and cell interactions.

Aiken: We have perfused prostacyclin in dogs at a rate of 15–30 ng/kg per min, which inhibits aggregation *in vivo* in the partially obstructed circumflex coronary artery. If we take a blood sample during the infusion we see a twofold shift in the dose–response curve to ADP.

Vane: Have you measured the concentration of prostacyclin in the arterial blood induced by that infusion?

Aiken: No, but we can calculate it from cardiac output; it's about 1–2 ng/ml.

Moncada: Another example of the methodological problem relates to a recent observation of ours that suggests that the doses of prostacyclin needed to increase the cutaneous bleeding time are smaller than those needed to inhibit '*ex vivo*' platelet aggregation. This tells us that small concentrations of prostacyclin could affect aggregation without our being able to detect this by conventional aggregation methods.

Gryglewski: Your data on the differential inhibition of cyclo-oxygenase are very interesting. May I add that it is difficult to inhibit the spontaneous generation of prostacyclin by the lungs when using typical cyclo-oxygenase inhibitors. In cats we had to use as much as 200 mg/kg of aspirin to reduce the arterio-venous difference in prostacyclin level. On the other hand, the same inhibitors are highly effective when the release of prostacyclin from the lungs is induced by methacholine (Mecholin).

Bakhle: Alternatively, the lung may be producing another prostacyclin-like material which is not derived via the cyclo-oxygenase pathway.

Herbaczyńska-Cedro: We studied the effect of hypoventilation, produced by a 50% reduction in rate and stroke volume of the respiratory pump, on prostacyclin-like activity bioassayed on the bovine coronary artery superfused with arterial blood in the dog. We found a huge relaxation of the isolated arterial strip during hypoventilation.

Hypoventilation produced in cats caused de-aggregation of platelets, as shown by a decrease in weight of the isolated collagen preparation superfused with arterial blood. Neither effect was inhibited by indomethacin or aspirin. Prostacyclin-like activity detected in the dog's arterial blood seemed to be more stable than prostacyclin. This suggests that apart from prostacyclin, which might have been released by hypoventilation and would account for such fast disaggregation, we may also have another substance (or substances) contributing to the relaxation of isolated arteries in the dog (Truskolaski et al 1979).

Vane: There are two possibilities: either the release of prostacyclin during hypoventilation is insensitive to aspirin-like drugs, or some different material is being released.

Herbaczyńska-Cedro: I would favour the second possibility, because the activity assessed by the delay-coil method seemed to be more stable than that of prostacyclin. However, the disaggregation of platelets seen during hypoventilation in cats suggests that prostacyclin might also have been released in these conditions.

Gryglewski: It is very difficult to assess the stability of a prostacyclin-like material being released *in vivo* by the delay-coil technique. Unstable prostacyclin should be decomposed during the passage through a 10-minute delay-coil. Decomposition certainly occurs when prostacyclin is slowly infused over a period of time into the coil; however, this is not the case when the same dose of prostacyclin is injected quickly into the coil. Bioassay is not the kind of technique that can differentiate between the type of release (slow or rapid) of prostacyclin *in vivo*. The delay-coil technique therefore has its limitations and one should be cautious in claiming stability of a disaggregatory or vasodilatory substance from the use of this technique only.

Vane: There are two stable anti-aggregating agents present *in vivo* that might be candidates for Dr Cedro's activity: one is adenosine. I don't know whether it has the same effects on the bovine coronary artery as prostacyclin. The other is 6-oxo-PGE_1. There is evidence that the chemical degradation product of prostacyclin, 6-oxo-$PGF_{1\alpha}$, is converted in the liver to 6-oxo-PGE_1, which is stable and is anti-aggregatory.

Moncada: One shouldn't rely on a single criterion for identifying prostacyclin. I would suggest at least three of the following: it should be an anti-aggregating compound, which is acid-labile and alkaline-stable, whose generation is inhibited by indomethacin or by lipid peroxides, is antagonized by specific antibodies, and relaxes a bovine coronary artery strip.

Ferreira: So the material released from the lung is not prostacyclin, because its generation is not inhibited by indomethacin?

Gryglewski: For the same reason it cannot be 6-oxo-PGE_1. Neither is it adenosine, since adenosine is 10 000–30 000 times less active than prostacyclin in the tendon assay. Physiological concentrations of adenosine in blood cannot be detected by this technique.

Herbaczyńska-Cedro: We tested the effect of adenosine on blood-superfused bovine coronary arteries. It relaxes the artery as prostacyclin does, but, as you say, the concentrations which evoked this effect are far from physiological.

Reid: Are we saying that there is a prostacyclin-like compound that has many of the vasodilator effects of prostacyclin, but is unidentified as yet?

Vane: Some of the evidence is pointing that way now.

Mellins: With respect to studies of the effects of hypo-and hyperventilation, these will need to be controlled very carefully for oxygen tension and pH for us to fully understand their physiological meaning. As the result of the studies Dr Stalcup will be presenting, we now know that angiotensin-converting enzyme activity, and hence the circulating levels of angiotensin II and bradykinin, are modulated by oxygen tension (p 293-311).

Vane: I am particularly interested in the concept of blood cells being 'modulated' by prostacyclin as they squeeze through the capillary; for instance, the deformability of the red blood cell membrane might be changed, although we have no evidence for this yet. But platelets are much too small to have to squeeze through the microcirculation, so the effect of prostacyclin on platelets must be mediated in some other way.

Moncada: In a study which compared platelet numbers in the arterial and venous circulation (see Crosby 1976) the platelet count was higher in the arterial blood. This was explained by the finding that some platelets on the venous side were returning to the lungs in groups of two or three. These small 'aggregates' would, when returning to the lung microcirculation, 'squeeze' their way through capillaries of 5–6 μm diameter. In this interaction release of prostacyclin would be induced and the platelet cyclic AMP level would increase; this would 'condition' the platelets to a decreased aggregability.

Gryglewski: The idea that platelets 'condition' the lungs to generate prostacyclin is a very nice one, but platelets are not essential in this respect since the isolated lungs of many animal species also generate prostacyclin when perfused with Krebs' solution. The perfused lung preparation used by Professor Woods and Professor Alberti would probably be in a more physiological situation than our pharmacological preparations. It would be interesting to see whether, in those physiological conditions, without any stimulation except for artificial ventilation, lungs spontaneously liberate prostacyclin.

Vane: I don't know how much 'damage' was done in the experiments by the Hammersmith group, but they showed a difference in arterial and venous prostacyclin levels in man, which suggests that prostacyclin was generated by those lungs (Hensby et al 1979).

Gryglewski: This experiment and any other experiment *in vivo* is not going to tell us whether prostacyclin is released from lungs as a result of stimulation of pulmonary endothelium by platelets or of spontaneous release of prostacyclin by the lung tissue.

Aiken: The idea of a local recharging of the cyclic AMP levels in the platelets as they go through the lungs could be very important, because there is suggestive evidence that the platelet cyclic AMP concentration is pushed down as platelets pass through capillary beds other than lung. For example, when we give an infusion or a bolus injection of prostacyclin and at the time of the peak effect, as determined by inhibition of aggregation in the dog coronary artery, take a blood sample and measure platelet cyclic AMP, the cyclic AMP level stays up in the sample for 10–15 minutes but the anti-aggregatory effects in the animal are reversed very quickly (five minutes). If we take a second blood sample as soon as aggregation resumes *in vivo*, the platelet cyclic AMP level has returned to normal. There appear to be factors related to the mechanics of blood flow which tend to bring the cyclic AMP concentration back down more rapidly *in vivo* than when a blood sample is withdrawn and allowed to sit relatively undisturbed.

Moncada: Salzman et al (1976) have demonstrated that platelet levels of cyclic AMP can be lowered by mechanical stimulation. In the blood *in vivo* the platelets are moving at high speed through different areas. This movement imposes flow conditions that will tend to lower the cyclic AMP level.

Ferreira: Is there a difference in the cyclic AMP levels in platelets from arterial and venous blood?

Moncada: We don't know.

Reid: What happens in the pulmonary circulation? One needs to know what effects changes in oxygen tension have here. In life, the lung capillary bed is fairly distensible and you can get a considerable range of capillary diameter: so the capillaries are a series of pulsating tubes.

Vane: We have no evidence that oxygen tension affects prostacyclin generation, except in so far as oxygen is needed for oxygenation of arachidonic acid. I don't know any work where venous and arterial endothelium have been compared in natural conditions for their prostacyclin-generating activity. Cyclic AMP levels in platelets at the different oxygen tensions haven't been measured either.

Junod: Have you observed any change in prostacyclin production, or in the cyclic AMP content of platelets, as a function of the type of flow used, continuous or pulsatile?

Vane: Dr Ten Hoor has perfused rat aorta and obtains prostacyclin production only when he pulsates the vessels (Ten Hoor et al 1980). So we come back to the concept that distortion of endothelial cells triggers prostacyclin release.

References

Aiken JW, Shebuski RJ, Gorman RR 1980 Blockage of partially obstructed coronary arteries with platelet thrombi: comparison between its prevention with cyclooxygenase inhibitors *versus* prostacyclin. In: Samuelsson B et al (eds) Advances in prostaglandin and thromboxane research. Raven Press, New York (4th Int Prostaglandin Conference, Washington DC) vol 8

Crosby WH 1976 Normal platelet numbers. Pulmonary-platelet interactions. Ser Haematol 8:89-97

Hensby CN, Dollery CT, Barnes PJ, Dargie H 1979 Production of 6-oxo-$PGF_{1\alpha}$ by human lung in vivo. Lancet 2:1162-1163

Moncada S, Korbut R, Bunting S, Vane JR 1978 Prostacyclin is a circulating hormone. Nature (Lond) 273:767-768

Salzman EW, Lindon NJ, Rodvien R 1976 Cyclic AMP in human blood platelets: relation to platelet prostaglandin synthesis induced by centrifugation or surface contact. J Cyclic Nucl Res 2:25-37

Smith JB, Ingerman CM, Silver MJ 1979 Normal bleeding times in rabbits containing antibodies that bind prostacyclin (PGI_2). Thromb Haemostasis 42:7p

Steer ML, MacIntyre DE, Levine L, Salzman EW 1980 Is prostacyclin a physiologically important circulating anti-platelet agent? Nature (Lond) 283:194-195
Ten Hoor F, De Dekere EAM, Haddeman E, Hornstra G, Quadt JFA 1980 Dietary manipulation of prostaglandin and thromboxane synthesis in heart, aorta and blood platelets of the rat. In: Samuelsson B et al (eds) Advances in prostaglandin and thromboxane research. Raven Press, New York (4th Int Prostaglandin Conference, Washington DC) vol 8:1771-1781
Truskolaski P, Herbaczyńska-Cedro K, Huszczuk A 1979 Blood from hypoperfused lungs contains biological activity which resembles PGI_2 and is not susceptible to prostaglandin synthetase inhibitors. Eur J Clin Invest 9:36 (abstr)

Regulation of pulmonary arachidonic acid metabolism by anti-inflammatory steroids

R.J. FLOWER

Department of Prostaglandin Research, Wellcome Research Laboratories, Langley Court, Beckenham, Kent, BR3 3BS, UK

Abstract Enzymes in cells from many tissues including the lung metabolize arachidonic acid to a variety of highly active local hormones such as prostaglandins and 'slow-reacting substances'. Many of these play a part in the inflammatory response which follows injury or trauma or, in the case of slow-reacting substance, asthmatic bronchoconstriction. Both non-steroidal and steroidal anti-inflammatory drugs inhibit the formation of some or all of these products. The non-steroidal drugs block prostaglandin formation but not the formation of products such as slow-reacting substances. The steroids block the formation of all products. Their mechanism of action, investigated in the guinea-pig perfused lung, involves inhibition of arachidonic acid liberation, probably by suppression of phospholipase activity. To achieve this steroids must first bind to receptors in lung tissue and initiate *de novo* RNA and protein synthesis. This culminates in the synthesis or secretion by some cells in the lung of a polypeptide of mol.wt. 10 000–15 000 with potent anti-phospholipase properties. The generation of this factor could partly explain why steroids are so effective in the treatment of many types of inflammatory disease, and in particular why they are so efficacious against asthma.

During the past decade we have come to appreciate the extraordinary range of biologically active compounds that can be generated from the seemingly innocuous C-20 polyunsaturated fatty acids. From just one member of this family—arachidonic acid—we can obtain, by the action of various enzymes, mediators of inflammation such as prostaglandin (PG) E (Van Dorp et al 1964, Bergström et al 1964), immensely potent modulators of platelet aggregation such as thromboxane or prostacyclin (Hamberg et al 1975, Moncada et al 1976, Johnson et al 1976), chemotactic agents such as 'HETE' (Hamberg & Samuelsson 1974a,b, Turner et al 1975) and 'slow-reacting substances' (SRS) such as leukotriene C (cf. Samuelsson et al 1979).

The discovery of these compounds and their biological activity is one of the

Metabolic activities of the lung
(Ciba Foundation symposium 78) p 185-201

most fascinating stories of recent years, but equally important has been the finding that the biosynthesis of all these agents is profoundly modified by anti-inflammatory agents. In this paper I discuss the ways in which the anti-inflammatory steroids interact with the biosynthesis of biologically active fatty acid derivatives, and indicate the therapeutic relevance of these findings.

It was the discovery by Vane and his colleagues in 1971 (Vane 1971, Ferreira et al 1971, Smith & Willis 1971) that non-steroidal drugs blocked the biosynthesis of PGs that stimulated research workers around the world to investigate the effect of other types of anti-inflammatory drug on PG production. The question most often formulated was quite simple: if the aspirin-like drugs owed their pharmacological activity to their ability to block PG biosynthesis, did other types of anti-inflammatory drugs have the same mode of action? Many investigators were interested in the steroids from this point of view. At the time of the original discovery the steroidal anti-inflammatory drugs were found to be without effect on the microsomal cyclo-oxygenase (which catalyses the biosynthesis of PGs), even in quite high concentrations (Ferreira et al 1971, Flower et al 1972, Smith & Willis 1971, Vane 1971). However, the steroids apparently shared several of the properties of the aspirin-like drugs which were thought to be due to inhibition of PG biosynthesis, and there was a lingering impression that the steroidal anti-inflammatory agents could in some way interfere with the PG biosynthetic pathways. Table 1 (based on data published in 1972) compares the anti-cyclo-oxygenase activity of four aspirin-like drugs with that of four anti-inflammatory steroids. Both types of drugs are effective in the anti-inflammatory (rat paw oedema) test, but only the aspirin-like drugs block the

TABLE 1

Differences in anti-enzyme activity between steroid and non-steroid anti-inflammatory drugs

Drug	*Cyclo-oxygenase*		*Rat paw oedema* ED_{50} *(mg/kg)*
	I_{50} *(μg/ml)*	*% inhibition at 100 μg/ml*	
Meclofenamic acid	0.03	100	15
Niflumic acid	0.03	100	47
Indomethacin	0.06	100	6
Mefenamic acid	0.17	100	68
Dexamethasone	–	10	$<$ 0.001
Triamcinolone acetonide	–	0	0.08
Fludrocortisone	–	5	$\simeq$ 0.15
Hydrocortisone	–	3	13

(Data from Flower et al 1972.)

cyclo-oxygenase. These findings posed a theoretical problem because the steroids are very powerful anti-inflammatory agents, and yet apparently had no effect on PG biosynthesis: did this mean they had a completely separate mode of action, or that PGs were not important in inflammation after all? Several papers were soon to be published which strongly suggested that steroids *could* block PG formation, although their mechanism of action was completely different from that of the aspirin-like drugs.

The first reports came from Herbaczyńska-Cedro & Staszewska-Barczak (1974) who showed that hydrocortisone reduced the release of PG-like substances into the venous effluent of the dog hind limb that occurs during muscular exercise. The mechanism of action was not elucidated, although other workers had been unable to inhibit PG production with hydrocortisone in tissue homogenates or other cell-free cyclo-oxygenase preparations, suggesting some mechanism of action other than a direct effect on the enzyme itself. Lewis & Piper (1975) studied ACTH-induced lipolysis in the fat pad of rabbits. In this system, lipolysis was accompanied by vasodilatation and the formation of PGs. An infusion of hydrocortisone, prior to ACTH, reduced the vasodilatation and PG release. Since the hydrocortisone neither prevented the formation of PGs in fat tissue homogenates, nor antagonized the vasodilatation induced by exogenous PGE_2, it was proposed that corticosteroids inhibited the *release* of PGs by preventing their transport from inside the fat cell to the extracellular space. However, other experiments suggested a different interpretation: Gryglewski and his colleagues (1975) found that two corticosteroids, hydrocortisone and dexamethasone, prevented the noradrenaline-induced release of PGs from the perfused mesenteric vascular bed of the rabbit, as well as the release of PGs from guinea-pig perfused lungs induced by antigen. However, the direct conversion of arachidonic acid in these preparations was unaffected by the steroids, indicating that the site of inhibition was not the cyclo-oxygenase or a 'release mechanism'. Indeed, these workers concluded that the corticosteroids acted by limiting substrate availability. This view was soon confirmed by Levine's group (Kantrowitz et al 1975, Tashjian et al 1975). Some elegant experiments published later by the same group (Hong & Levine 1976, Tam et al 1977) using cell cultures labelled with tritiated arachidonic acid added considerable experimental support to this idea, as did the work of other groups (cf. Floman & Zor 1977, Parente et al 1978).

What follows is an account of the pharmacological activity of anti-inflammatory steroids in one model system—the guinea-pig perfused lung. This review is based on experimental results published by my co-workers and myself (Nijkamp et al 1976, Blackwell et al 1978, Flower & Blackwell 1979).

THE GUINEA-PIG LUNG AS A MODEL SYSTEM FOR EXAMINING THE EFFECTS OF STEROIDS

Since the experiments of Piper & Vane (1969) the guinea-pig perfused lung used in conjunction with a bioassay cascade has been a favourite preparation in our laboratory for studying the generation and release of prostaglandins. The idea of the preparation is simple: oxygenated Krebs' solution at 37°C is perfused at 5–10 ml/min through the pulmonary artery of the isolated lung of a guinea-pig. The pulmonary venous effluent is diverted over a selection of bioassay tissues in cascade. For the detection of prostaglandin endoperoxides and thromboxanes, a typical choice of tissues would be a rabbit aortic strip, plus a rat stomach strip, a rat colon, guinea-pig trachea, or chick rectum. The specificity of the tissues for prostaglandin products is further increased by the infusion into the pulmonary venous effluent of antagonists to other smooth muscle contractile substances.

In 1976 we used this preparation to determine the activity of 'rabbit aorta contracting substance—releasing factor' (RCS-RF), a low molecular weight principle extracted from the effluent of lung that had been shocked. Injection into the pulmonary artery of purified RCS-RF results in the liberation from the lungs of smooth muscle contractile substances (which may be identified by differential bioassay and other techniques as a mixture of PG endoperoxides and thromboxane A_2). Indomethacin, and other aspirin-like drugs, inhibit this generation, as expected; but while looking at the inhibitory activity of some other types of drugs we noticed that the anti-inflammatory steroid dexamethasone prevented the effect of RCS-RF but did not inhibit the conversion of arachidonic acid to PG products by the lung.

The lack of effect of dexamethasone on the conversion of arachidonic acid by the lung clearly showed that this drug did not inhibit the cyclo-oxygenase. Other steroids were tested and it was soon discovered that almost all the anti-inflammatory agents were effective against RCS-RF-induced release and that, furthermore, their rank order and ratio of potency against RCS-RF was very similar to their anti-inflammatory activity (see Table 2). Another interesting point emerged: the I_{50} concentration for each steroid depended on the duration of the infusion. This meant, for example, that an infusion of 1 μg/ml dexamethasone for long periods of time produced the same inhibition as, or greater inhibition than, 20 μg/ml infused for much shorter periods. In any case there was a time delay of 15–30 min before the onset of the effect. Further experiments quickly established that steroids also inhibited the releasing activity of histamine and serotonin.

TABLE 2

Effect of some anti-inflammatory steroids on the release of PG endoperoxides and TXA_2 from perfused guinea-pig lungs in response to injections of RCS-RF

Steroid	I_{50}[a] *(μg/ml)*	*Relative potency*[b]	*Relative anti-inflammatory potency*[b]
Dexamethasone	1.4	31.2	25
Betamethasone	1.4	31.2	25
Triamcinolone	4.2	10.4	5
Fludrocortisone	5.1	8.5	10
Prednisolone	6.4	6.8	4
Corticosterone	33.6	1.3	0.4
Cortisone	43.5	1	0.8
Hydrocortisone	43.8	1	1

[a]Expressed as base.
[b]Hydrocortisone = 1.

MODE AND SITE OF ACTION OF STEROID BLOCKADE

How and where were the steroids acting? When arachidonic acid was injected or infused into the pulmonary artery of the guinea-pig lung preparation it was immediately converted into hydroxy-acids and prostaglandin endoperoxide transformation products (that this was a conversion and not a release was easily demonstrated using labelled arachidonate). We therefore inferred that the availability of the substrate was an important rate-limiting step in prostaglandin generation by this preparation. If so, releasing agents such as RCS-RF might act by releasing substrate from some intracellular store. We decided to test this hypothesis by measuring the release of arachidonate from lungs during challenge by these agents. Unfortunately, the lungs avidly metabolize arachidonate. We prevented this by infusing into the lungs 5,8,11,14-eicosatetraynoic acid (TYA), an acetylenic arachidonic acid analogue that inhibits both the lipoxygenase and cyclo-oxygenase pathways (Hamberg & Samuelsson 1974). Control experiments using labelled arachidonate demonstrated that TYA at 20 μg/min completely inhibited the metabolism of arachidonate by the lungs. During the infusion of TYA an injection of RCS-RF was made and the perfusate collected. This was extracted and methylated, the methyl arachidonate was isolated by thin-layer chromatography, and the amount was estimated by gas–liquid chromatography. In each case injections of RCS-RF caused the (variable) release of arachidonic acid from the lungs. When steroids were infused this action was blocked, but it was restored when the steroid infusion was stopped.

It seemed that the anti-inflammatory steroids somehow prevented the release of substrate from an intracellular lipid store—but which one? Free arachidonic acid is present in rather small amounts in cells (Haye et al 1973, Kunze & Vogt 1971, Samuelsson 1972) but occurs in large amounts in phospholipids, mono-, di-, or triglycerides, or cholesterol esters. Most attention has been focused on the first of these possibilities. We have demonstrated in spleen and platelets that the majority of the arachidonic acid substrate utilized for prostaglandin biosynthesis is derived from the phosphatide fraction (Flower & Blackwell 1976, Blackwell et al 1977). A conceptual advantage of the phosphatide fraction as a source of the arachidonate is that it provides a ready explanation for the ability of so many membrane-linked events to trigger the generation of prostaglandins. If the cellular source of arachidonate *is* the phosphatide pool, it follows that a phospholipase plays an important role. In the particular case of arachidonic acid (which is generally esterified in the 2′ position), phospholipase A_2 is presumably the hydrolytic enzyme.

Do PG-releasing agents, such as RCS-RF, stimulate phospholipase and, if so, is this the enzymic step which is steroid sensitive? To try to answer these questions we devised a method for assaying phospholipase activity in perfused lungs. This depends on the hydrolysis by the lung of a specifically labelled phosphatide. A sample of a mixture of 2′-[^{3}H-oleoyl]phosphatidylcholine and [^{14}C]oleic acid was injected as a bolus through the lungs and the effluent was collected and extracted with hexane. The ^{14}C/^{3}H ratio was determined and the hydrolysis of the phosphatide was calculated. We found that the timing of these experiments was critical; when the lung preparation was first perfused, the basal (i.e. unstimulated) hydrolysis was very high; but this soon declined (within about 30 min), reaching a relatively stable level (which was maintained for approximately two hours), after which the basal hydrolysis rapidly began to rise. In our experience, this second phase (which occurs after about three hours) is irreversible, and may be connected with cytolysis and cell death. All the experiments described below were performed during the relatively stable ‘plateau’ phase.

The background hydrolytic activity of the lung was blocked by several agents, such as mepacrine (I_{50} 20 μg/ml perfusing fluid), chlorpromazine (I_{50} 33.5 μg/ml), and procaine (I_{50} 73.4 μg/ml). Aspirin and indomethacin had I_{50} values of 400 μg/ml or even greater, demonstrating that these drugs are virtually inactive against this enzyme. The steroids betamethasone, dexamethasone and hydrocortisone were very active (I_{50} values of 1.4, 1.5 and 48 μg/ml, respectively). Aldosterone was inactive at concentrations of up to 80 μg/ml.

Unlike mepacrine, chlorpromazine and procaine, the steroids did not act against phospholipase A_2 activity in cell-free lung homogenates, and their mode of inhibition differs from that of the non-steroids in a temporal sense too. When phosphatide hydrolysis was measured every 10 min before, during and after an infusion of dexamethasone (2 μg/ml) the rate of hydrolysis began to fall soon after the infusion was begun and reached almost nil after about 50 min. As soon as the infusion was terminated, hydrolysis began to increase again and had returned to control values 40–50 min later.

The basal hydrolysis could be stimulated as well as inhibited. A variety of agents 'activated' phospholipase A_2 activity, the most potent being mechanical trauma (in this case equivalent to 15 seconds of gentle mechanical vibration of the lung parenchyma with an electrical vibrator). This observation corresponds well with the earlier finding that a massive release of prostaglandin endoperoxide occurs after mechanical vibration of the lung. The phospholipase-stimulating activity of histamine, RCS-RF and antigen was blocked in a dose-dependent fashion by both mepacrine and dexamethasone.

THE 'SECOND MESSENGER' THEORY OF STEROID ACTION

We had shown that the anti-inflammatory steroids prevented the release of thromboxanes by preventing arachidonic acid mobilization secondary to stimulation of phospholipase. How exactly did they accomplish this, and why did they work only in intact cells?

In many types of target cells a corticosteroid must first combine with a cytosolic receptor protein. This drug–receptor complex is then translocated to the nucleus where it initiates protein synthesis, ultimately resulting in a biological effect (Buller & O'Malley 1976, Chan & O'Malley 1976, Baxter & Tomkins 1971). In the lung a similar situation seems to obtain: we were able to demonstrate that guinea-pig lung contains proteinaceous glucocorticoid receptors capable of binding [^{3}H]dexamethasone. Interestingly, cortexolone, a glucocorticoid analogue which prevents the combination of dexamethasone with the receptor in these binding assays, also inhibits the anti-phospholipase action of dexamethasone in the perfused lung. Our experiments do not enable us to say definitely that the steroid–receptor complex migrates to the nucleus, but presumably it does, because we also found that inhibition of RNA synthesis (by actinomycin D) or protein synthesis (by puromycin), or inhibition of both (by cycloheximide), reduced or abolished the anti-phospholipase activity of dexamethasone in the perfused lungs (see also the work of Danon & Assouline 1978, Di Rosa & Persico 1979, Russo-Marie et al

1979). These findings strongly suggested that (short latency of action nothwithstanding) the steroids produce their inhibitory effect on phospholipase by initiating transcriptional and translational activity within the target cells of the lung.

Presumably the steroids were initiating the *de novo* biosynthesis (or secretion) of an anti-phospholipase factor. In a further series of experiments we provided strong evidence for this hypothesis. To do this we used two lungs perfused in series. Effluent from one perfused lung (called the generator lung) was re-oxygenated and pumped directly through another perfused lung (test lung) which also received cycloheximide to render it insensitive to steroids. Anti-inflammatory steroids were infused either through the generator lung or into the effluent leaving the generator lung. Thus, the only difference in the effluent perfusing the test lung was whether or not the steroid has passed through the first lung. Bioassay or radiochemical assays were done to determine phopholipase activity.

When steroids were infused directly into the test lung they did not affect phospholipase activity. When steroids were infused into the generator lung, however, phospholipase activity of the test lung (estimated by either technique) was greatly reduced. This experiment and others of a similar nature convinced us that the steroids caused the liberation by some cell type in the lung of a potent inhibitor of phospholipase-dependent PG biosynthesis. Unknown to us at that time, a similar conclusion had been reached by Di Rosa and his colleagues in Naples (Carnuccio et al 1980), using a rat leucocyte system in which steroids also powerfully inhibit PG formation. They demonstrated that a non-dialysable heat-labile inhibitor was responsible for the effect of the steroids in this model.

Since the discovery of this second messenger the Naples group and our group have collaborated in experiments to try to identify the inhibitor. Although the work is unfinished it seems that it is a polypeptide having a molecular weight of about 10 000–15 000.

SIGNIFICANCE OF THESE FINDINGS

We have known for many years that steroids are effective against a wide range of inflammatory disorders. There is considerable evidence that prostaglandins and other products of arachidonic acid metabolism are important in inflammation and probably other clinical conditions, such as asthma. In this paper I have described experiments which link the action of steroids to an action on the phospholipase—a key enzyme in the supply of substrates for biosynthesis of these lipid products. *In vitro* at least, the action of steroids seems to be mediated by a second messenger—a polypeptide—synthesized or secreted by cells in response to the steroid. We do not know yet whether this polypeptide is responsible for the actions of the steroid *in vivo* but, if it is, this opens up new vistas of anti-inflammatory chemotherapy. Perhaps this compound or an analogue will have many of the anti-inflammatory effects of steroids with few of the side-effects that make long-term therapy so undesirable.

References

Baxter JD, Tomkins GM 1971 Specific cytoplasmic glucocorticoid hormone receptors in hepatoma tissue culture cells. Proc Natl Acad Sci USA 68:932-937

Bergström S, Danielsson H, Samuelsson B 1964 The enzymatic formation of prostaglandin E_2 from arachidonic acid. Prostaglandins and related factors. 32. Biochim Biophys Acta 90: 207-210

Blackwell GJ, Duncombe WG, Flower RJ, Parsons MF, Vane JR 1977 The distribution and metabolism of arachidonic acid in rabbit platelets during aggregation and its modification by drugs. Br J Pharmacol 59:353-366

Blackwell GJ, Flower RJ, Nijkamp FP, Vane JR 1978 Phospholipase A_2 activity of guinea pig isolated perfused lungs: stimulation and inhibition by anti-inflammatory steroids. Br J Pharmacol 62:79-89

Buller RE, O'Malley BW 1976 The biology and mechanism of steroid hormone receptor interaction with the eukaryotic nucleus. Biochem Pharmacol 25:1-12

Carnuccio R, Di Rosa M, Persico P 1980 Hydrocortisone induced inhibitor of prostaglandin biosynthesis in rat leucocytes. Br J Pharmacol 68:14-16

Chan L, O'Malley BW 1976 Mechanism of action of the sex steroid hormones. N Engl J Med 294: 1372-1379

Danon A, Assouline G 1978 Inhibition of prostaglandin biosynthesis by corticosteroids requires RNA and protein synthesis. Nature (Lond) 273:552-554

Di Rosa M, Persico P 1979 Mechanism of inhibition of prostaglandin biosynthesis by hydrocortisone in rat leucocytes. Br J Pharmacol 66:161-163

Ferreira SH, Moncada S, Vane JR 1971 Indomethacin and aspirin abolish prostaglandin release from the spleen. Nat New Biol 231:237-239

Floman N, Zor U 1977 Mechanism of steroid action in ocular inflammation: inhibition of prostaglandin production. Invest Ophthalmol Visual Sci 16:69-73

Flower RJ, Blackwell GJ 1976 The importance of phospholipase A_2 in prostaglandin biosynthesis. Biochem Pharmacol 25:285-291

Flower RJ, Blackwell GJ 1979 Anti-inflammatory steroids induce biosynthesis of a phospholipase A_2 inhibitor which prevents prostaglandin generation. Nature (Lond) 278:456-459

Flower RJ, Gryglewski R, Herbaczyńska-Cedro K, Vane JR 1972 The effect of anti-inflammatory drugs on prostaglandin biosynthesis. Nat New Biol 238:104-106

Gryglewski RJ, Panczenko B, Korbut R, Grodzinska L, Ocetkiewicz A 1975 Corticosteroids inhibit prostaglandin release from perfused mesenteric blood vessels of rabbit and from perfused lungs of sensitized guinea-pigs. Prostaglandins 10:343-355

Hamberg M, Samuelsson B 1974a Prostaglandin endoperoxides. Novel transformations of arachidonic acid in human platelets. Proc Natl Acad Sci USA 71:3400-3404

Hamberg M, Samuelsson B 1974b Prostaglandin endoperoxides. VII. Novel transformations of arachidonic acid in guinea-pig lung. Biochem Biophys Res Commun 16:942-949

Hamberg M, Svensson J, Samuelsson 1975 Thromboxanes: a new group of biologically active compounds derived from prostaglandin endoperoxides. Proc Natl Acad Sci USA 72:2994-2998

Haye B, Champion S, Jacquemin C 1973 Control by TSH of a phospholipase A_2 activity, a limiting factor in the biosynthesis of prostaglandins in the thyroid. FEBS (Fed Eur Biochem Soc) Lett 30:253-260
Herbaczyńska-Cedro K, Staszewska-Barczak J 1974 Adrenocortical hormones and the release of prostaglandin-like substances (PLS). Abstracts of II Congress of Hungarian Pharmacological Society p 19, Budapest
Hong S-CL, Levine L 1976 Inhibition of arachidonic acid release from cells as the biochemical action of anti-inflammatory steroids. Proc Natl Acad Sci USA 73:1730-1734
Johnson RA, Morton DR, Kinner JH, Gorman RR, McGuire JR, Sun FF, Whittaker N, Bunting S, Salmon JA, Moncada S, Vane JR 1976 The chemical structure of prostaglandin X (prostacyclin). Prostaglandins 12:915-928
Kantrowitz F, Robinson DC, McGuire MB, Levine L 1975 Corticosteroids inhibit prostaglandin production by rheumatoid synovia. Nature (Lond) 258:737-739
Kunze H, Vogt W 1971 Significance of phospholipase A for prostaglandin formation. Ann NY Acad Sci 180:123-125
Lewis GP, Piper PJ 1975 Inhibition of release of prostaglandins as an explanation of some of the actions of anti-inflammatory steroids. Nature (Lond) 254:308-311
Moncada S, Gryglewski R, Bunting S, Vane JR 1976 An enzyme isolated from arteries transforms prostaglandin endoperoxides to an unstable substance that inhibits platelet aggregation. Nature (Lond) 263:663-665
Nijkamp FP, Flower RJ, Moncada S, Vane JR 1976 Partial purification of rabbit aorta contracting substance-releasing factor and inhibition of its activity by anti-inflammatory steroids. Nature (Lond) 263:479-482
Parente L, Ammendola G, Persico P, Di Rosa M 1978 Glucocorticosteroids, prostaglandins and the inflammatory process. Pol J Pharmacol Pharm 30:141-155
Piper PJ, Vane JR 1969 Release of additional factors in anaphylaxis and its antagonism by anti-inflammatory drugs. Nature (Lond) 233:29-35
Russo-Marie F, Paing M, Duval D 1979 Involvement of glucocorticoid receptors in steroid-induced inhibition of prostaglandin secretion. J Biol Chem 254:8498-8504
Samuelsson B 1972 Biosynthesis of prostaglandins. Fed Proc 31:1442-1450
Samuelsson B, Borgeat P, Hammarström S, Murphy RC 1979 Introduction to a nomenclature: leukotrienes. Prostaglandins 17:785-787
Smith JB, Willis AL 1971 Aspirin selectively inhibits prostaglandin production in human platelets. Nat New Biol 231:235-237
Tam S, Hong S-CL, Levine L 1977 Relationships among the steroids of anti-inflammatory properties and inhibition of prostaglandin production and arachidonic acid release by transformed mouse fibroblasts. J Pharmacol Exp Ther 203:162-168
Tashjian AH, Voelkel EF, McDonough J, Levine L 1975 Hydrocortisone inhibits prostaglandin production by mouse fibrosarcoma cells. Nature (Lond) 258:739-741
Turner SR, Tainer JA, Lynn WS 1975 Biogenesis of chemotactic molecules by the arachidonate lipoxygenase system of platelets. Nature (Lond) 257:680-681
Van Dorp DA, Beerthuis RK, Nugteren DH, Vonkeman H 1964 The biosynthesis of prostaglandins. Biochim Biophys Acta 90:204-207
Vane JR 1971 Inhibition of prostaglandin synthesis as mechanism of action for aspirin-like drugs. Nat New Biol 231:232-235

Discussion

Stubbs: I am intrigued to learn that phospholipids are a source of prostaglandins, particularly since phospholipid production can be modified by a variety of factors. Is there any suggestion that the rate of production of prostaglandins is limited by the formation of phospholipids? I am thinking particularly here of situations where lung phospholipid may be depleted, such as the respiratory distress syndrome in the neonate.

Flower: I don't know of any evidence suggesting that PG synthesis is limited by the rate of phospholipid formation. Rather, it is limited by the rate of release of suitable substrates from the phospholipids.

Vane: The rate-limiting step in prostaglandin biosynthesis is undoubtedly the release of arachidonic acid, because if you infuse arachidonic acid into animals or add it to whole-organ preparations these compounds are immediately generated. So the enzyme that cyclizes arachidonic acid is waiting for the substrate to come along.

Ferreira: I believe that arachidonic acid goes into the general pool for phospholipids. If not, all arachidonic acid would be transformed to prostaglandins!

Vane: Yes, but what gets to the cyclo-oxygenase is immediately transformed.

Soffer: Steroids don't inhibit phospholipase A_2 in a cell-free system; does your inhibitor inhibit this enzyme in a cell-free system?

Flower: We haven't tested this yet. One problem is that there are many phospholipases in the cell, and we aren't sure which are the most relevant.

Soffer: This isn't important physiologically, but it is important for understanding what is going on at the molecular level. Do you think that the agent you have isolated acts directly as an inhibitor of phospholipase A_2, or by some indirect mechanism which may influence the reaction catalysed by the enzyme?

Flower: We don't know yet. The polypeptide needn't be an inhibitor of the enzyme itself to have an effect. Many phospholipases are calcium dependent and the inhibitor might act by altering calcium movement, thereby blocking enzyme activity indirectly.

Morishige: Does the inhibitor bind calcium? Could the inhibitor be calmodulin, which sequesters calcium?

Flower: That's a very interesting idea, but I think that in most systems (for example, platelets: Wong & Cheung 1979) calmodulin *stimulates* the phospholipase A_2 and thus *increases* prostaglandin formation.

Ballard: The time course of this process interests me. I know of no other system involving *de novo* synthesis of both RNA and protein that shows a maximum effect at 1–2 hours. This is very rapid and suggests that a different mechanism may be operating. Would you also comment on the dose–response properties of the system to steroid?

Flower: The perfused lungs are rather an unsatisfactory system for establishing dose–response relationships to steroids. I used doses of dexamethasone of 1 μg/ml in most experiments, but I obtained the same effect if the concentration was reduced by a factor of 10 or even more; however, the latency of the effect was much longer in that case. In similar experiments with rat macrophages Di Rosa and his colleagues have also shown the release of a phospholipase inhibitor by steroids, and this phenomenon is also blocked by cycloheximide, actinomycin etc. (Carnuccio et al 1980). These cells behave much more 'physiologically' than perfused lungs; responses are obtained with doses of hydrocortisone down to 10^{-7}M; the latency of the effect is also quite short in this system. Effects are obtained within 30 min and are completely prevented by adding cycloheximide for 10 minutes before the steroid. There are other reports of such rapid effects of steroids (cf. Divakaran & Friedmann 1976, Foster & Perkins 1977, Baxter & Tomkins 1970). The time for half-maximal block in our lung system is about 45 minutes.

Gryglewski: A lot of prostanoid is released in anaphylactic shock in cats. However, 10–15 minutes after the injection of hydrocortisone semisuccinate (50 mg/kg), prostanoids disappear from blood and the blood pressure rises (Gryglewski et al 1977). Also, *in vitro*, Dr Brune demonstrated that high concentrations of steroids inhibit the generation of prostanoids by macrophages within 10–15 minutes and that this inhibition is not prevented by cycloheximide (Brune & Rainsford 1979). Could these rapid effects perhaps be mediated through an alternative pathway? Maybe stabilization of membranes by steroids could be important when they are used at high pharmacological concentrations.

Vane: What does stabilization of membranes really mean?

Gryglewski: It could mean that phospholipids were not so easily hydrolysed by phospholipase A_2, as the result of a physicochemical interaction between 'pharmacological' concentrations of steroids and biological membranes of target cells of steroids.

Flower: To me that would imply that if you give an anti-inflammatory dose of dexamethasone to a rat (about 100 μg) there are enough molecules to 'stabilize' all the membranes of all the cells in the body and somehow block the hydrolysis of phospholipids. That doesn't seem a tenable hypothesis. What I am suggesting is entirely different, because combination of the steroid with a receptor initiates a cascade of biochemical events. In other words, there is a 'biological amplifier' at work!

Woods: There are enzymes that are very rapidly induced. The inducing effects of tryptophan on tryptophan pyrrolase in the isolated perfused liver are demonstrable within an hour, and this can be inhibited by cycloheximide and other blockers of protein synthesis, so that the system responds in as short a time as Dr Flower has been describing (Green et al 1976).

Ballard: The increase in tryptophan pyrrolase activity is felt to be a post-transcriptional event (pseudoinduction), involving increased association of apoenzyme and cofactor which stabilizes this relatively short-lived enzyme.

Flower: This short time course puzzled me too, but this is not the only system where such a short latency has been documented. It is also possible that we are not getting a *de novo* synthesis of this polypeptide, but rather a release by steroids of an inhibitor that is already formed.

Soffer: Does the agent you have isolated have anti-inflammatory properties?

Flower: We haven't yet got enough of it to test this exciting possibility.

Said: Is anything known about this polypeptide that would elucidate its mode of action?

Flower: We know its molecular weight (c. 10 000–15 000) and various physicochemical properties but little else, I'm afraid. Its effect on lung cells and other cells is indistinguishable from that of the corticosteroids, except that it has a very fast onset time.

Said: Incidentally, I am rather pleased to see that a peptide regulates the entire arachidonate cascade!

Aiken: Does cortexolone, which inhibits the anti-phospholipase effect of steroids in lung, also block the anti-inflammatory effects of steroids?

Flower: Yes.

Collier: A possible supplementary explanation of the corticosteroid effect you describe arises from our observation that corticosteroids administered in a single dose to rats increase quite considerably the level of plasma inhibitors of prostaglandin synthesis (Saeed et al 1977).

Flower: I was certainly not proposing that this is the exclusive mechanism of steroid action; the activity of steroids is difficult to understand because just about every nucleated cell in the body responds to them. As you say, there may be more than one mechanism involved. The anti-inflammatory effect of dexamethasone in the rat is expressed within 30 min to one hour.

Collier: The rise in endogenous inhibitors of prostaglandin synthesis in plasma is detectable about 4 h after a single intraperitoneal dose of 24 mg/kg dexamethasone in the rat and reaches a plateau by about 24 h. This time course seems to be in line with clinical experience.

Vane: One of my initial questions was: which cell types in the lungs release prostaglandins or thromboxanes, and does the migration of cells or platelets play any role? Do macrophages or fibroblasts in the lungs contribute to thromboxane release, for example?

Flower: We did culture some lung epithelial cells; they produced thromboxane at first but lost this ability during successive passages.

Bakhle: Human lung perfused with arachidonic acid, guinea-pig SRS-A or the calcium ionophore (A23187) produces no thromboxane A_2-like activity (Al-Ubaidi & Bakhle 1980).

Piper: We found the same in chopped human lung subjected to various stimuli, with one exception: thromboxane synthesis was turned on by vibrating or agitating the tissue. Evidently there has to be some form of mechanical distortion or damage, but not by anaphylaxis or any mediator that we have injected.

Bakhle: Theories of the mediators of asthma have been based on the production of thromboxane A_2 by guinea-pig lung after a variety of stimuli (see Mathé et al 1977); if that material is *not* produced in human lung, we shall have to change our theories.

Reid: It has been implied that endothelial cells produce prostacyclin and other prostaglandins. Ryan & Ryan (1977) have obtained histochemical evidence of some synthetic activity in the alveolar wall. From their illustrations, the enzyme appears to be located in an interstitial cell, in either a fibroblast or a myofibroblast. If that is confirmed it indicates that there is prostaglandin synthetase in the interstitium.

Gryglewski: We proposed compartmentalization of the production of eicosanoids by lungs on a pharmacological basis. Histamine-contracted guinea-pig trachea produced PGE_2 and not TXA_2, whereas the pulmonary strip produced TXA_2 and not PGE_2. We inferred that different histamine-sensitive contractile elements are responsible for the generation of PGE_2 and TXA_2 in lungs. To my knowledge there is *no* good histochemical method for the detection and cellular localization of cyclo-oxygenase or prostacyclin synthetase in tissues.

Said: I agree. The methods are not specific enough. Similarly, the prostaglandin-degrading enzyme (PG dehydrogenase) has not been shown convincingly in the lung by histochemical techniques.

Bakhle: There clearly are tissue inhomogeneities; PG dehydrogenase doesn't seem to be present in endothelial cells, since cultured endothelial cells don't metabolize prostaglandins; and you don't get thromboxane A_2 out of endothelial cells. So thromboxane production and PG inactivation must occur in cell types other than endothelial cells.

Burri: What is your 'releasing factor', Dr Flower, and where do you obtain it?

Flower: Priscilla Piper and John Vane first described 'Rabbit aorta contracting substance–releasing factor' (RCS-RF) in the effluent from guinea-pig perfused lungs which had been challenged after sensitization to albumin (Piper & Vane 1969). This causes a massive release of pharmacologically active mediators; from the effluent you obtain an agent that has powerful PG-releasing activity and is apparently not SRS-A. The structure of an SRS has now been described by Samuelsson and his colleagues. It consists of a peptide linked to a fatty acid (cf. Hammerström et al 1979 and this volume p 203-215).

Piper: It is very interesting that SRS-A has the same prostaglandin-releasing power as the releasing factor (RCS-RF), and is blocked by corticosteroids; this makes me question the distinction between the releasing factor and SRS-A. We couldn't repeat your experiments.

Flower: We did some paper chromatography on extracts from perfused lung and showed that guinea-pig ileum contracting activity was found in two zones of the chromatogram, whereas the 'releasing' activity was present only in one; we called the latter RCS-RF and we presumed that the former was SRS-A (Nijkamp et al 1976).

Bakhle: Dr Piper, you showed that SRS-A releases PG-like substances from unsensitized lung, and that you can block that release with betamethasone; didn't you (Engineer et al 1978) then find that an infusion of arachidonate restored the release by SRS-A, even when betamethasone was present?

Piper: We obtain an apparent restoration of the release, but it only happens once and we cannot obtain the restoration in every experiment.

Bakhle: If that were confirmed it would suggest a mechanism of SRS-A action quite different from the phospholipase activation usually postulated.

Slater: An interesting group of substances derived from the peroxidation of polyunsaturated fatty acids (such as arachidonic acid) are the hydroxyaldehydes like 4-hydroxyoct-2-en-1-al (for review see Schauenstein et al 1977). These substances can react non-enzymically with thiols like glutathione to yield several types of adduct: products formed by Michael addition or the thiazolidine-4-carboxylic acid derivatives are important in this respect. Reaction of the 4-hydroxyalkenals with glutathione can yield products rather similar to the structures proposed for leukotriene C and SRS-A. Perhaps some of these 4-hydroxyalkenals (and their adducts with thiols) should be examined pharmacologically. They are certainly very reactive biochemically and can inhibit important enzyme reactions at low concentrations (see Schauenstein & Esterbauer 1979). One extremely active compound in this respect is 4-hydroxynon-2-en-1-al, recently isolated and identified from peroxidizing liver microsomes (Benedetti et al 1979a). Such compounds react readily with primary amines like the polyamines (White & Slater 1974) and can cyclize with thiols to yield thiazolidine-4-carboxylic acid derivatives. The latter materials are currently of interest in the experimental chemotherapy of cancer (e.g. Conroy et al 1977, Brugarolas & Gosalvez 1980).

The 4-hydroxyalkenals, such as 4-hydroxypentenal, 4-hydroxynonenal and related ketoaldehydes, have inhibitory actions on several membrane-linked enzymes, including glucose-6-phosphatase and cytochrome *P*-450 (see Dianzani 1979, Benedetti et al 1979a). They also have effects on capillary permeability and red cell fragility (Ugazio et al 1976, Benedetti et al 1979b). Some of the toxic effects are considerably attenuated by prior reaction with thiols like glutathione.

Moncada: So they might be more toxic if they *don't* react with glutathione or another amino acid?

Slater: Yes. High, localized concentrations of the 4-hydroxyalkenals (or ketoaldehydes) can be expected to react with neighbouring primary amino and thiol groups; some of these will be essential for enzyme activity. If the hydroxyaldehyde is combined first with cysteine or glutathione to form an adduct, the acute toxicity is considerably reduced (see Conroy et al 1977). The adducts of 4-hydroxyalkenals with thiol groups exist in equilibrium with the parent substances (aldehyde + cysteine $\rightleftharpoons$ adduct); injection of the adduct results in a considerably lower local concentration of the aldehyde and this is reflected in lower toxicity in general (see Schauenstein et al 1977).

Moncada: The reaction with glutathione or cysteine might be a protective mechanism—a kind of detoxification mechanism of the body. The 5,6-epoxide intermediate might then be a very reactive molecule. Is the reaction with glutathione or cysteine a known mechanism of protection? If what you are saying is right, it is probable that the pharmacologically important compounds, or the pathologically important compounds, are the intermediates and not these stable end-products. This is known for other areas of arachidonic acid metabolism, like thromboxane A_2 and thromboxane B_2. [See p 211 for further discussion.]

References

Al-Ubaidi F, Bakhle YS 1980 Differences in biological activation of arachidonic acid in perfused lungs from guinea-pig, rat and man. Eur J Pharmacol 62:89-96

Baxter JD, Tomkins GM 1970 The relationship between glucocorticoid binding and tyrosine aminotransferase induction in hepatoma tissue culture cells. Proc Natl Acad Sci USA 65:709-715

Benedetti A, Esterbauer H, Comporti M 1979a In: 15th Congresso della Società Italiana di Patologia, Sorrento, p 167

Benedetti A, Casini AF, Ferrali M, Comporti M 1979b In: 15th Congresso della Società Italiana di Patologia, Sorrento, p 165

Brugarolas A, Gosalvez M 1980 Treatment of cancer by an inducer of reverse transformation. Lancet 1:68-70

Brune K, Rainsford KD 1979 Prostaglandin release from macrophages: modulation by anti-inflammatory drugs. In: Rainsford KD, Ford-Hutchinson AW (eds) Prostaglandins and inflammation. Birkhäuser Verlag, Basel, AAS6:159-165

Carnuccio R, Di Rosa M, Persico P 1980 Hydrocortisone-induced inhibitor of prostaglandin biosynthesis in rat leucocytes. Br J Pharmacol 68:14-16

Conroy PJ, Nodes JT, Slater TF, White GW 1977 The inhibitory effects of a 4-hydroxy-pentenal: cysteine adduct against sarcoma 180 cells in mice. Eur J Cancer 13:55-63

Dianzani MU 1979 Biological activity of methylglyoxal and related aldehydes. In: Submolecular biology and cancer. Excerpta Medica, Amsterdam (Ciba Found Symp 67) p 245-265

Divakaran P, Friedmann N 1976 A fast *in vitro* effect of glucocorticoids on hepatic lipolysis. Endocrinology 98:1550-1553

Engineer DM, Morris HR, Piper PJ, Sirois P 1978 The release of prostaglandins and thromboxanes from guinea-pig lung by slow reacting substance of anaphylaxis and its inhibition. Br J Pharmacol 64:211-218

Foster SJ, Perkins JP 1977 Glucocorticoids increase the responsiveness of cells in culture to prostaglandin E_1. Proc Natl Acad Sci USA 74:4816-4820

Green AR, Woods HF, Joseph MH 1976 Tryptophan metabolism in the isolated perfused liver of the rat: effects of tryptophan concentration, hydrocortisone and allopurinol on tryptophan pyrrolase activity and kynurenine formation. Br J Pharmacol 57:103-114

Gryglewski RJ, Korbut R, Grodzińska L, Dembińska-Kieć A 1977 Effect of glucocorticosteroids on the release of prostaglandin-like substances in anaphylaxis. In: Bonta IL (ed) Recent developments in the pharmacology of inflammatory mediators (Agents and Actions, Suppl 2) Birkhäuser Verlag, Basel, p 68-76

Hammarström S, Murphy RC, Samuelsson B, Clark DA, Mioskowski C, Corey EJ 1979 Structure of leukotriene C: identification of the amino acid part. Biochem Biophys Res Commun 91: 1266-1272

Mathé AA, Hedqvist P, Strandberg K, Leslie CA 1977 Aspects of prostaglandin function in the lung. N Engl J Med 296:850-855 and 910-914

Nijkamp FP, Flower RJ, Moncada S, Vane JR 1976 Partial purification of rabbit aorta contracting substance–releasing factor and inhibition of its activity by anti-inflammatory steroids. Nature (Lond) 263:479-482

Piper PJ, Vane JR 1969 Release of additional factors in anaphylaxis and its antagonism by anti-inflammatory drugs. Nature (Lond) 233:29-35

Ryan US, Ryan JW 1977 Correlations between the fine structure of the alveolar capillary unit and its metabolic activities. In: Bakhle YS, Vane JR (eds) Metabolic functions of the lung (Lung biology in health and disease, vol 4) Dekker, New York, p 197-232

Saeed SA, McDonald-Gibson WJ, Cuthbert J, Copas JL, Schneider C, Gardiner PJ, Butt NM, Collier HOJ 1977 Endogenous inhibitor of prostaglandin synthetase. Nature (Lond) 270:32-36

Schauenstein E, Esterbauer H 1979 Formation and properties of reactive aldehydes. In: Submolecular biology and cancer. Excerpta Medica, Amsterdam (Ciba Found Symp 67) p 225-241

Schauenstein E, Esterbauer H, Zollner H 1977 Aldehydes in biological systems. Pion/Academic, London (Gore PH, transl)

Ugazio G, Torrielli MV, Burdino M, Sawyer BC, Slater TF 1976 Long-range effects of products of carbon-tetrachloride stimulated lipid peroxidation. Biochem Soc Trans 4:353-356

White GW, Slater TF 1974 The reaction of polyamines with aldehydic products of lipid peroxidation. Abstracts of 9th FEBS Meeting, Budapest, abstr 367

Wong PYK, Cheung WY 1979 Calmodulin stimulates human platelet phospholipase A_2. Biochem Biophys Res Commun 90: 473:480

Slow-reacting substances and their structural elucidation

PRISCILLA J. PIPER, MARWA N. SAMHOUN, J.R. TIPPINS, H.R. MORRIS* and G.W. TAYLOR*

*Department of Pharmacology, Institute of Basic Medical Sciences, Royal College of Surgeons of England, Lincoln's Inn Fields, London WC2A 3PN and *Department of Biochemistry, Imperial College, London SW7, UK*

Abstract For more than forty years since their discovery, the structure of a group of closely related materials known collectively as slow-reacting substances has been unknown. These substances are released from a variety of tissues in response to immunological or non-immunological stimulation. A slow-reacting substance is believed to be implicated in hypersensitivity reactions such as asthma; in order to fully understand its bronchoconstrictor role, the structural elucidation of these materials has been a necessary (albeit difficult) task.

Studies on both immunologically generated slow-reacting substance of anaphylaxis (SRS-A) and other slow-reacting substances (SRSs) have indicated a precursor role for arachidonic acid in their biosynthesis; this, coupled with enzymic and chemical activity destruction data, gave an insight into the structure of these moieties.

In order to define the structure of these materials homogeneous SRS-A was required; a purification scheme was developed relying on the high resolution separative capability of reverse-phase high pressure liquid chromatography, resulting in extensively purified SRS-A. It was then possible to demonstrate that SRS-A possessed a characteristic ultraviolet spectrum, allowing us for the first time to define a major structural moiety in the molecule (conjugated triene).

To complement studies on, and to act as a model for the more pathologically relevant SRS-A, a slow-reacting substance was produced from rat basophilic leukaemia (RBL-1) cells. The structure of this biologically active species has been determined by mass spectrometric examination of the *intact* molecule as a derivative, together with analytical protein chemical studies, and shown to be the novel peptidolipid 5-hydroxy-6-cysteinylglycinyl-7,9,11,14-eicosatetraenoic acid.

In 1938 Feldberg and Kellaway described a material with smooth muscle contracting activity, released from perfused guinea-pig lung on treatment with cobra venom. Two years later Kellaway & Trethewie (1940) reported the liberation of a 'slow-reacting smooth muscle-stimulating substance in anaphylaxis' from perfused sensitized guinea-pig lung in response to antigen

Metabolic activities of the lung
(Ciba Foundation symposium 78) p 203-215

challenge. In 1960, with the development of anti-histamine drugs, Brocklehurst was able to separate the contractile activity of this material from that of histamine and described the substance as slow-reacting substance of anaphylaxis (SRS-A). The structure of SRS-A has until recently remained a mystery (Morris et al 1980a).

A number of similar materials from a range of tissues and dispersed cells have been described in recent years, released either immunologically or non-immunologically (e.g. with calcium ionophore, see Bach & Brashler 1974, Jakschik et al 1977, Murphy et al 1979). The pharmacological and physicochemical properties of these various slow-reacting substances (SRSs) have been described as being similar to those of SRS-A.

We have, in the past few years, been active in the study of the slow-reacting substances, and can now announce the first structure of a naturally occurring SRS based on definitive mass spectrometric data.

In our laboratory slow-reacting substances have been prepared from two sources: SRS-A was released by antigen challenge of isolated perfused lung from guinea-pigs sensitized to ovalbumin; SRS was released from the rat basophilic leukaemia (RBL-1) cells dispersed in a suitable medium by stimulation with the calcium ionophore A23187. These stimuli both trigger the mobilization of arachidonic acid by a calcium-dependent phospholipase A_2 and its subsequent metabolism; there is strong evidence, given below, that SRS-A and SRSs are derived from this fatty acid.

The modulation of the release of SRS-A has been studied in guinea-pig chopped lung; this enables test and control experiments to be performed using tissue from one animal, which is necessary where quantities of the compound under examination are limited. Using this method we have been able to show that the release of SRS-A from the guinea-pig lung is potentiated by indomethacin, which inhibits the metabolism of arachidonic acid via the cyclo-oxygenase pathway, and by a number of unsaturated fatty acids, especially arachidonic acid and eicosapentaenoic acid (Fig. 1). These fatty acids may increase the release of SRS-A by acting as substrates for the synthesis of SRS-A or by displacing endogenous arachidonic acid, thus causing increased generation of SRS-A (Piper et al 1979). We have also shown that compounds which inhibit the action of lipoxygenase (eicosatetraynoic acid and nor-dihydroguaiaretic acid) also inhibit the release of SRS-A (Piper et al 1979). We have suggested that the potentiation of SRS-A release by compounds that block the cyclo-oxygenase pathway is the result of a redirection of arachidonic acid metabolism via the lipoxygenase pathway (Hamberg 1976). In fact, arachidonic acid may be metabolized by a number of lipoxygenases and Murphy et al (1979) have suggested that a lipoxygenase which converts arachidonic

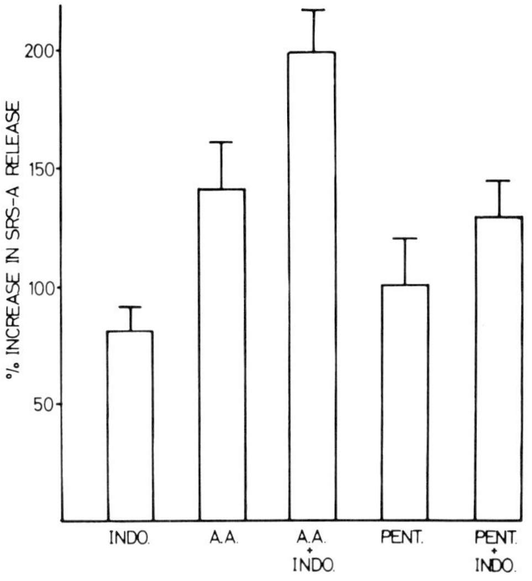

FIG. 1. The effect of indomethacin (Indo., 1 μg/ml), arachidonic acid (10 μg/ml) and 5,8,11,14, 17-eicosapentaenoic acid (Pent., 10 μg/ml) on SRS-A release from guinea-pig chopped lung. (From Morris et al 1980c, by permission of the Editor of *Prostaglandins*.)

acid to a 5-hydroperoxy intermediate is involved in the production of an SRS from the murine mastocytoma cells. Thus it appears that SRS-A and SRSs are metabolites of arachidonic acid; radiolabelled arachidonic acid has been incorporated into RBL-1 SRS (Jakschik et al 1978), although we were unable to incorporate [^{14}C] arachidonic acid into SRS-A from guinea-pig chopped lung (Morris et al 1979a). Potentiation of SRS release by a variety of thiols has been observed by Bach & Brashler (1978) and Orange & Chang (1975) from mononuclear cells and human lung fragments respectively, suggesting that these compounds might be incorporated into the SRS molecule. Indeed we have demonstrated the presence of a thioether linkage in SRS-A from guinea-pig lung (Morris et al 1979a).

The slow-reacting substances produced in our laboratory were purified as described (Morris et al 1978, Morris et al 1979a). The purification procedure is shown in Table 1, and was developed to maximize data on the physicochemical properties of SRSs while being fully applicable to the high-yield purification of minute quantities of biologically active molecules (e.g. salt-free buffers are used for compatibility with bioassay, mass spectrometry, etc.). The final high pressure liquid chromatography (HPLC) step resolves partially purified material into four ultraviolet-absorbing compounds (Fig.2a). Compound I (λ_{max}^{MeOH} 280 nm) fulfils all the criteria for SRS-A

TABLE 1

Purification of SRS-A

Lung effluent collected on ice
Charcoal adsorption, elution with 80% ethanol, rotary evaporation
Gel filtration on Sephadex G-15 in methanol:ammonia:water
Ether extraction from pH 3 acetic acid (5 °C)
HPLC-1 methanol:water
HPLC-2 propanol:acetic acid:water

and has the characteristic u.v. spectrum originally described in 1978 for the conjugated triene moiety in SRS-A (Morris et al 1978); compound II has a spectrum resembling that of compound I but shifted hypsochromically by 3 nm and with a reduced biological activity (this probably represents a *cis/trans* isomerization of compound I); compound III has a u.v. spectrum typical of a conjugated triene with a λ_{max}^{MeOH} of 270 nm; it is biologically inactive on the guinea-pig ileum and has subsequently been identified by mass spectrometry as 5,12-dihydroxy-6,8,10,14-eicosatetraenoic acid (Morris et al 1979a); compound IV (λ_{max}^{MeOH} 268 nm) is probably related to compound III by an isomerization (Fig.2b). At all stages of purification the SRSs were monitored by their ability to contract the isolated superfused guinea-pig ileum longitudinal smooth muscle in the presence of mepyramine and hyoscine. All SRS-like activity was checked for antagonism by FPL 55712, a specific SRS antagonist.

The release of SRS-A from perfused lung from guinea-pigs sensitized to ovalbumin was originally studied using this sytem as a model of the situation that arises in humans in pathological conditions such as asthma. However, SRS-A has proved to be an extremely potent material biologically but is only released from the lungs in vanishingly small quantities; this had made the structural elucidation of material from this source extremely difficult. The SRS from RBL-1 cells was therefore also studied, as this has the same biological (Table 2), physicochemical and chromatographic properties as SRS-A but is released with far fewer impurities from RBL-1 cultures and in much larger quantities. We have used RBL-1 SRS as a model to optimize the conditions for our mass spectrometric studies on the more pathologically relevant SRS-A.

At all stages of purification, SRS from various sources (e.g. perfused guinea-pig lung, RBL-l cells, human lung fragments, and rat peritoneal cells) co-eluted. This indicated to us that these SRSs were closely related, if not actually chemically identical (Morris et al 1979b, 1980a).

Structural analysis of SRS-A and SRS has involved three major methods: chemical and enzymic degradation, analytical protein chemistry and mass

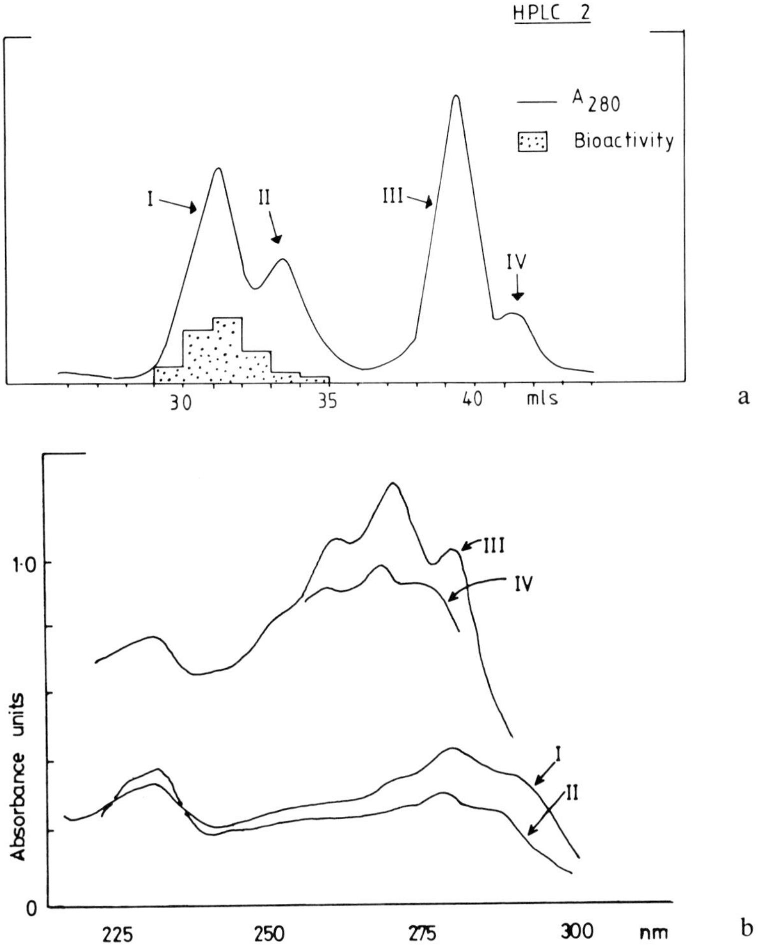

FIG.2.(a) Elution profile of SRS-A from guinea-pig lung after HPLC 2. (From Piper et al 1979a, by permission of Birkhäuser Verlag.)
(b) Full u.v. absorbance spectra of compound I–IV. (From Piper et al 1979a, by permission of Birkhäuser Verlag.)

spectrometry. We have monitored biological activity after brief exposure of SRS or SRS-A to various reagents; this has indicated the presence of various functional groups, namely α-amino (short acetylation), thioether (cyanogen bromide) and carboxyl (methylation). The presence of an α-amino group in the structure enabled us to use this as a marker label in the mass spectrometric work.

TABLE 2

Comparison of biological properties of slow-reacting substances

Property	*Guinea-pig*	*Human SRS-A*	*Rat SRS*	*RBL1-SRS*	*Mouse mastocytoma SRS*
Contracts guinea-pig ileum	+ (2)	+ (2)	+ (2)	+ (1)	+ (1)
Contracts human bronchus, guinea-pig trachea	+ (2)[a]	+ (1)	+ (1)	+ (2)[a]	NT
Releases PGs, thromboxane	+ (2)	+ (1)	+ (1)	+ (1)	+ (1)
Antagonized by FPL 55712	+ (2)	+ (2)	+ (2)	+ (1)	+ (1)

(1), ex-charcoal material used.
(2), material from all stages of purification used.
NT, not tested.
[a]Not tested on human bronchus.

The presence of a *cis*, *cis*-1,4-pentadiene unit in SRS-A was suggested by our early work on lipoxygenase inactivation of SRS-A (Engineer et al 1978).

Turning now to our model RBL-1 SRS system, amino acid analysis of fractions collected across the peak of biological activity showed the presence of only two amino acids, glycine and cysteine. Amino-terminal analysis (dansylation, Hartley 1970) indicated the presence of cysteine only, thus defining the amino acid portion of RBL-1 SRS as the dipeptide cysteinylglycine; this is linked to the hydrocarbon part of the molecule through a thioether linkage (CNBr data). Mass spectrometric analysis of a derivative of the intact SRS then enabled us to define the full covalent structure of this material as 5-hydroxy-6-cysteinylglycinyl-7,9,11,14-eicosatetraenoic acid (Morris et al 1980b) (Fig.3). The derivative chosen for mass spectrometric analysis of this SRS was the trimethylsilyl ether of the *N*-acetyl methyl ester, and was suggested by the known physicochemical properties of SRS (see above). To enable easy identification of SRS ions, and to differentiate such ions from

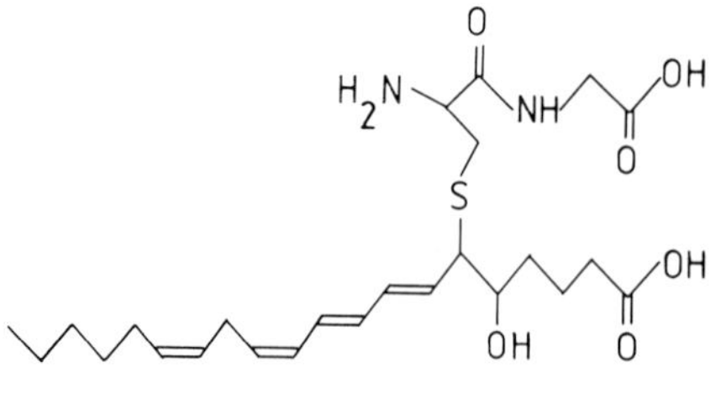

FIG.3. 5-Hydroxy-6-cysteinylglycinyl-7,9,11,14-eicosatetraenoic acid. (From Morris et al 1980b, by permission of the Editor of *Prostaglandins*.)

background, the 1:1 d_3:h_3 *N*-acetyl derivative was prepared, leading to characteristic 'doublets', three mass units apart, in the mass spectrum (Morris et al 1980b) (Fig.4).

The mass spectrum defines the molecular weight of the SRS derivative (m/e 638 (M+) m/e (M+ $-CH_3$) m/e 607 (M+ $-OCH_3$)), cleavage of the peptide portion (m/e 404/405 and m/e 314/15 (−TMSOH)), and the existence and position of a hydroxyl group as a trimethylsilyl derivative (m/e 548 (M+ −TMSOH), m/e 203 ($TMSO^+ = CH(CH_2)_3COOCH_3$). The detailed interpretation of the mass spectrum will be reported elsewhere. This spectrum also allows us to say what is not present in the SRS molecule. We can discount the presence of a sulphate moiety in the molecule (widely expected as a result of arylsulphatase inactivation: Orange et al 1974); the mass spectrum clearly shows the absence of amide or similar carboxy-terminal blocking groups in RBL-SRS.

We also note that the structure we propose for the major biologically active species of RBL-1 SRS could arise as part of the glutathione detoxification pathway, involving nucleophilic attack of glutathione or cysteinylglycine on a 5,6-oxido-eicosatetraenoic acid. Further steps on this pathway would lead to the cysteinyl and the *N*-acetylcysteinyl products.

It is interesting that detoxification should lead to the generation of such a potent biologically active substance; this suggests that its precursor(s) are even more potent.

After HPLC we have occasionally observed small amounts of biologically

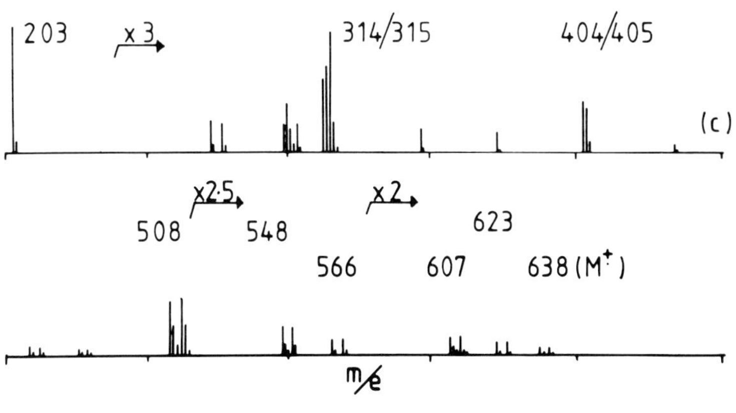

FIG. 4. Electron impact mass spectrum of the trimethylsilyl ether of the *N*-acetyl (CH_3CO:CD_2CO1:) methyl ester of compound I from RBL-1 SRS (~ 1000 units) at 250 °C, showing the 1:1 isotope labelling pattern. (From Morris et al 1980b, by permission of the Editor of *Prostaglandins*.)

active material eluting before compound I (16 ml elution volume), and inactive compounds with conjugated triene u.v. spectra eluting much later (less polar); these SRS-related compounds are currently under investigation. The first demonstration, given here, that a mass spectrum can be produced from undegraded SRS, forms the basis for unequivocal identification of all these substances, using the derivatives described. The mass spectrum can further be used for future accurate comparisons of SRSs from different sources and will also be of importance as a basis for quantitative studies.

These studies have now been extended to immunologically generated SRS-A and have allowed us for the first time to define the structure of this important molecule (Morris et al 1980a). An understanding of the structure and genesis of SRS-A reveals new horizons in the study of asthma and related pathological conditions, and opens the way for the development of potentially useful drugs.

References

Bach MK, Brashler JR 1974 *In vivo* and *in vitro* production of a slow-reacting substance in the rat upon treatment with calcium ionophore. J Immunol 113:2040-2044

Bach MK, Brashler JR 1978 Stimulated production of slow-reacting substances by mercaptans from ionophore A23187-induced mononuclear cells: mercaptan structure–activity studies. Life Sci 23:2119-2126

Brocklehurst WE 1960 The release of histamine and formation of a slow-reacting substance (SRS-A) during anaphylactic shock J Physiol (Lond) 151:416-435

Engineer DM, Morris HR, Piper PJ, Sirois P 1978 Release of prostaglandins and thromboxanes from guinea-pig lung by slow-reacting substance of anaphylaxis and its inhibition. Br J Pharmacol 64:211-218

Feldberg W, Kellaway CH 1938 Liberation of histamine and formation of a lecithin-like substance by cobra venom. J. Physiol (Lond) 94:187-226

Hamberg M 1976 On the formation of thromboxane B_2 and 12-L-hydroxy-5,8,14-eicosatetraenoic acid (12 ho.20:4) in tissues from the guinea-pig. Biochim Biophys Acta 431:651-654

Hartley BS 1970 Strategy and tactics in protein chemistry. Biochem J 119:805-822

Jakschik BA, Kulczycki A, MacDonald HH, Parker CW 1977 Release of slow-reacting substance (SRS) from rat basophil leukemia (RBL-1) cells. J Immunol 119:618-622

Jakschik BA, Lee LH, Shuffer A, Parker CW 1978 Arachidonic acid metabolism in rat basophil leukemia (RBL-1) cells. Prostaglandins 16:773-748

Kellaway CH, Trethewie ER 1940 The liberation of a slow-reacting smooth muscle stimulating substance in anaphylaxis. Q J Exp Physiol 30:121-145

Morris HR, Taylor GW, Piper PJ, Sirois P, Tippins JR 1978 Slow-reacting substance of anaphylaxis: purification and characterisation. FEBS (Fed Eur Biochem Soc) Lett 87:203-206

Morris HR, Piper PJ, Taylor GW, Tippins JR 1979a Slow-reacting substance of anaphylaxis: studies on purification and characterisation. In: Rainsford KD, Ford-Hutchinson AW (eds) Prostaglandins and inflammation. Birkhäuser Verlag, Basel. Agents & Actions Suppl 6:27-36

Morris HR, Piper PJ, Taylor GW, Tippins JR 1979b Comparative studies on immunologically produced slow-reacting substances from man, guinea-pig and rat. Br J Pharmacol 67:179-184

Morris HR, Taylor GW, Piper PJ, Tippins JR 1980a Structure of slow-reacting substance of anaphylaxis from guinea-pig lung. Nature (Lond) 285:104-106
Morris HR, Taylor GW, Piper PJ, Samhoun MN, Tippins JR 1980b Slow-reacting substances (SRSs): the structure identification of SRSs from rat basophil leukaemia (RBL-1) cells. Prostaglandins 19:185-201
Morris HR, Piper PJ, Taylor GW, Tippins JR 1980c The role of arachidonate lipoxygenase in the release of SRS-A from guinea-pig chopped lung. Prostaglandins 19:371-383
Murphy RC, Hammarström S, Samuelsson B 1979 Leukotriene C: A slow-reacting substance from murine mastocytoma cells. Proc Natl Acad Sci USA 76:4275-4279
Orange RP, Change PL 1975 The effect of thiols on immunologic release of slow-reacting substance of anaphylaxis. I. Human lung. J Immunol 115:1072-1077
Orange RP, Murphy RC, Austen KF 1974 Inactivation of slow-reacting substance of anaphylaxis (SRS-A) by arylsulphatases. J Immunol 113:316-322
Piper PJ, Tippins JR, Morris HR, Taylor GW 1979 Arachidonic acid metabolism and SRS-A. In: Brune K, Baggiolini M (eds) Arachidonic acid metabolism in inflammation and thrombosis. Birkhäuser Verlag, Basel. Agents & Actions Suppl. 4:37-48

Discussion

Vane: May we take up the point about the origin of slow-reacting substance (SRS) through detoxification by glutathione? Are you concurring with the view that a 5,6-epoxy compound might be the real villain in asthma?

Piper: Yes, because the addition of thiol side-chain is a familiar way of detoxifying potent substances that are not wanted free in the circulation.

Vane: Have you been able to look at the biological activity of the synthetic compound?

Piper: Unfortunately not.

Vane: If SRS from basophils has all the biological activity of SRS-A, where is the detoxification?

Flower: It might be a case of 'lethal synthesis'; you have an epoxide to which glutathione has been attached, perhaps as a routine detoxification step, but which in this case is unfortunately more toxic than the original compound.

Vane: We can't say yet whether SRS is more or less potent than the 5,6-epoxide.

Moncada: It is possible that the unstable intermediate, the epoxide, is really the active material, and that the biological activity we see with SRS is small compared with that of this epoxide. Peroxides in general are very reactive, damaging substances. We know that they increase bronchial reactivity and increase mediator release in isolated lung during anaphylactic shock (Adcock et al 1978a,b, Adcock & Garland 1980).

Vane: And we discovered those unstable intermediates by using continuous on-line bioassay, and yet by the same bioassay SRS-A does not lose activity if you re-test it after its initial release; so, if this concept is right, the 5,6-epoxide must be detoxified rapidly even before it gets into the effluent from the guinea-pig lung.

Piper: SRS-A is stable in a Krebs-perfused system; we don't know what happens in the circulation. We might have a very different picture there.

Collier: I should like to make three comments. First, on your suggestion that SRS-A is a by-product of detoxification, SRS-A is itself surely rather harmful, and nature might be expected to have done better in detoxifying the epoxide than to produce SRS-A! Secondly, it seems paradoxical that lipoxygenase both liberates and destroys SRS-A. Perhaps it is a question of differences in time and place? Thirdly, I believe that Berry and I were the first to demonstrate experimentally a special relationship between arachidonic acid and SRS-A. In 1964 we found that, of all fatty acids tested, only arachidonic acid resembles SRS-A in having a bronchoconstrictor action in the guinea-pig that was blocked by aspirin (Berry 1966, Collier 1976).

Piper: SRS-A is inactivated by the lipoxygenase extracted from soya beans, but I think it unlikely that all lipoxygenases do this. We don't know enough about the mammalian lipoxygenases to say this yet.

Vane: Perhaps the destruction of SRS-A is by the addition of another hydroperoxy group?

Aiken: Another way of looking at the 5,6-epoxide is not that it is more toxic than SRS but that it has a different function. The 5,6-epoxide might react in a membrane with proteins and thereby anchor them in certain locations; it might be a way of bringing proteins together in certain configurations in membranes. It may be toxic only if it gets free from the membrane. The conversion to SRS might be a detoxification of the free epoxide, whereas in a membrane the epoxide might have some function in determining membrane structure.

Vane: Why is SRS-A, or its precursor, liberated in anaphylactic shock? Is this a diversion of a pathway, or exposure of an enzyme, or what?

Piper: In the experimental production of SRS-A we are directing metabolism of arachidonic acid via the lipoxygenase pathway, because we always have indomethacin present, which inhibits the cyclo-oxygenase pathway. SRS-A is produced after challenge with ovalbumin, but less than in the presence of indomethacin.

Gryglewski: In anaphylactic shock, guinea-pig lung produces prostacyclin, prostaglandins, thromboxane and SRS-A, so all pathways of arachidonic acid metabolism are stimulated. Can you increase the generation of SRS-A in indomethacin-treated anaphylactic lungs by adding cysteine or glutathione to the perfusing medium?

Piper: Cysteine increases the output of SRS-A; I have no evidence about the effect of added glutathione.

Vane: For those not familiar with this field, there has been a tremendous race to find the structure of SRS, or SRS-A. Samuelsson announced the structure of 'an SRS' at a meeting as 5-hydroxy-6-cysteine-eicosatetraenoic acid; he later published an amended structure, that of 5-hydroxy-6-glutathione-eicosatetraenoic acid (Hammarström et al 1979). Now Dr Piper is saying that SRS is the cysteinylglycine derivative.

Piper: Samuelsson did not claim to have found the structure of SRS-A; he said 'an SRS'. People have been saying that he claimed that the structure of SRS-A is the same as that of leukotriene C, which he did not. We certainly have no evidence that leukotriene C appears in SRS-A at all.

Vane: Perhaps over the next few years you will find a whole family of SRSs, all containing some sulphur amino acids.

Piper: I think so. I am not disputing Samuelsson's structure for his material, but ours is different. As you say, there may be a whole family of related substances.

Slater: To revert to the topic of detoxification: if a highly reactive lipophilic intermediate (such as a free radical) is produced within the membranes of the endoplasmic reticulum, its high chemical reactivity will greatly restrict its diffusion radius. In other words, a highly reactive species will be restricted to its microenvironment (Slater 1976). Products of the primary reactions of such an excited intermediate (i.e. secondarily derived species) will have considerably lower chemical reactivity in general, and will have a correspondingly increased average diffusion radius. This may ensure biological disturbances occurring at a considerable distance from the initial locus of formation of the primary species: disturbances due to the secondary, or even tertiary, derived products. In this sense we have something of a paradox: the primary, highly reactive species may form secondary products of intrinsically lower chemical reactivity, and this may be viewed as a detoxification. However, the detoxified material may be able to manifest disturbances at sites far removed from the initial site of excitation or activation, at sites inaccessible to the primary excited species. In this sense, 'detoxification' must be clearly defined in each particular context.

Another aspect of the enzymic formation of highly reactive species in the endoplasmic reticulum is that often this results in destruction of the enzymes responsible for the activation process: the primary species may destroy the enzyme system responsible for their own formation. An example of this is the activation of CCl_4 by the liver NADPH–cytochrome *P*-450 electron transport chain. The formation of $CCl_3^{\cdot}$ and $CCl_3O_2^{\cdot}$ free radicals is accompanied by destruction of cytochrome *P*-450 and NADPH (Recknagel & Glende 1973, Slater et al 1964).

Alberti: What does SRS-A do in the human, apart from its effects on the bronchus?

Vane: The only human experiments I know are on isolated human bronchial tissue, which it contracts. During anaphylaxis in animals there is release of histamine, bradykinin, possibly 5-HT, various prostaglandins (E_2 and $F_{2\alpha}$), SRS-A and thromboxane A_2. The release of prostaglandins E_2 and $F_{2\alpha}$ and TXA_2 can be antagonized by aspirin but that doesn't help in most patients with asthma. Giving antagonists to the H_1 and H_2 receptors for histamine doesn't improve asthma either, so the general assumption is that only one substance is left as the mediator which contracts human bronchial tissue in asthma or promotes anaphylaxis in experimental models, and that is SRS-A. That assumption may be invalid.

Alberti: Has SRS-A been isolated from human lung?

Piper: Yes. We have compared human SRS-A with SRS-A from guinea-pig lung and found that they co-elute after high pressure liquid chromatography and have the same biological actions (Morris et al 1979).

SRS-A increases permeability in skin, certainly in the guinea-pig.

Vane: It can be released from cat paws, either by scalding or by drugs (Anggard et al 1963, Strandberg 1971).

Piper: Some indirect evidence suggests that SRS increases mucus production, which would be relevant to asthma. It also interferes with the transport of mucus up the airways.

Bakhle: Do you have enough of your SRS to be able to assess its potency, in terms of moles per bioassay unit?

Piper: Our unit of SRS-A is equivalent to 4–6 ng of pure material. This was determined by bioassay on guinea-pig ileum and u.v. absorbance.

References

Adcock JJ, Garland LG 1980 A possible role for lipoxygenase products as regulators of airway smooth muscle reactivity. Br J Pharmacol 69:167-169

Adcock JJ, Garland LG, Moncada S, Salmon JA 1978a Enhancement of anaphylactic mediator release from guinea-pig perfused lungs by fatty acid hydroperoxides. Prostaglandins 16:163-188

Adcock JJ, Garland LG, Moncada S, Salmon JA 1978b The mechanism of enhancement by fatty acid hydroperoxides of anaphylactic mediator release. Prostaglandins 16:179-187

Anggard E, Bergqvist U, Hogberg B, Johansson K, Thon IL, Uvnas B 1963 Biologically active principles occurring on histamine release from cat paw, guinea pig lung and isolated rat mast cells. Acta Physiol Scand 59:97-110

Berry PA 1966 Slow-reacting substance in anaphylaxis (SRS-A), its release, actions and antagonism. PhD Thesis. Council of National Academic Awards, London, p 91-92

Collier HOJ 1976 Role of the kallikrein–kinin system in lung diseases. In: Pisano JJ, Austen KF (eds) Chemistry and biology of the kallikrein–kinin system in health and disease. (Fogarty Int Center Proc no. 27) US Govt Printing Office, Washington DC, p 495-503

Hammarström S, Murphy RC, Samuelsson B, Clark DA, Mioskowski C, Corey EJ 1979 Structure of leukotriene C: identification of the amino acid part. Biochem Biophys Res Commun 91:1266-1272

Morris HR, Piper PJ, Taylor GW, Tippins JR 1979 Comparative studies on immunologically and non-immunologically produced slow-reacting substances from man, guinea-pig and rat. Br J Pharmacol 67:179-184

Recknagel RO, Glende EA 1973 CRC Crit Rev Toxicol 2:263-297

Slater TF 1976 In: Dianzani MU et al (eds) Recent advances in biochemical pathology: toxic liver injury. Minerva Medica, Turin, p 99-108

Slater TF, Straüli UD, Sawyer BC 1964 Changes in liver nucleotide concentrations in experimental liver injury. I. Carbon tetrachloride poisoning. Biochem J 93:260-266

Strandberg K 1971 Efflux of slow reacting substance (SRS) and prostaglandins from cat paws perfused with *d*-tubocurarine and *n*-octylamine. Acta Physiol Scand 82:509-520

The lung in relation to vasoactive polypeptides

SAMI I. SAID*†, VIKTOR MUTT** and ERVIN G. ERDÖS†

Dallas Veterans Administration Medical Center and Departments of Internal Medicine and Pharmacology, University of Texas Southwestern Medical School, Dallas, Texas, USA, and Biochemistry Department, Karolinska Institutet, Stockholm, Sweden***

Abstract Among the metabolic functions of the lung are the formation, release, activation and inactivation of biologically active peptides. The following peptides may be present or formed in normal lung: vasoactive intestinal peptide or a peptide closely related to it, a spasmogenic peptide not yet fully identified, bradykinin, substance P, a bombesin-like peptide (especially in fetal and neonatal lung), and eosinophil-chemotactic peptides. These peptides are found in special neuroendocrine cells, in neurons, or in mast cells. Normal lung also inactivates bradykinin and activates angiotensin; both processes are catalysed by the same enzyme (kininase II or angiotensin-converting enzyme), located in pulmonary vascular endothelium.

Pulmonary tumours and certain non-tumorous lesions can produce and release a variety of peptide hormones that are not normally generated by the lung in substantial amounts. This 'ectopic' secretion of hormones may be detectable only by sensitive assays or may result in specific clinical syndromes.

Mammalian lung can generate, degrade, activate and, especially in certain pathological states, release into the circulation a variety of active polypeptides. These peptides, in turn, can influence the functions of the lung, as well as of other organs. We review here these aspects of the metabolic–endocrine functions of the lung, with special reference to two recently discovered vasoactive peptides occurring in normal lungs.

BIOLOGICALLY ACTIVE PEPTIDES IN NORMAL LUNG

Evidence for the presence of vasoactive peptides in extracts of normal lungs was reported in the late 1960s (Said 1967, Said & Mutt 1969). Efforts to purify, isolate and identify these peptides have been continued since then. So far, two such peptides have been partially purified and characterized—one

Metabolic activities of the lung
(Ciba Foundation symposium 78) p 217-237

that relaxes a variety of vascular and non-vascular smooth muscles, and another that contracts these smooth muscles (Said & Mutt 1977). Although the chemical identities of these two peptides remain to be established, the relaxant peptide is closely related to, if not identical with, the vasoactive intestinal peptide (VIP) that occurs widely in the nervous system and the gastrointestinal tract (Said 1980a). From its unique spectrum of biological activity the spasmogenic peptide is probably distinct from other known peptides with similar actions (Said & Mutt 1977).

Vasodilator, smooth-muscle relaxant, VIP-like peptide

Purification and isolation. Initially, the sole bioassay used in the extraction and purification of the VIP-like peptide was based on its ability to dilate the femoral vascular bed and to lower systemic arterial blood pressure in anaesthetized dogs (Said & Mutt 1969). With the adoption of the system of superfused, isolated smooth muscle organs as an additional bioassay (Vane 1964) it became apparent that the most active vasodilator fractions contained not one but at least two vasoactive peptides, having opposing actions on most smooth muscles.

The procedures for obtaining highly purified preparations of smooth-muscle relaxing peptide from porcine lung extracts have been briefly described (Said & Mutt 1977) and are outlined in Table 1. The use of high pressure liquid chromatography has recently permitted the separation of the purest peptide fractions from earlier purification steps into several fractions. One of these exhibited smooth-muscle effects and chromatographic characteristics like those of VIP. Its possible identity to the latter peptide has not been established by sequence analysis.

Actions. Purified peptide fractions rich in this peptide relax a variety of isolated bioassay organs, including trachea, lung, pulmonary artery and gall bladder of guinea-pig; stomach strip and colon of rat; and chick rectum (Fig. 1a). These actions are independent of adrenergic or cholinergic receptors

TABLE 1

Steps in the isolation of VIP-like peptide from lung

1. Methanol extraction of crude peptide preparation
2. Chromatography on Sephadex-G column
3. Chromatography on carboxymethyl–cellulose column
4. Counter-current distribution
5. High pressure liquid chromatography

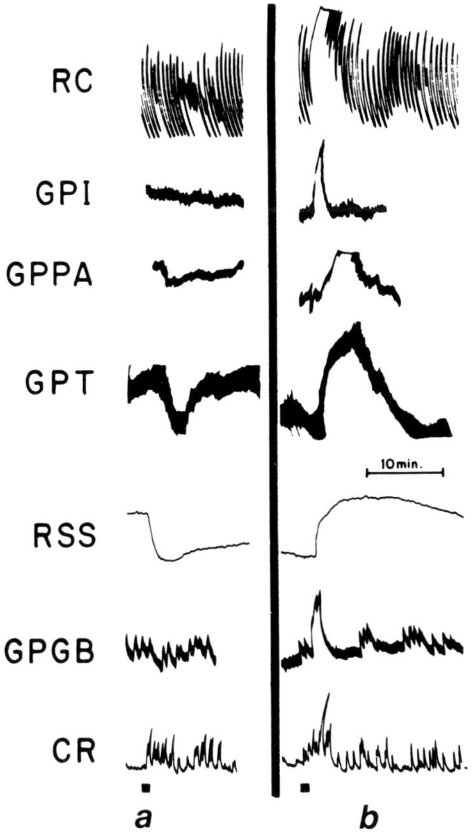

FIG. 1. Responses of isolated, superfused smooth-muscle organs to 125 μg per ml of (a) relaxant and (b) spasmogenic lung peptide fractions, infused at 1 ml per min (data from two experiments). RC, rat colon; GPI, guinea-pig ileum; GPPA, guinea-pig pulmonary artery; GPT, guinea-pig trachea; RSS, rat stomach strip; GPGB, guinea-pig gall bladder; CR, chick rectum. Assay organs had been pretreated with a mixture of pharmacological blockers containing: 10^{-7} g/ml mepyramine maleate, 2×10^{-7} g/ml methysergide bimaleate, 2×10^{-6} g/ml propranolol HCl, 10^{-7} g/ml phenoxybenzamine HCl, and 10^{-7} g/ml of hyoscine HBr. Peptide solutions were infused at mark below. Upward movement is contraction and downward movement relaxation. (Reproduced with permission from Said & Mutt 1977.)

and resemble the smooth-muscle effects of the vasoactive intestinal peptide (VIP). The latter was isolated and characterized by us (Said & Mutt 1970, 1972, Mutt & Said 1974) in the course of our investigation of the lung peptide. This lung peptide has an immunological determinant in common with VIP since it binds well with antibodies to VIP in radioimmunoassay (Said & Mutt 1977) and in immunofluorescence studies (Uddman et al 1978, Dey & Said 1980).

Because of the scarcity of highly purified preparations of this peptide its pharmacological effects beyond vasodilatation and smooth-muscle relaxation have not yet been determined. Since, as indicated, this peptide is closely related to VIP, it is likely to share at least some of the other actions of that peptide, such as stimulation of adenylate cyclase activity and promotion of water and ion secretion from mucosal surfaces.

Localization. Immunohistochemical techniques, using antibodies against VIP, localize the pulmonary VIP-like peptide in mast cells (Cutz et al 1978) and in nerve cell bodies and nerve fibres in the walls of bronchi (Uddman et al 1978) and pulmonary vessels (Dey & Said 1980). Within the bronchial walls, nerves with VIP-like immunofluorescence occur in relation to the secretory glands and smooth muscle. VIP-positive nerves are also present in bronchial vessels and in ganglion-like structures in peribronchial connective tissue (Dey & Said 1980).

The predominantly neural distribution of this peptide in the lung thus appears to parallel that of VIP elsewhere in the body (Said 1980a).

Release. The strong immunological cross-reactivity between the VIP isolated from intestinal extracts and the VIP-like peptide in lung extracts has provided a means of assessing the release of this peptide from the lung in experimental and clinical conditions. Such release has been demonstrated experimentally in pulmonary perfusate and alveolar fluid during anaphylactic shock (A.R. Johnson, E.G. Erdös & S.I. Said, unpublished), in alveolar foam and pulmonary lymph during hypervolaemic and alloxan-induced pulmonary oedema (N. Hara & S.I. Said, unpublished), and after the instillation of hydrochloric acid in the airways (M. Aoyagi & S.I. Said, unpublished). As discussed later, immunoreactive VIP levels in the plasma are increased in some patients with bronchogenic tumours, presumably as a result of its release by these tumours (see p 228).

Spasmogenic lung peptide

Purification. The procedures for obtaining purified preparations of the spasmogenic peptide are as summarized above for the VIP-like peptide (Table 1). The spasmogenic activity is concentrated in the last peptide fraction eluted from chromatography on carboxymethyl–cellulose, just following the fraction that is richest in the VIP-like peptide. Recently, this biological activity has been further purified by means of high pressure liquid chromatography.

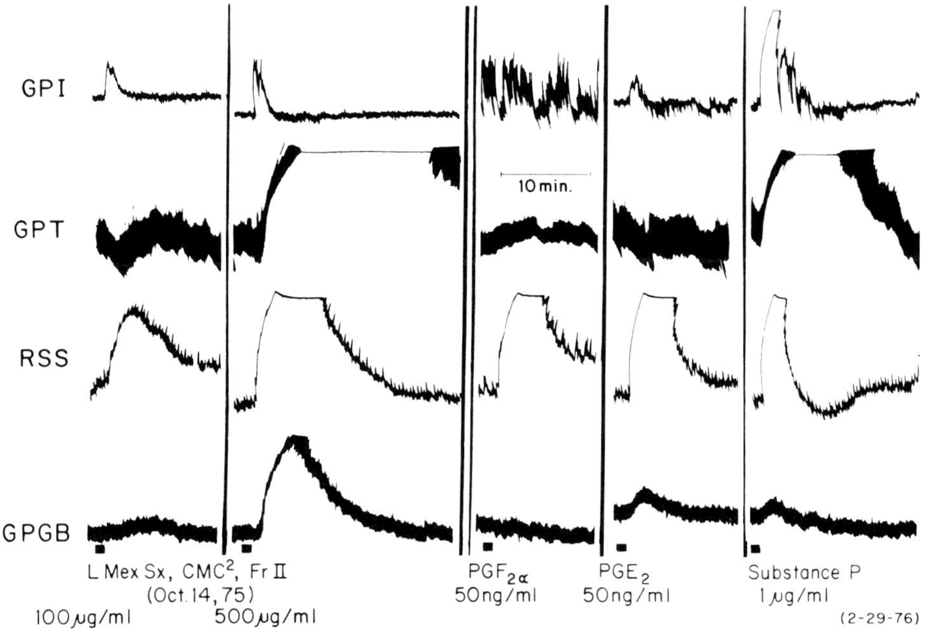

a

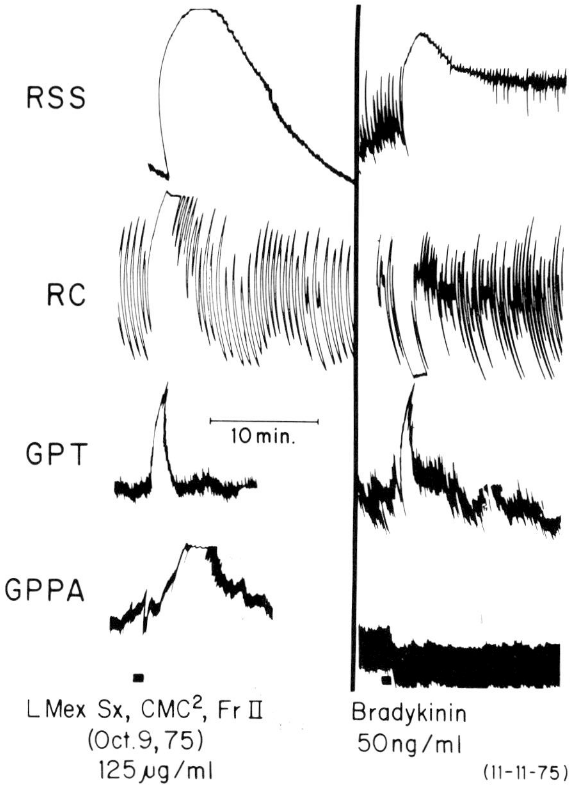

b

FIG. 2. (a) Responses of guinea-pig ileum (GPI), guinea-pig trachea (GPT), rat stomach strip (RSS), and guinea-pig gall bladder (GPGB) to two doses (100 and 500 μg/ml) of spasmogenic lung peptide fraction and to prostaglandin $F_{2\alpha}$ (50 ng/ml), prostaglandin E_2 (50 ng/ml) and substance P (1 μg/ml). All agents were dissolved in Krebs' solution and infused at 1 ml/min.

(b) Responses of RSS, rat colon (RC), GPT and guinea-pig pulmonary artery (GPPA) to same spasmogenic peptide fraction (125 μg/ml) (left) and to bradykinin (50 ng/ml) (right). (Reproduced with permission from Said & Mutt 1977.)

Actions. The known biological actions of this peptide are limited to peripheral vasodilatation and contraction of isolated smooth muscle organs. The peptide contracts a variety of smooth muscles, as outlined above and illustrated in Figs.1b and 2. In contrast to the VIP-like peptide the spasmogenic lung peptide does not cross-react with antibodies to VIP.

Substance P

The discovery that extracts of equine brain and intestine elicited atropine-resistant contraction of rabbit jejunum, and hypotension, was attributed by von Euler & Gaddum (1931) to the presence of an active compound that came to be known as substance P. Years later, Chang & Leeman (1971) isolated substance P from bovine hypothalamus and identified it as an 11-residue peptide. Studer et al (1973) isolated an identical peptide from horse intestine. Through the use of specific antibodies this peptide has been localized more precisely by radioimmunoassay and immunofluorescence techniques in the central and peripheral nervous systems and the gut. It has also been found in the lung, where it occurs in nerve fibres in the smooth muscle of the tracheobronchial tree and in the walls of pulmonary arteries and veins (Nilsson et al 1977, Sundler et al 1977).

Substance P has multiple actions on vascular and non-vascular smooth muscle, contracting the stomach strip and duodenum of rat, the jejunum of rabbit, and the ileum and gall bladder of guinea-pig (Fig.2a). This peptide also induces systemic hypotension and promotes salivary secretion.

There is little or no information on the possible release of substance P from the lung in physiological or pathological states.

Bradykinin

In addition to being inactivated by pulmonary endothelium (see below), this potent nonapeptide may also be generated by the lung and other tissues. Liberation of bradykinin results from the action of kallikrein or other proteolytic enzymes on kininogens, protein substrates in plasma or tissues.

The biological effects of bradykinin have been extensively investigated. They include peripheral vasodilatation, increased systemic vascular permeability, contraction of rat stomach strip, relaxation of rat colon, contractions of guinea-pig trachea, ileum and gall bladder (Fig.2b), and pain. Some of the effects of bradykinin, including contraction of tracheal smooth muscle, can be abolished by pretreatment with inhibitors of prostaglandin synthesis (Fig.3). Bradykinin stimulates prostaglandin biosynthesis and

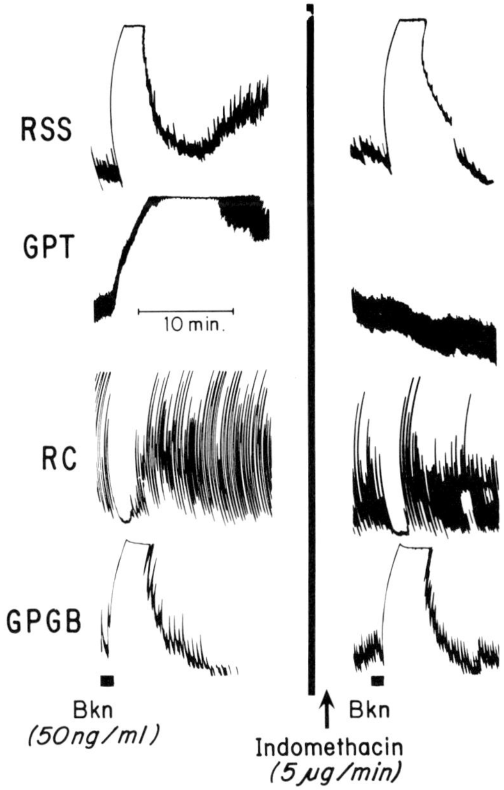

FIG.3. Responses of rat stomach strip (RSS), guinea-pig trachea (GPT), rat colon (RC), and guinea-pig gall bladder (GPGB) to bradykinin (Bkn, 50 ng/ml), given before (left) and after (right) the assay tissues were treated with indomethacin (5 μg/ml).

release by a number of organs and tissues, including the lungs (McGiff et al 1972, Palmer et al 1973, Terragno et al 1975, Needleman et al 1975), by stimulating the generation of arachidonic acid (Vargaftig & Dao Hai 1972, Damas & Bourdon 1974, Hsueh et al 1977), and possibly also by stimulating the conversion of arachidonic acid to prostaglandins (Nasjletti & Malik 1979). The released prostaglandins may mediate or accentuate the actions of bradykinin (Ferreira et al 1973, Nasjletti & Malik 1979).

Bombesin

The 14-residue peptide named bombesin was isolated from amphibian skin (Erspamer & Melchiori 1973). Bombesin-like immunoreactivity has been found in mammalian gastrointestinal organs and brain, and in fetal and neonatal lung (Wharton et al 1978).

Bombesin influences gastrointestinal, cardiovascular, metabolic, endocrine and other functions. It contracts a variety of smooth muscles, including rat stomach strip; guinea-pig lung, pulmonary artery and gall bladder; and chick rectum (Fig.4).

Eosinophil-chemotactic factors

The lung can form and release several peptide moieties that are chemotactic for white blood cells. These peptide factors include (a) two related

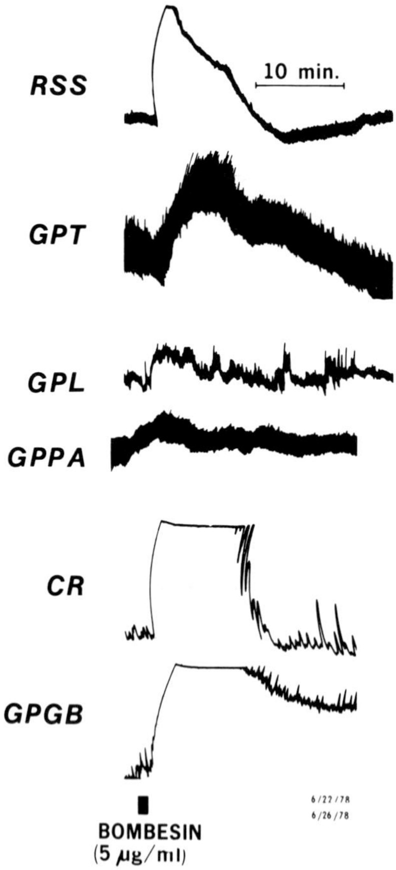

FIG.4. Contractile responses of rat stomach strip (RSS), guinea-pig trachea (GPT), guinea-pig lung (GPL), guinea-pig pulmonary artery (GPPA), chick rectum (CR), and guinea-pig gall bladder (GPGB) to bombesin (5 μg/ml). Data from two experiments.

tetrapeptides (Ala-Gly-Ser-Glu and Val-Gly-Ser-Glu), of low molecular weight (300–400), that have the activity of the *Eosinophil-Chemotactic Factor of Anaphylaxis (ECF-A)*; and (b) other eosinophil-chemotactic peptides of higher molecular weight (1200–2500) (Lewis & Austen 1977).

Peptide-containing cells in the lung

Peptides may be located in and secreted by endocrine cells or neurons (cf. Said 1980b). In the lung, cells with morphological features suggesting endocrine function (Hage 1972, Cutz & Orange 1977, Said 1979) are known by a variety of names: Feyrter cells, Kulchitsky cells, neuroendocrine or neurosecretory cells, pulmonary argyrophil cells, argyrophil-fluorescent-granulated cells, or APUD cells. The latter acronym is derived from a set of cytochemical features (*a*mine content, amine-*p*recursor *u*ptake, and *d*ecarboxylation). Cells belonging to the APUD system occur in many apparently unrelated organs including the pituitary, thyroid (C cells), pancreatic islets, adrenal medulla, stomach and small intestine (Pearse 1968).

These cells are more plentiful in fetal and newborn lungs than in mature lungs. They occur either as single elements or as clusters of cells within the bronchial and bronchiolar epithelium (the clusters are called 'neuroepithelial bodies': Lauweryns et al 1973). They contain argyrophilic, serotonin-rich granules that are depleted when exposed to hypoxia. The likely neuroendocrine role of these clusters of cells is emphasized by their rich efferent and afferent innervation.

Whereas bombesin has been localized in pulmonary endocrine cells (Wharton et al 1978), the VIP-like peptide and substance P appear to be principally contained in neurons (see above), and the eosinophil-chemotactic factors in mast cells (Lewis & Austen 1977).

PULMONARY METABOLISM OF ACTIVE PEPTIDES

The lung has the only capillary bed in the body through which the entire blood flow passes. This makes the pulmonary circulation uniquely suited for exercising a controlling influence on the metabolism of blood-borne hormonal substances (Said 1968, 1973, Bakhle & Vane 1974, Junod 1975). Among the substances that are actively metabolized during their passage through the lung are two vasoactive peptides, bradykinin and angiotensin.

Inactivation of bradykinin and activation of angiotensin

Ferreira & Vane (1967) showed that 80% of the bradykinin introduced into the venous blood was removed in one passage through cat lungs. Similarly effective inactivation of bradykinin by the lung has been demonstrated in several other mammalian species. In the same year Ng & Vane (1967) reported that conversion of the relatively inactive angiotensin I into the potent vasopressor angiotensin II occurred more rapidly in the lung than in blood or other tissues.

The enzymic inactivation of bradykinin can be achieved by at least two kininases. The first to be characterized, kininase I, or carboxypeptidase N (also called arginine carboxypeptidase, EC 3.4.17.3, by the Enzyme Commission, although it also cleaves carboxy terminal lysine in many substrates), is a plasma enzyme that inactivates bradykinin by removing the carboxy terminal arginine (Erdös & Sloane 1962). The second enzyme, kininase II, or dipeptidyl carboxypeptidase (EC 3.4.15.1), is principally a membrane-bound enzyme occurring in the lung and elsewhere, that breaks peptidyl–dipeptide bonds from the carboxy terminal end (Erdös & Yang 1966, Yang & Erdös 1967).

Kininase II (angiotensin-converting enzyme)

Angiotensin I-converting enzyme was discovered in plasma by Skeggs and co-workers (1956). This enzyme removes the carboxy terminal dipeptide, histidyl-leucine, from angiotensin I, converting it to the octapeptide angiotensin II. Several observations suggested the possibility that pulmonary inactivation of bradykinin and conversion of angiotensin I to angiotensin II might be catalysed by one and the same enzyme. For example: (a) the respective enzyme activities were present in high concentrations in the pulmonary circulation; (b) peptides from the venom of *Bothrops jararaca* and other snakes both potentiated the action of bradykinin and inhibited the conversion of angiotensin I; (c) the activities of the two enzymes were found in the same crude preparations of lung homogenates; and (d) purification of one activity resulted in concomitant purification of the other (Bakhle & Vane 1974).

On the other hand, certain apparent differences between the two enzyme activities (e.g., the requirement of chloride for angiotensin conversion but not for bradykinin hydrolysis) created some scepticism about attributing both activities to the same enzyme. Yang and co-workers (1970, 1971), first using partially purified enzyme preparations and specific inhibitors, and later with antibody to the enzyme and homogeneous enzyme, established the identity of angiotensin I-converting enzyme with kininase II (Erdös 1979a).

Properties and localization. The enzyme is a zinc-containing glycoprotein that releases carboxy terminal dipeptides from its substrates, which include angiotensin I and bradykinin (Soffer et al 1974). Other endogenous substrates are the enkephalins (Erdös et al 1978) and insulin (at least *in vitro*). Peptides that are not hydrolysed by this enzyme include those with a penultimate proline residue (e.g., angiotensin II), those lacking a free carboxy terminal carboxyl group, and those smaller than a tripeptide (Cushman et al 1979). Angiotensin-converting enzyme is located in pulmonary vascular endothelium (Ryan et al 1976), and to some extent in the endothelium of peripheral vascular beds (Caldwell et al 1976). The enzyme also occurs in some epithelial cells, such as the brush border of the renal proximal tubule (Ward et al 1977) and intestinal mucosa (Ward et al 1980). Low levels of kininase II activity are found in plasma and other biological fluids (Yang & Erdös 1967). This activity is elevated in sarcoidosis, but not in tuberculosis (Lieberman 1975), and the increase may result from increased enzyme activity in lymph nodes. Acute hypoxia decreases pulmonary kininase II activity in dogs (Stalcup et al 1979), and the enzyme is released from perfused lungs of sensitized rats during anaphylactic shock (Erdös 1975).

Beginning with the snake venom peptides referred to above, other inhibitors have now been prepared. These have greater specificity and potency (Cushman et al 1979, Erdös 1979b), and include one, captopril, that is effective by mouth. These inhibitors are now under active investigation for their usefulness as antihypertensive drugs.

The development of techniques for growing endothelial cells in culture (Gimbrone et al 1974) has provided a useful model for investigating peptide metabolism in vascular endothelial cells from lung and elsewhere (Johnson & Erdös 1977a, Stalcup et al 1979). Johnson & Erdös (1977b) have reported that substance P is inactivated by cultured endothelial cells from human umbilical cord (though pulmonary inactivation of this peptide is ineffective).

Metabolism of other peptides

There is evidence that, in contrast to bradykinin, several other naturally occurring, biologically active peptides undergo little or no inactivation in the pulmonary circulation. These peptides include: substance P, oxytocin, vasopressin, angiotensin II (Bakhle & Vane 1974) and VIP (Kitamura et al 1975).

FORMATION AND RELEASE OF PEPTIDE HORMONES BY LUNG TUMOURS

Tumours and occasionally non-neoplastic lesions of the lung may form and

TABLE 2

Secretion of peptide hormones by pulmonary tumours and other lesions

Hormone	*Syndrome*	*Lesion*
Adrenocorticotrophic hormone & related peptides	Hypokalaemic alkalosis, oedema, Cushing's syndrome	Oat-cell carcinoma, adenoma
Antidiuretic hormone (arginine vasopressin)	Hyponatraemia, syndrome of inappropriate secretion of antidiuretic hormone	Oat-cell carcinoma, adenoma; tuberculosis, pneumonia, aspergillosis
Parathyroid hormone or related peptide	Hypercalcaemia	Bronchogenic carcinoma other than oat-cell variety
Gonadotropins	Gynaecomastia (adults), precocious puberty (children)	Large-cell carcinoma
Calcitonin	No clinical findings	Bronchogenic carcinoma; inflammatory & other lesions
Vasoactive intestinal peptide or related peptide	Watery diarrhoea or no symptoms	Bronchogenic carcinoma of all cell types
Growth hormone	Hypertrophic osteoarthropathy	Squamous-cell carcinoma
Insulin-like peptide	Hypoglycaemia	Mesenchymal tumours
Glucagon or related peptide	Diabetes	Fibrosarcoma
Prolactin	Galactorrhoea or no symptoms	Undifferentiated carcinoma
Combination of two or more peptides	Multiple syndromes or no symptoms	Undifferentiated carcinoma

release a broad variety of peptide hormones. This hormonal secretion is estimated to occur in at least 10% of patients with bronchogenic cancer. Since this is now the leading cancer in men and the second commonest in women, the 'ectopic' secretion of hormones is by no means a rare phenomenon.

The particularly high potential of pulmonary tumours (and other pathological lesions) for producing peptide hormones is unexplained. The liberated hormones are largely indistinguishable from, or close variants of, the normal hormones secreted by their respective endocrine glands.

Hormonal secretion by the lung (or other organs not normally considered endocrinologically active, such as the kidney) is often asymptomatic, but it may result in a variety of endocrine 'paraneoplastic' syndromes (Hall 1974, Said 1974, Blackman et al 1978, Odell & Wolfsen 1978). The commonest peptides of 'ectopic' origin are ACTH (adrenocorticotropin), antidiuretic hormone (vasopressin) and parathyroid hormone. The effects of these and other tumour-associated hormones, and the underlying anatomical lesions, are outlined in Table 2.

ACKNOWLEDGEMENTS

This work was supported in part by Lung Center Award HL-14187 from the National Heart, Lung & Blood Institute, by Research Grant CA-21570 from the National Cancer Institute, US Public Health Service, and by Swedish Medical Research Council Grant 13X01010. We thank Mrs Vicky Roe for typing the manuscript.

References

Bakhle YS, Vane JR 1974 Pharmacokinetic function of the pulmonary circulation. Physiol Rev 54:1007-1045

Blackman MR, Rosen SW, Weintraub BD 1978 Ectopic hormones. Adv Intern Med 23:85-113

Caldwell PRB, Seegal BC, Hsu KC, Das M, Soffer RL 1976 Angiotensin-converting enzyme: vascular endothelial localization. Science (Wash DC) 191:1050-1051

Chang MM, Leeman SE 1970 Isolation of a sialogogic peptide from bovine hypothalamic tissue and its characterization as substance P. J Biol Chem 245:4784-4790

Cushman DW, Cheung HS, Sabo EF, Rubin B, Ondetti MA 1979 Development of specific inhibitors of angiotensin I converting enzyme (kininase II). Fed Proc 38:2778-2782

Cutz E, Orange RP 1977 Mast cells and endocrine (APUD) cells of the lung. In: Lichtenstein LM et al (eds) Asthma: physiology, immunopharmacology and treatment. Academic Press, New York, p 51-76

Cutz E, Chan W, Track NS, Goth A, Said SI 1978 Release of vasoactive intestinal polypeptide in mast cells by histamine liberators. Nature (Lond) 275:661-662

Damas J, Bourdon V 1974 Libération d'acide arachidonique par la bradykinine. CR Séances Soc Biol Fil 168:1445-1448

Dey RD, Said SI 1980 Immunocytochemical localization of VIP-immunoreactive nerves in bronchial walls and pulmonary vessels. Fed Proc 39:1062

Erdös EG 1975 Angiotensin I converting enzyme. Circ Res 36:247-255

Erdös EG 1979a Kininases. In: Erdös EG (ed) Bradykinin, kallidin and kallikrein: supplement. Springer-Verlag, Berlin (Handbook of Experimental Pharmacology 25, Suppl) p 427-487

Erdös EG 1979b Inhibitors of kininases. Fed Proc 38:2774-2777

Erdös EG, Sloane EM 1962 An enzyme in human blood plasma that inactivates bradykinin and kallidins. Biochem Pharmacol 11:585-592

Erdös EG, Yang HYT 1966 Inactivation and potentiation of the effects of bradykinin. In: Erdös EG et al (eds) Hypotensive peptides. Springer-Verlag, Berlin, p 235-250

Erdös EG, Johnson AR, Boyden NT 1978 Hydrolysis of enkephalin by cultured human endothelial cells and by purified peptidyl dipeptidase. Biochem Pharmacol 27:843-848

Erspamer V, Melchiori P 1973 Active polypeptides of the amphibian skin and their synthetic analogues. Pure Appl Chem 35:463-494

Ferreira SH, Vane JR 1967 The disappearance of bradykinin and eledoisin in the circulation and vascular beds of the cat. Br J Pharmacol Chemother 30:417-424

Ferreira SH, Moncada S, Vane JR 1973 Prostaglandins and the mechanism of analgesia produced by aspirin-like drugs. Br J Pharmacol 49:86-97

Gimbrone MA, Jr, Cotran RS, Folkman J 1974 Human vascular endothelial cells in culture. Growth and DNA synthesis. J Cell Biol 60:673-684

Hage E 1972 Endocrine cells in the bronchial mucosa of human foetuses. Acta Pathol Microbiol Scand 80:225-234

Hall TC 1974 Paraneoplastic syndromes. Ann NY Acad Sci 230:5-577

Hsueh W, Isakson PC, Needleman P 1977 Hormone selective lipase activation in the isolated rabbit heart. Prostaglandins 13:1073-1091

Johnson AR, Erdös EG 1977a Metabolism of vasoactive peptides by human endothelial cells in culture. J Clin Invest 59:684-695

Johnson AR, Erdös EG 1977b Inactivation of substance P by cultured human endothelial cells. In: von Euler US, Pernow P (eds) Substance P. Raven Press, New York

Junod AF 1975 Metabolism, production, and release of hormones and mediators in the lung. Am Rev Respir Dis 112:93-107

Kitamura S, Yoshida T, Said SI 1975 Vasoactive intestinal polypeptide: inactivation in liver and potentiation in lung of anesthetized dogs. Proc Soc Exp Biol Med 148:25-29

Lauweryns JM, Cokelaere M, Theunynck P 1973 Serotonin-producing neuroepithelial bodies in rabbit respiratory mucosa. Science (Wash DC) 180:410-413

Lewis RA, Austen KF 1977 Nonrespiratory functions of pulmonary cells: The mast cell. Fed Proc 36:2676-2683

Lieberman J 1975 Elevation of serum angiotensin-converting-enzyme (ACE) level in sarcoidosis. Am J Med 59:365-372

McGiff JC, Terragno NA, Malik KU, Lonigro AJ 1972 Release of prostaglandin E-like substance from canine kidney by bradykinin. Circ Res 31:36-43

Mutt V, Said SI 1974 Structure of the porcine vasoactive intestinal octacosapeptide: The amino-acid sequence. Use of kallikrein in its determination. Eur J Biochem 42:581-589

Nasjletti A, Malik KU 1979 Relationships between the kallikrein–kinin and prostaglandin systems. Life Sci 25:99-110

Needleman P, Key SL, Denny SE, Isakson PC, Marshall GR 1975 Mechanism and modification of bradykinin-induced coronary vasodilation. Proc Natl Acad Sci USA 72:2060-2063

Ng KKF, Vane JR 1967 The conversion of angiotensin I to angiotensin II. Nature (Lond) 216:762-766

Nilsson G, Dahlberg K, Brodin E, Sundler F, Strandberg K 1977 Distribution and constrictor effect of substance P in guinea pig tracheobronchial tissue. In: von Euler US, Pernow B (eds) Substance P. Raven Press, New York, p 75-81

Odell WD, Wolfsen AR 1978 Humoral syndromes associated with cancer. Annu Rev Med 29:379-406

Palmer MA, Piper PJ, Vane JR 1973 Release of rabbit aorta contracting substance (RCS) and prostaglandins induced by chemical or mechanical stimulation of guinea-pig lungs. Br J Pharmacol 49:226-242

Pearse AGE 1968 Common cytochemical and ultrastructural characteristics of cells producing polypeptide hormones (the APUD series) and their relevance to thyroid and ultimobranchial C cells and calcitonin. Proc R Soc Lond B Biol Sci 170:71-80

Ryan US, Ryan JW, Whitaker C, Chiu A 1976 Localization of angiotensin converting enzyme (kininase II). II. Immunocytochemistry and immunofluorescence. Tissue & Cell 8:125-145

Said SI 1967 Vasoactive substance in the lung. In: Proceedings of the Tenth Aspen Emphysema Conference, Aspen, Colorado, June 7-10, 1967. US Public Health Service Publication 1787, p 223-228

Said SI 1968 The lung as a metabolic organ. N Engl J Med 279:1330-1334
Said SI 1973 The lung in relation to vasoactive hormones. Fed Proc 32:1973-1976
Said SI 1974 Endocrine role of the lung in disease. Am J Med 57:453-465
Said SI 1979 Metabolic and endocrine functions of the lung. Current Concepts (A Scope publication) Upjohn, Kalamazoo, Michigan
Said SI 1980a Vasoactive intestinal peptide (VIP): isolation, distribution, biological actions, structure–function relationships, and possible functions. In: Glass GBJ (ed) Gastrointestinal hormones. Raven Press, New York p 245-273
Said SI 1980b Peptides common to the nervous system and the gastrointestinal tract. In: Martini L, Ganong WF (eds) Frontiers in neuroendocrinology. Raven Press, New York, vol 6:293-331
Said SI, Mutt V 1969 Long-acting vasodilator peptide from lung tissue. Nature (Lond) 224:699-700
Said SI, Mutt V 1970 Polypeptide with broad biological activity: Isolation from small intestine. Science (Wash DC) 169:1217-1218
Said SI, Mutt V 1972 Isolation from porcine intestinal wall of a vasoactive octacosapeptide related to secretin and to glucagon. Eur J Biochem 28:199-204
Said SI, Mutt V 1977 Relationship of spasmogenic and smooth muscle relaxant peptides from normal lung to other vasoactive compounds. Nature (Lond) 265:84-86
Skeggs LT, Kahn JR, Shumway NP 1956 The preparation and function of the hypertensin-converting enzyme. J Exp Med 103:295-299
Soffer RL, Reza R, Caldwell PRB 1974 Angiotensin-converting enzyme from rabbit pulmonary particles. Proc Natl Acad Sci USA 71:1720-1724
Stalcup SA, Lipset JS, Woan J-M, Leuenberger P, Mellins RB 1979 Inhibition of angiotensin converting enzyme activity in cultured endothelial cells by hypoxia. J Clin Invest 63:966-976
Studer RO, Trzeciak H, Lergier W 1973 Isolierung und Aminosäuresequenz von Substanz P aus Pferdedarm. Helv Chim Acta 56:860-866
Sundler F, Alumets J, Brodin E, Dahlberg K, Nilsson G 1977 Perivascular substance P-immunoreactive nerves in tracheobronchial tissue. In: von Euler US, Pernow B (eds) Substance P. Raven Press, New York, p 271-273
Terragno DA, Crowshaw K, Terragno NA, McGiff JC 1975 Prostaglandin synthesis by bovine mesenteric arteries and veins. Circ Res 36 (Suppl I): 76-80
Uddman R, Alumets J, Densert O, Håkanson R, Sundler F 1978 Occurrence and distribution of VIP nerves in the nasal mucosa and tracheobronchial wall. Acta Oto-laryngol 86:443-448
Vane JR 1964 The use of isolated organs for detecting active substances in the circulating blood. Br J Pharmacol Chemother 23:360-373
Vargaftig BB, Dao Hai N 1972 Selective inhibition by mepacrine of the release of 'rabbit aorta contracting substance' evoked by the administration of bradykinin. J Pharm Pharmacol 24:159-161
von Euler US, Gaddum JH 1931 An unidentified depressor substance in certain tissue extracts. J Physiol (Lond) 72:74-87
Ward PE, Schultz W, Reynolds RC, Erdös EG 1977 Metabolism of kinins and angiotensins in the isolated glomerulus and brush border of rat kidney. Lab Invest 36:559-606
Ward PE, Sheridan MA, Hammon KJ, Erdös EG 1980 Angiotensin I converting enzyme (kininase II) of the brush border of human and swine intestine. Biochem Pharmacol 29:1525-1529
Wharton J, Polak JM, Bloom SR, Ghatei MA, Solcia E, Brown MR, Pearse AGE 1978 Bombesin-like immunoreactivity in the lung. Nature (Lond) 273:769-770
Yang HYT, Erdös EG 1967 Second kininase in human blood plasma. Nature (Lond) 215:1402-1403
Yang HYT, Erdös EG, Levin Y 1970 A dipeptidyl carboxypeptidase that converts angiotensin I and inactivates bradykinin. Biochim Biophys Acta 214:374-376
Yang HYT, Erdös EG, Levin Y 1971 Characterization of a dipeptide hydrolase (kininase II: angiotensin I converting enzyme). J Pharmacol Exp Ther 177:291-300

Discussion

Vane: We may now be in a position to answer the question raised earlier (p 179) of whether the indomethacin-resistant, muscle-relaxing activity that appears during hypoventilation is due to prostacyclin or to something else, because there are several indications from Dr Said's paper that vasoactive peptides might be secreted in certain conditions and, if so, they would cause relaxation of the coronary arteries. I don't much like the idea of indomethacin resistance for the basal secretion of prostacyclin but not for its stimulated secretion; and we know instances of peptides and prostaglandins being released at the same time. We also know that Professor Gryglewski finds less prostacyclin activity measuring 6-oxo-$PGF_{1\alpha}$ by mass spectrometry than by bioassay, and we find the same discrepancy using blood-bathed organs and radioimmunoassay in experiments in dogs (Mullane et al 1980). The hypothesis therefore is that the excess biological activity is due to secretion of VIP-like peptide at the same time as prostacyclin. Can we test this?

Said: We have looked at the release of VIP-like peptide from the lung using radioimmunoassay (with antibody raised against VIP itself). In experimental anaphylaxis this peptide is released into the alveolar fluid and perfusate. It is also released in pulmonary oedema, induced in several ways (see p 220), and after instillation of HCl in the airways, a model of the 'aspiration pneumonia' that follows aspiration of gastric contents after heavy intake of alcohol or other depressant drugs. Acid aspiration into the airways causes severe lung injury which we have shown to be associated with VIP release (as well as with release of thromboxane A_2, prostacyclin and $PGF_{2\alpha}$).

Vane: Have you tried the effect of hypoxia?

Said: We don't have enough information yet on the possible release of VIP by hypoxia.

Herbaczyńska-Cedro: We observed relaxation of the isolated, blood-superfused bovine coronary artery in conditions in which pulmonary artery pressure was increased, as in hypoventilation. Is this likely to be accounted for by the release of VIP-like peptide? What is its effect on platelets?

Said: It is possible, but I can't say without more specific evidence.

Vane: A necessary corollary to the hypothesis is that the VIP-like peptide disaggregates platelets.

Said: We have tried VIP itself on platelets; unfortunately it does *not* prevent the aggregating effect of ADP or thrombin.

Gryglewski: We found the same lack of effect of VIP on platelet disaggregation *in vivo* (Gryglewski et al 1980).

Alberti: Would you expect a neurotransmitter to affect platelets?

Said: This peptide stimulated cyclic AMP accumulation in every preparation in which this effect was examined (Laburthe et al 1978), which did not include platelets. On the assumption that whatever stimulates cyclic AMP production should also inhibit platelet aggregation, we were surprised by the lack of a disaggregatory effect for VIP, but we don't know yet whether it promotes cyclic AMP accumulation in platelets.

Reid: You sent us some vasoactive peptide to test in organ cultures of bronchial glands. We were surprised to find that at low concentration it inhibits basal mucus production by about 40% (Coles et al 1980).

Said: VIP stimulates water and electrolyte secretion from the intestine (Schwartz et al 1974, Krejs et al 1978) and airways (Hutto et al 1979). I don't know how to reconcile this with the inhibition of bronchial mucus secretion that you see.

Reid: VIP has a different effect in the lung from the periphery. Incidentally, the VIP did not affect the secretory cells of surface bronchial epithelium, only the mucous and serous cells of the submucosal glands (Coles & Reid 1980).

Woods: Have you been able to look at tumour material or body fluids from patients with pulmonary carcinoid tumours who also have crippling diarrhoea, where it is sometimes very difficult to find the cause? I have two such patients who had pulmonary tumours, said to be carcinoma of the bronchus, removed several years previously, who now have widespread metastases and crippling diarrhoea.

Said: The principal clinical condition associated with hypersecretion of VIP is 'pancreatic cholera', in which there is severe watery diarrhoea, associated with islet cell tumours, or sometimes neurogenic tumours, and occasionally lung tumours (Said & Faloona 1975). We have found increased immunoreactive VIP in such tumours as well as in the plasma. In the few patients with carcinoid whom we have examined, we have not found elevated plasma VIP levels.

Woods: Neither of our patients has increased levels of immunoreactive VIP in the plasma.

Moncada: Do these patients have any osteolysis?

Woods: No, nor do they have secondaries in bone. One has secondary tumours in the brain and the other in the liver.

Ballard: The question has arisen whether the ACTH molecule from ectopic lung tumours is formed from the same gene as pituitary ACTH. Miller et al (1980) recently reported that tryptic digests of the precursor molecule from tumour and pituitary yield identical peptides, suggesting that ectopic and pituitary ACTH do arise from the same gene.

Stubbs: May we turn to the smooth muscle properties of peptides and their possible relevance to asthma? It is well recognized that opioids such as morphine can precipitate asthma. During studies on the hormonal and metabolic effects of an enkephalin analogue ([H-Tyr-D-Ala-Gly-MePhe-Met(o)-ol]enkephalin; Sandoz, FK 33 824), which has opiate-like activity, I noticed the development of a transient wheeze in some subjects.

For many years it has been known that some diabetics develop a characteristic facial flush when they drink alcohol (chlorpropamide-alcohol-flush, or CPAF). Leslie & Pyke (1978) showed that CPAF occurs in non-diabetics and is blocked by the opiate antagonist naloxone (Leslie et al 1979). Recently Leslie et al (1980) have also shown that CPAF may be accompanied by naloxone-reversible bronchoconstriction, which suggests opioid mediation of this form of asthma. Some of the peptides you discussed may have opioid activity; are any of their effects on smooth muscle antagonized by naloxone?

Said: We have not found any inhibition of the blood pressure-lowering effect of VIP or of its smooth muscle relaxant effects with naloxone.

Stubbs: Have you tried antihistamine drugs—H_1 or H_2 blockers? Histamine may have a role in the production of opioid-like activity in animals (Glick & Crane 1978).

Said: H_1 and H_2 blockers don't inhibit the effects of the vasoactive lung peptides.

Mellins: Have you looked at patients with mesothelioma of the pleura for the presence of vasoactive chemical mediators? As you know, with very little or no overt pulmonary disease these patients develop pronounced clubbing of the fingers, suggesting the possibility that there are increased levels of circulating vasoactive substances.

Said: I haven't; that would be worth investigating.

Alberti: Has somatostatin been found in the lung?

Said: I haven't seen any reports of this, but I would not be surprised if several further peptides were to be found in the lung.

Alberti: You discussed the enzyme dipeptidyl carboxypeptidase (kininase II; converting enzyme) and you mentioned that insulin is also a substrate; this might make a difference to my results, depending on which two amino acids were removed! What is known about this? Is insulin still immunoreactive after the dipeptide is removed?

Soffer: This enzyme removes Lys-Ala from the carboxyl terminus of the B chain of insulin (Igic et al 1972). It is assumed that the entire insulin molecule can serve as a substrate because it inhibits the reaction, but the actual demonstration of removal of Lys-Ala was done with isolated B chain. Nobody knows the upper size limit for substrates for converting enzyme. I don't know whether the product of this reaction has insulin-like activity.

Alberti: We measure total immunoreactivity and the metabolic effects that we have been looking at; in terms of total immunoreactivity insulin has a half-life of four hours. If the enzyme just removed a couple of residues one would probably retain biological activity.

Bakhle: Geddes et al (1979) studied insulin clearance through the pulmonary circulation of dogs and found no arterio-venous differences in the resting state, though after an injection of insulin in the pulmonary artery, aortic levels were higher and then lower than mixed venous levels.

Stubbs: Rubenstein et al (1968) showed a 10–18% clearance of insulin by the lungs in five out of six patients undergoing cardiopulmonary bypass.

Reid: Can you tell us more about the liberation of these vasoactive peptides, Dr Said?

Said: We studied the release of VIP on stimulation of isolated guinea-pig trachea. With pulse stimulations of 1 ms and higher we produce a relaxation that is resistant to atropine and propranolol. This has been described as the non-adrenergic, non-cholinergic inhibitory system, which has been found in the airways and gut. This relaxation was blocked by tetrodotoxin, which inhibits neuronal transport. At the same time as the relaxation, levels of VIP were increased in the medium, so perhaps VIP mediates the non-adrenergic, non-cholinergic inhibitory system in the airways. That would be an important physiological role for this peptide.

Vane: Dr Flower, when you stimulate the guinea-pig lung with bradykinin and get a release of thromboxane, is this sensitive to steroids?

Flower: Not in the perfused guinea-pig lung, but *in vivo* in the rabbit bradykinin stimulates the release of prostacyclin, and this is a steroid-sensitive step.

Vane: Bradykinin causes release of thromboxane and other prostaglandin-like substances in lungs, yet it doesn't cause platelet aggregation. Is it causing the release of arachidonate through a different enzyme from phospholipase A_2?

Said: I don't know. It could be stimulating the formation of two products that cancel each other out on the platelet.

Piper: Have you tried the effect of naloxone against VIP-like peptide?

Said: We have tested the possible inhibitory effect of naloxone against three actions of VIP: its ability to increase femoral blood flow while reducing arterial blood pressure, its relaxation of rat gastric smooth muscle, and relaxation of guinea-pig trachea smooth muscle. Naloxone did not significantly reduce or prevent any of these effects. Similarly, naloxone did not reverse the inhibition of electrically induced contractions of mouse vas deferens by VIP

(Kastin et al 1978). On the other hand, naloxone blunted the plasma prolactin response of rats to VIP (Kato et al 1978). So, any possible interactions between VIP and the opioid peptides have not yet been clearly identified.

Piper: It would be a tempting idea if so, because substance P has been shown to interact with the enkephalins elsewhere.

Stubbs: Failure to show naloxone blockade doesn't necessarily mean an absence of opioid activity. There may be more than one type of opioid receptor, some of which are relatively insensitive to naloxone antagonism (Lord et al 1977).

Vane: Is the converse true, that naloxone blockade doesn't necessarily mean opioid activity?

Said: According to Hans Kosterlitz, to establish that an effect that is blocked by naloxone is related to opioid receptors one must show the failure of the stereoisomer of naloxone to have the same effect.

Stubbs: There is evidence that naloxone may have pharmacological actions unrelated to opiate receptor blockade (Sawynok et al 1979), as Dr Vane and Dr Said intimated.

Collier: On this question of a relationship to opioids, Beubler & Lembeck (1979) showed that VIP as well as E prostaglandins produce fluid accumulation in the intestinal lumen and diarrhoea, both of which are antagonized by morphine, and that this antagonism is in turn blocked by naloxone.

Said: VIP is far more effective than E prostaglandins in increasing secretion from the gut.

Collier: As a footnote to Dr Stubbs' comments on the effects of ethanol on bronchoconstiction on patients on chlorpropamide (p 234), Herxheimer & Stresemann (1963) showed that asthmatic volunteers who had responded moderately to bradykinin with bronchoconstriction, after having several drinks suffered from severe bronchoconstriction when they inhaled bradykinin again. They attributed this to the potentiation by ethanol of bradykinin-induced bronchoconstriction.

Stubbs: And it is now being suggested that some of the intoxicant effects of ethanol in humans may be reversed by naloxone (Jeffcoate et al 1979)!

References

Beubler E, Lembeck F 1979 Inhibition of stimulated fluid secretion in the rat small and large intestine by opiate agonists. Naunyn-Schmiedebergs Arch Pharmacol 306:113-118

Coles SJ, Reid L, Said SI 1980 Effect of vasoactive intestinal polypeptide on glycoprotein secretion by submucosal gland and surface epithelium of human airway *in vitro*. In: Sturgess JM (ed) Perspectives in cystic fibrosis. Imperial Press, Canada (Proc 8th int cystic fibrosis congress) p 9a

Geddes DM, Blackburn JP, Bailey JS, Muller PJ 1979 Effects of pulmonary circulation on blood levels of insulin and glucagon in ambulant dogs. J Appl Physiol 46:593-598

Glick SD, Crane LA 1978 Opiate-like and abstinence-like effects of intracerebral histamine administration in rats. Nature (Lond) 273:547-549

Gryglewski RJ, Spławiński J, Korbut R 1980 Endogenous mechanisms that regulate prostacyclin release. In: Samuelsson B et al (eds) Advances in prostaglandin and thromboxane research. Raven Press, New York (4th Int Prostaglandin Conference, Washington DC) vol 7:777-787

Herxheimer H, Stresemann E 1963 Bradykinin and ethanol in bronchial asthma. Arch Int Pharmacodyn Ther 144:315-318

Hutto R, Granger DN, Taylor AE 1979 Effects of vasoactive intestinal polypeptide on potential and short-circuit current in isolated dog tracheal epithelial sheets. Physiologist 22:59

Igic R, Yeh HSJ, Sorrells K, Erdös EG 1972 Cleavage of active peptides by a lung enzyme. Experientia (Basel) 28:135-136

Jeffcoate WJ, Herbert M, Cullen MH, Hastings AG, Walder CP 1979 Prevention of effects of alcohol intoxication by naloxone. Lancet 1:1157-1159

Kastin AJ, Coy DH, Schally AV, Meyers CA 1978 Activity of VIP, somatostatin and other peptides in the mouse vas deferens assay. Pharmacol Biochem Behav 9:673-676

Kato Y, Iwasaki Y, Iwasaki J, Abe H, Yanaihara N, Imura H 1978 Prolactin release by vasoactive intestinal polypeptide in rats. Endocrinology 103:554-558

Krejs GJ, Barkley RM, Read NW, Fordtran JS 1978 Intestinal secretion induced by vasoactive intestinal polypeptide. J Clin Invest 58:1337-1345

Laburthe M, Bataille D, Rousset M, Besson J, Broer Y, Zweibaum A, Rosselin G 1978 The expression of cell surface receptors for VIP, secretin and glucagon in normal and transformed cells of the digestive tract. In: Nicholls P (ed) Membrane proteins. Pergamon Press, Oxford (FEBS, Federation of European Biochemical Societies, 11th Meeting, Copenhagen, 1977) vol 45:271-290

Leslie RDG, Pyke DA 1978 Chlorpropamide-alcohol flushing: a dominantly inherited trait associated with diabetes. Br Med J 2:1519-1521

Leslie RDG, Pyke DA, Stubbs WA 1979 Sensitivity to enkephalin as a cause of non-insulin dependent diabetes. Lancet 1:341-343

Leslie RDG, Bellamy D, Pyke DA 1980 Asthma induced by enkephalin. Br Med J 1:16-18

Lord JAH, Waterfield AA, Hughes J, Kosterlitz HW 1977 Endogenous opioid peptides: multiple agonists and receptors. Nature (Lond) 267:495-499

Miller WL, Baxter JD, Roberts JL 1980 The processing of human ACTH. Clin Res 28:70A (abstr)

Mullane KM, Moncada S, Vane JR 1980 Prostacyclin release induced by bradykinin may contribute to the antihypertensive action of angiotensin converting enzyme inhibitors. In: Samuelsson B et al (eds) Advances in prostaglandin and thromboxane research. Raven Press, New York (4th Int Prostaglandin Conference, Washington DC) vol 7:1159-1161

Rubenstein AH, Zwi S, Miller K 1968 Insulin and the lung. Diabetologia 4:236-238

Said SI, Faloona GR 1975 Elevated plasma and tissue levels of vasoactive intestinal polypeptide in the watery-diarrhea syndrome due to pancreatic, bronchogenic and other tumours. N Engl J Med 293:155-160

Sawynok J, Pinsky C, Labella FS 1979 Minireview on the specificity of naloxone as an opiate antagonist. Life Sci 25:1621-1632

Schwartz CJ, Kimberg DV, Sheerin HE, Field M, Said SI 1974 Vasoactive intestinal peptide stimulation of adenylate cyclase and active electrolyte secretion in intestinal mucosa. J Clin Invest 54:536-544

Endocrine influences on aspects of lung biochemistry

WALTER K. MORISHIGE

Department of Physiology, John A. Burns School of Medicine, University of Hawaii, Honolulu, Hawaii 98622, USA

Abstract Evidence is presented that the postnatal rat lung is receptive to several hormones. Experimental diabetes caused a significant depression in lung glucose oxidation rate which was normalized by exogenous insulin therapy. Diabetes also depressed the rate of amino acid incorporation into lung protein; *in vitro*, insulin stimulated synthesis of selective protein species by the diabetic lung. These results, together with the demonstration of pulmonary receptor sites for insulin and the observation that diabetes selectively affects the ultrastructure of only two cell types in the lung, suggest that insulin may be an important regulator of lung function. That androgens and oestrogens may also exert an effect on the lung is suggested by the presence of distinct receptor activities for these hormones, which appear to be influenced by serum titres of the gonadal steroids. The lung is capable of generating a considerable amount of cyclic GMP *in vitro*. This ability appears to be dependent upon continued protein synthesis and is influenced by the endocrine state of the animal. Certain steroid hormones are capable of altering cyclic GMP production by the lung when introduced *in vitro*.

The fetal lung has been a focus of interest of many endocrinologists since 1969, when Liggins suggested that glucocorticoids promote fetal lung maturation and thereby accelerate the appearance of lung surfactant. The significance of this suggestion was in its relationship to the respiratory distress syndrome of the newborn. The postnatal lung, on the other hand, has been relatively neglected, perhaps because there are no documented lung malfunctions that can be specifically attributed to any given endocrine malady. In spite of this, we have examined the possibility that the metabolically active postnatal lung may be a target site for several hormones.

INSULIN AND THE LUNG

Adult male rats were rendered diabetic by a single subcutaneous injection of

Metabolic activities of the lung
(Ciba Foundation symposium 78) p 239-250

streptozotocin (75 mg/kg). Diabetes mellitus in these rats was evident by the second day after treatment, when the blood glucose level was maximal and serum insulin concentration was minimal. Coincident with these changes was a prominent decline in the ability of the lung to oxidize glucose, which by the third post-treatment day represented a decrease of 57%. A single subcutaneous injection of protamine zinc insulin (PZI) to these rats was followed by a transient normalization of lung glucose oxidation rate at the time when the circulating insulin level was maximal, although hyperglycaemia was evident throughout the 24-hour observation period. Two consecutive injections of PZI restored the rate of glucose oxidation to normal, and tended to suppress the hyperglycaemic condition. The depression in the rate of glucose utilization in the diabetic rat was due to a significant decrease in V_{max}, without an alteration in either K_m or in the hexose monophosphate shunt activity, the major pathway of glucose oxidation in lung tissue (Salisbury-Murphy et al 1966). These results suggested that glucose transport into lung tissue was impaired in the absence of insulin (Morishige et al 1977).

Although we were able to demonstrate that exogenous insulin treatment of the diabetic rat normalized the rate of lung glucose oxidation, we were unable to observe this effect after *in vitro* addition of the hormone, thus confirming an earlier observation (Felts 1964). The *in vitro* presence of insulin also failed to stimulate glucose incorporation into lung lipids (Salisbury-Murphy et al 1966, Moxley & Longmore 1975); however, perfusion of the intact lung with buffer containing insulin has been shown to stimulate glucose utilization (Weber & Visscher 1969, Stubbs et al 1977, Kerr et al 1979). It thus appears that under certain conditions a response of the lung to insulin is demonstrable *in vitro*.

We also observed that the diabetic rat lung incorporated [^{3}H]leucine into protein at a significantly reduced rate, which amounted to a reduction of 24% below the normal rate (Morishige et al 1977). Incubation of diabetic rat lung cells with 10 nM-insulin *in vitro* stimulated the incorporation of leucine into selected protein species when examined by polyacrylamide gel electrophoresis (Fig. 1). These results are in contrast to those reported recently by Rannels et al (1979), who found normal rates of protein synthesis in the lung of streptozotocin-diabetic rats. The reason for this discrepancy is not evident; however, insulin has been shown to increase the rate of amino acid uptake (Gregorio & Massaro 1977) and to decrease the rate of protein degradation (Thet et al 1977) in the normal rat lung.

Two lines of evidence provide additional support for the suggestion that insulin exerts an important influence on the lung. First, the rat lung contains high affinity receptor sites for insulin. These receptors are associated with the

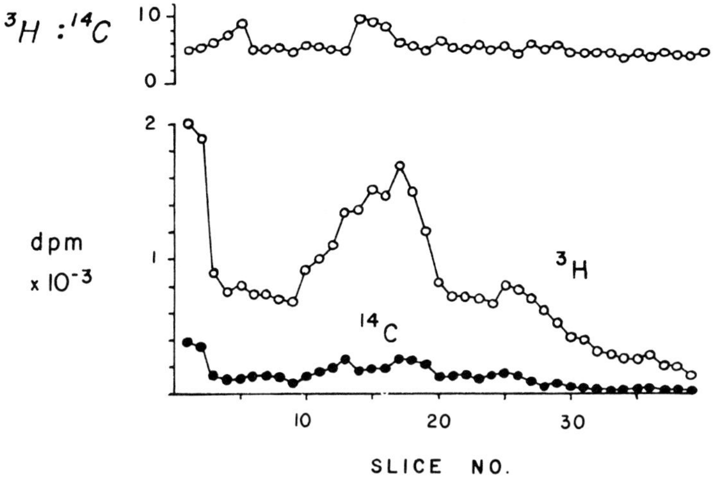

FIG. 1. Effect of insulin on lung protein synthesis *in vitro*. Lungs of streptozotocin-diabetic rats were perfused with Joklik-MEM, and infused via the trachea with Joklik-MEM containing 1 mM-Ca^{2+}, 1% bovine albumin, 0.4% collagenase and 18 units/ml elastase. After 15 minutes the lung tissue was briefly minced, shaken in Joklik-MEM containing 1 mM-Ca^{2+} and 1% bovine albumin (JCB), filtered through three sizes of nylon cloth, and centrifuged through Percoll and Ficoll gradients. The resultant dispersed cell preparation was then divided into two tubes. To one tube was added JCB containing 10% diabetic rat serum and 5 μCi/ml [^{14}C]leucine. To the second tube was added JCB containing 10% diabetic rat serum, 10 nM-porcine insulin and 20 μCi/ml [^{3}H]leucine. The tubes were incubated for 6 h at 37°C, after which the pelleted cells from both tubes were combined, sonicated in 0.05% EDTA, and co-electrophoresed in 7% polyacrylamide gels, essentially as described by Katzenellenbogen & Gorski (1972).

membrane fraction of lung homogenate, and are specific for insulin (Morishige et al 1977). Second, examination of the lung by transmission electron microscopy revealed that streptozotocin diabetes resulted in substantive ultrastructural changes in two cell types: the type II pneumonocyte (Plopper & Morishige 1978) and the Clara cell (Plopper & Morishige 1979). In the former cell type, a striking dilatation of the granular endoplasmic reticulum was seen in the presence of unaltered numbers of lamellar bodies. In the Clara cell, the number of ovoid secretory granules decreased, while that of rod-shaped granules increased. Exogenous insulin therapy (1 unit PZI/rat per day for 2 or 7 days) normalized the ultrastructure of both cell types.

SEX STEROIDS AND THE LUNG

Sucrose density gradient centrifugation of rat lung cytosol revealed the presence of distinct receptor activities for androgenic and for oestrogenic steroids. Both activities possessed high affinity for their respective ligands, and were present in lungs of both sexes and at all postnatal ages examined (Days 10 to 100). The androgen receptor had almost equal affinity for dihydrotestosterone (DHT) and testosterone; however, after incubation of lung tissue with testosterone, DHT was the predominant androgen found in lung nuclei, suggesting that testosterone undergoes 5α-reduction before translocation to the nucleus.

During postnatal development in male rats the level of androphilic receptors was fairly constant between 10 and 41 days of age, ranging from 4 to 7 fmol/mg protein. During the peri-pubertal period of 42 to 46 days, however, a marked increase in receptor concentration occurred, attaining a level of 14.5 fmol/mg protein on Day 46, the day in which all rats showed external signs of the onset of puberty. Androphilic receptor levels remained elevated at least up to Day 67, but tended to be slightly diminished at 100 days of age. In contrast, oestrophilic receptor activity was elevated before puberty and rapidly decreased to low levels after the onset of puberty. These changes in receptor level relate well to the reported changes in blood levels of androgens and oestrogen during this period (Dohler & Wuttke 1975, Moger 1977) and suggest a possible homologous hormonal regulation of sex steroid receptor levels in lung.

In adult female rats, the level of both androphilic and oestrophilic receptor activities appeared to be influenced by the oestrous cycle. Both receptor activities were significantly higher during oestrus than during di-oestrus. As in the male, it is conceivable that the sex steroid receptors are influenced by the hormones which they bind (Morishige & Uetake 1978).

CYCLIC GUANOSINE 3′:5′-MONOPHOSPHATE (CYCLIC GMP) GENERATION BY THE LUNG

Cyclic GMP and the enzyme which catalyses its formation, guanylate cyclase, are present in higher concentration in the lung than in any other mammalian tissue (Hardman & Sutherland 1969). The significance of this is still unclear; however, in contrast to adenylate cyclase, there appears to be no reproducible evidence that guanylate cyclase activity in any tissue is directly influenced by hormones (Steiner et al 1972, Goldberg & Haddox 1977). In spite of this, we have examined the influence of hormones on lung cyclic GMP levels, because of some interesting observations in preliminary experiments.

Slices of lung, liver, heart and kidney were preincubated in a synthetic medium (Joklik–MEM containing 1 mM-Ca^{2+} and 1% bovine albumin (JCB)) at 37°C for 30 minutes, and then incubated at that temperature for four hours in JCB containing 1 mM-methylisobutylxanthine (MIX), a phosphodiesterase inhibitor. Aliquots of the incubation medium were taken at hourly intervals and assayed for cyclic GMP by radioimmunoassay. The results, shown in Table 1, confirm earlier observations (Steiner et al 1972) on the elevated levels of cyclic GMP in lung tissue, and further indicate that the lung is capable of generating a considerable amount of this nucleotide *in vitro*.

TABLE 1
In vitro generation of cyclic GMP by slices of lung, heart, liver and kidney of the rat

Incubation time at 37°C (h)	*Cyclic GMP in medium (fmol mg^{-1}ml^{-1})*			
	Lung	*Heart*	*Liver*	*Kidney*
1	106 ± 4[a]	73 ± 3	46 ± 4	71 ± 7
2	181 ± 3	126 ± 1	59 ± 5	107 ± 11
3	957 ± 45	171 ± 4	76 ± 7	126 ± 13
4	2153 ± 109	207 ± 5	95 ± 5	150 ± 12

[a]Mean ± SEM.
Immature male rats of the Wistar strain were anaesthetized with Nembutal and perfused via the inferior vena cava with Joklik-MEM for approximately 3 min. The tissues were sliced at 1 mm with a McIlwain chopper, preincubated in JCB for 30 minutes at 37°C and incubated for 4 h at 37°C in JCB containing 1 mM-MIX under an atmosphere of 95% O_2 – 5% CO_2. Aliquots of the medium were removed at hourly intervals and assayed for cyclic GMP by radioimmunoassay. Mean of 4 experiments.

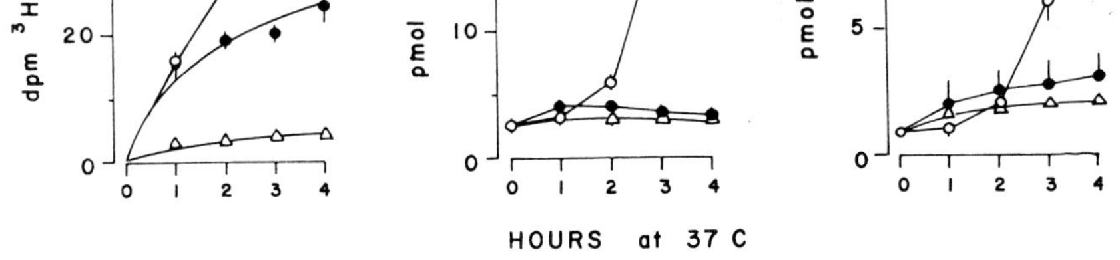

FIG. 2. Effect of inhibitors of protein synthesis on lung protein synthesis and cyclic GMP generation *in vitro*. Lung cells (see legend to Fig. 1) from normal adult male rats were incubated in JCB-MIX containing 0.5 μCi/ml [^{3}H]leucine in the presence or absence of cycloheximide (100 μg/ml) or of actinomycin D (10 μg/ml). At the indicated time intervals the cells were pelleted by centrifugation and the specific radioactivity in the trichloroacetic acid-insoluble cell fraction was determined. Cyclic GMP concentration in both the cell pellet and medium was determined by radioimmunoassay. Mean of 5 experiments. ○, no inhibitor; ●, actinomycin D; △, cycloheximide.

When either lung slices or dispersed lung cells were incubated in JCB-MIX, the rate of [^{3}H]leucine incorporation into lung protein proceeded linearly during a four-hour incubation period at 37°C. This was accompanied by an exponential increase in both tissue (or cellular) and medium cyclic GMP levels (Fig. 2). The presence of cycloheximide (100 μg/ml) or of actinomycin D (10 μg/ml) in the incubation medium inhibited the rate of [^{3}H]leucine incorporation; however, these agents also markedly impaired the ability of the lung to generate cyclic GMP (Fig. 2), suggesting that its production by the lung is dependent upon continued synthesis of proteins.

When rats were rendered hypothyroid (by dietary iodine deficiency plus propylthiouracil), diabetic (by streptozotocin treatment), or adrenal insufficient (by surgical adrenalectomy), the capacity of the lung to generate cyclic GMP *in vitro* was significantly enhanced (Table 2). Treatment of the

TABLE 2
In vitro generation of cyclic GMP by hormonally deficient lung slices: effect of *in vivo* hormone treatment

Treatment group	*Cyclic GMP in medium (fmol mg^{-1} ml^{-1})*
1. Intact control (6)	2085 ± 249[a]
Hypothyroid[b] (6)	3635 ± 301**
Hypothyroid + T_3 (6)	1873 ± 216
(25 μg T_3/100 g per day, × 3 days)	
2. Intact control (4)	2426 ± 241
Diabetic[c] (4)	5412 ± 597**
Diabetic + PZI (4)	2813 ± 261
(1 unit PZI/rat per day, × 2 days)	
3. Intact control (9)	2126 ± 145
Adrenalectomized[d] (9)	3454 ± 302**
Adrenalectomized + dexamethasone (9)	3217 ± 200**
(100 μg/100 g per day, × 3 days)	

[a]Mean ± SEM.
[b]Fed Remington diet (with vitamins) containing 0.25% propyl thiouracil for 21–30 days, *ad libitum*.
[c]Streptozotocin-treated (75 mg/kg); killed on the third post-treatment day.
[d]Bilaterally adrenalectomized 5 days before sacrifice; given 1% saline to drink.

**Significantly different from intact control ($P<0.01$).

All rats were 48–60-day-old male Wistars and were littermate-matched in each treatment group. One mm lung slices were incubated in JCB-MIX for 4 h at 37°C and the concentration of cyclic GMP in the medium was determined.

hypothyroid rats with three daily injections of triiodothyronine (T_3) (25 μg/100 g body weight per day) restored lung cyclic GMP production rate to normal, as did two daily injections of PZI (1 unit/rat per day) to the diabetic rats. In contrast, treatment of the adrenalectomized rats with dexamethasone (100 μg/100 g body weight per day for three days) had no effect (Table 2). The normalizing effects of T_3 and insulin seen after whole-animal treatment were

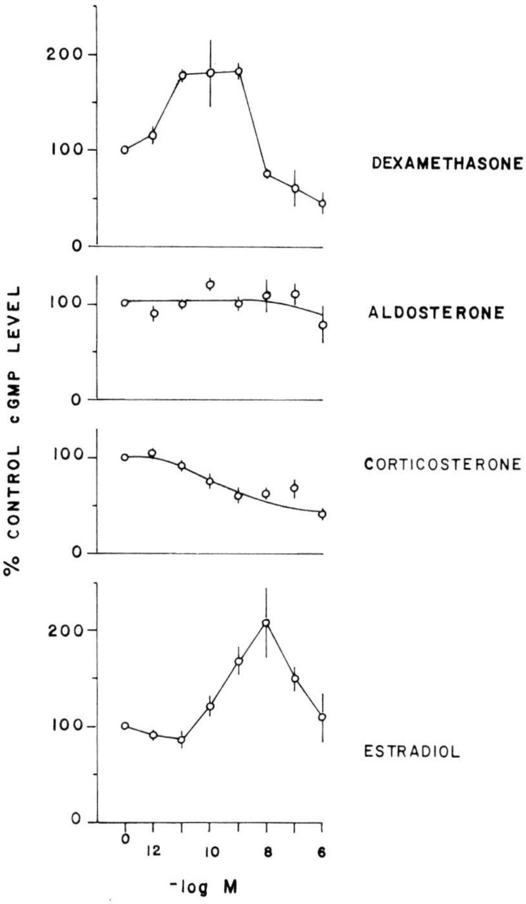

FIG. 3. *In vitro* effects of steroid hormones on cyclic GMP generation by the lung of adrenalectomized-gonadectomized rats. Prepubertal male rats (38–42-day-old) were bilaterally adrenalectomized and gonadectomized 24–72 h before sacrifice. One mm slices of the perfused lungs were preincubated for 30 min at 37°C in JCB and incubated for 4 h at that temperature in JCB-MIX containing the steroid hormones at the indicated concentrations. Aliquots of the medium were assayed for cyclic GMP. The results are expressed as % of cyclic GMP levels generated in the absence of steroids. Abscissa values represent the negative logarithm of the molar concentration of the steroid. Mean of 3 experiments.

not observed when these hormones were tested *in vitro* (data not shown); however, the addition of steroid hormones to slices of adrenalectomized–gonadectomized rat lung did influence *in vitro* production of cyclic GMP by the lung, although different effects were seen with different steroids (Fig. 3). Dexamethasone exerted a biphasic effect, being stimulatory at low concentrations and inhibitory at higher concentrations. Corticosterone, the natural glucocorticoid of the rat, was inhibitory at concentrations of 100 pM or higher, while aldosterone was without apparent effect. Interestingly, oestradiol markedly enhanced cyclic GMP generation, although only at very high concentrations (Fig. 3). These results provide the first demonstration of hormonal effects on lung levels of cyclic GMP, although their significance in relation to the overall physiology of the lung is unclear and must await future experiments.

CONCLUSIONS

The postnatal lung appears to be responsive to the actions of several hormones: insulin, androgens, oestrogens, thyroid hormone, and glucocorticoids. Future experiments will very possibly uncover a number of other hormones which, either alone or in combination, regulate the diversified biochemical processes of this heterogeneous cell population.

ACKNOWLEDGEMENTS

I am indebted to Dr Charles Plopper for his excellent collaboration in some of these studies, and gratefully acknowledge the expert technical assistance of Ms C. Uetake, Mr J. Akaka and Mrs N. Joun. These investigations were supported by NIH-NHLBI Grants HL-16949 and HL-19195. I am supported by NIH-NHLBI Research Career Development Award K04-HL-00216.

References

Dohler KD, Wuttke W 1975 Changes with age in levels of serum gonadotropins, prolactin, and gonadal steroids in perpubertal male and female rats. Endocrinology 97:898-907

Felts JM 1964 Biochemistry of the lung. Health Phys 10:973-979

Goldberg ND, Haddox MK 1977 Cyclic GMP metabolism and involvement in biological regulation. Annu Rev Biochem 46:823-896

Gregorio CA, Massaro D 1977 Influence of insulin on amino acid uptake by lung slices. J Appl Physiol Respir Environ Excercise Physiol 42:216-220

Hardman JG, Sutherland EW 1969 Guanyl cyclase, an enzyme catalyzing the formation of guanosine 3′,5′-monophosphate from guanosine triphosphate. J Biol Chem 244:6363-6370

Katzenellenbogen BS, Gorski J 1972 Estrogen action *in vitro*: induction of the synthesis of a specific uterine protein. J Biol Chem 247:1299-1305

Kerr JS, Baker NJ, Bassett DJP, Fisher AB 1979 Effect of perfusate glucose concentration on rat lung glycolysis. Am J Physiol 236:E229-E233

Liggins GC 1969 The foetal role in the initiation of parturition in the ewe. In: Foetal autonomy. Churchill, London (Ciba Found Symp) p 218-231
Moger WH 1977 Serum 5α-androstane-3α,17β-diol, androsterone, and testosterone concentrations in the male rat. Influence of age and gonadotropin stimulation. Endocrinology 100: 1027-1032
Morishige WK, Uetake C 1978 Receptors for androgen and estrogen in the rat lung. Endocrinology 102:1827-1837
Morishige WK, Uetake C, Greenwood FC, Akaka J 1977 Pulmonary insulin responsivity: *in vivo* effects of insulin on the diabetic rat lung and specific insulin binding to lung receptors in normal rats. Endocrinology 100:1710-1722
Moxley MA, Longmore WJ 1975 Studies of the effects of alloxan and streptozotocin induced diabetes on lipid metabolism in the isolated perfused rat lung. Life Sci 17:921-926
Plopper CG, Morishige WK 1978 Alterations in granular (type II) pneumocyte ultrastructure by streptozotocin-induced diabetes in the rat. Lab Invest 38:143-148
Plopper CG, Morishige WK 1979 Alterations in the ultrastructure of non-ciliated bronchiolar epithelial (Clara) cells by streptozotocin-induced diabetes in rats. Am Rev Respir Dis 120: 1137-1143
Rannels DE, Sahms RH, Watkins CA 1979 Effects of starvation and diabetes on protein synthesis in lung. Am J Physiol 236:E421-E428
Salisbury-Murphy S, Rubinstein D, Beck JC 1966 Lipid metabolism in lung slices. Am J Physiol 211:988-992
Steiner AL, Pagliara AS, Chase LR, Kipnis DM 1972 Radioimmunoassay for cyclic nucleotides. II. Adenosine 3′,5′-monophosphate and guanosine 3′,5′-monophosphate in mammalian tissues and body fluids. J Biol Chem 247:1114-1120
Stubbs WA, Morgan I, Lloyd B, Alberti KGMM 1977 The effect of insulin on lung metabolism in the rat. Clin Endocrinol 7:181-184
Thet LA, Delaney MD, Gregorio CA, Massaro D 1977 Protein metabolism by rat lung: influence of fasting, glucose and insulin. J Appl Physiol Respir Environ Exercise Physiol 43:463-467
Weber KC, Visscher MB 1969 Metabolism of the isolated canine lung. Am J Physiol 217: 1044:1052

Discussion

Vane: You showed a very rapid rise in cyclic GMP which started after about two hours of incubation (Fig. 2, p 243). Has the lung tissue changed, or has something been produced which stimulates cyclic GMP formation?

Morishige: We wondered about that, and we thought it might be due to an influence of preincubation. We therefore varied our preincubation time from 30 minutes to three hours and, in the presence of methylisobutylxanthine from time zero, the same thing happened. It might be a reflection of the rate of diffusion of this phosphodiesterase inhibitor into the cell, although my understanding is that it is freely diffusible and enters rapidly.

Vane: Have you added arachidonic acid to these cultures?

Morishige: Yes. However, it seemed to be toxic to the cells. Perhaps the concentrations were too high. Indomethacin had no effect on cyclic GMP production by these lung cells.

Junod: What do the cyclic GMP changes signify? Do they represent primarily the direct effect of these hormones, or are they related to something else, and are only secondary events?

Morishige: This is not known. The significance of even the existence of cyclic GMP is unknown. There is some evidence fo. .nediation of some of the secondary or tertiary effects of hormones by cyclic GMP, but it does not seem to participate as a direct second messenger as cyclic AMP does (Goldberg & Haddox 1977). Klass (1978, 1979) has done a good study of the possible influence of cyclic GMP on lung. He observed that after a brief period of hyperventilation of rat lung there was an increased efflux of phospholipids into the lavage fluid, and this was attended by an increase in the cyclic GMP level of the lung. When he perfused rat lung with dibutyryl cyclic GMP, a synthetic analogue of cyclic GMP which enters the cell more readily, phospholipid efflux also increased. Taking these results together, he suggests that cyclic GMP causes increased surfactant release.

Ayuso-Parrilla: What were the experimental conditions under which you showed an effect of insulin on protein synthesis? I ask this because we have done some experiments using isolated rat lung cells which indicate that glucose stimulates protein synthesis through some mechanism that requires glucose breakdown. Since insulin increases glucose utilization, I wonder whether the stimulation of protein synthesis in lung cells by insulin would be secondary to its effect on glucose utilization.

I should also like to know whether the effect of insulin on leucine incorporation reflects an increased synthesis of bulk protein or only of some specific proteins.

Morishige: We haven't done a detailed analysis of the different types of lung proteins which respond to insulin, although our double-label study would suggest that insulin does not have a uniform effect on all protein species in lung. As to glucose stimulation, we have only used a single concentration of 5 mM.

Parrilla: In our experiments on isolated lung cells glucose is virtually undetectable within the cell. This means that the main rate-limiting step on glucose utilization in this preparation of isolated lung cells must be transport across the plasma membrane. Above 4 mM-glucose the system is saturated; we don't find any further increase in glucose utilization by isolated cells. If we extrapolate this to the whole animal it means that under physiological conditions (~ 8 mM plasma glucose), utilization of glucose by lung cells would be expected to be saturated. According to your findings in perfused lung and to our unpublished experiments on isolated lung cells, insulin changes the V_{max} of the system for glucose utilization, which allows us to conclude that so far insulin is the only known modulator that controls the rate of glucose utilization in lung cells *in vivo*.

Alberti: We see increasing glucose uptake by lung cells up to 8mM-glucose; I'm not sure whether uptake is saturated or not at physiological concentrations in our experiments.

I agree with you, Dr Morishige, on how difficult it is to achieve normoglycaemia in a streptozotocin-diabetic rat. We had to give four units of PZI per day to achieve this, which is a high dose for a 200 g rat. Dr Rasch finds that by using a very special heat-treated long-acting insulin she can achieve normoglycaemia much more easily (Rasch 1979).

Finally, have you compared the numbers and properties of insulin receptors in lung and in other tissues?

Morishige: We have compared lung, liver and adipose tissue. The total binding capacity of lung tissue for insulin is much less than that of adipose tissue and liver, but the apparent K_d seems to be similar in all three tissues.

Alberti: That would fit in with the biological effects of insulin.

Parrilla: When you make rats diabetic with streptozotocin the glucagon-producing cells remain and the diabetic syndrome and insulin requirements are completely different from those in diabetic pancreatectomized rats.

Morishige: Yes. We haven't studied pancreatectomized animals.

Vane: Dr Soffer spoke earlier about the content of insulin in the lungs, and it is now clear that there are insulin receptors in lung tissue. Were you really saying that the lungs synthesize insulin?

Soffer: Rosenzweig et al (1980) have recently detected insulin by radioimmunoassay and bioassay in a number of tissues, as well as in cultured lymphocytes and fibroblasts. This surprised me, because I thought insulin was made exclusively in the pancreas. Apparently its ubiquitous distribution has been suspected for some time, but nobody knows its function in extra-pancreatic tissues. The content is much lower than in the pancreas, and it isn't clear whether it is synthesized in these tissues or not, although the evidence seems to suggest that it is. The purpose of the paper was perhaps to stimulate investigators to consider this extra-pancreatic insulin in their studies of metabolism in isolated tissues.

Ballard: Regarding oestradiol binding by lung cells, did you look at competition with diethylstilboestrol? Mendelson et al (1980) reported that human fetal lung has binding sites with relatively low affinity for oestradiol compared to what you find in the adult lung. Also, diethylstilboestrol did not compete effectively for the human binding sites.

Morishige: The oestrogen-binding protein in fetal lung described by Mendelson and associates is probably similar to α-fetoprotein, which does not mediate any biological effects of steroids but may be important in retaining the steroids at high concentration within the cell. This binding protein didn't show any biological specificity.

Ballard: Does this suggest that fetal lung doesn't have a true receptor and that the adult lung may have one?

Morishige: Not necessarily. Receptors for oestrogen may be present in the fetal lung but at a concentration which is too low to be detectable in the presence of the very high level of non-receptor oestrophiles.

Bakhle: The oestradiol-binding proteins that you look at are in the cytosol. Is there any evidence for binding of oestradiol to membrane fragments?

Morishige: Many people have found this, but we have worked on the cytosol and nuclear fractions only.

Ballard: Did you take account of receptors in the nucleus when you studied variation over the oestrous cycle?

Morishige: We haven't done a quantitative analysis of nuclear receptor levels, although we did do a pulse-chase analysis on lung perfused *in situ* with labelled oestradiol or dihydrotestosterone, followed by an excess concentration of unlabelled steroid, and found much more radioactivity in the nucleus than in the cytosol. This suggested translocation of the steroid–receptor complex to the nucleus.

References

Goldberg ND, Haddox MK 1977 Cyclic GMP metabolism and involvement in biological regulation. Annu Rev Biochem 46:823-896

Klass DJ 1978 Lung tissue guanosine 3′,5′-monophosphate: effects of ventilation and anesthesia. J Appl Physiol Respirat Environ Exercise Physiol 45:487-494

Klass DJ 1979 Dibutyryl cyclic GMP and hyperventilation promote rat lung phospholipid release. J Appl Physiol Respirat Environ Exercise Physiol 47:285-289

Mendelson CR, MacDonald PC, Johnston JM 1980 Estrogen binding in human fetal lung tissue cytosol. Endocrinology 106:368-374

Rasch R 1979 Control of blood glucose levels in streptozotocin diabetic rats using a long-acting heat-treated insulin. Diabetologia 16:185-190

Rosenzweig J, Havrankova J, Lesniak MA, Brownstein M, Roth J 1980 Insulin is ubiquitous in extrapancreatic tissues. Proc Natl Acad Sci USA 77:572-576

Hormonal influences during fetal lung development

PHILIP L. BALLARD

Department of Pediatrics and Cardiovascular Research Institute, University of California, San Francisco, California 94143, USA

Abstract Maturation of the fetal lung is accelerated by *in utero* treatment with corticosteroids and thyroid hormones. Other agents such as catecholamines, thyrotropin-releasing hormone, oestradiol, heroin and cyclic AMP also influence pulmonary phospholipid metabolism. Glucocorticoids cause precocious development of both lung morphology and the surfactant system in type II cells, resulting in more stable lungs with increased air space. The properties of glucocorticoid action are consistent with enzyme induction mediated by interaction of steroid with cytoplasmic glucocorticoid receptors. Receptors are present in lung of many species, including the human fetus, and in both pulmonary fibroblasts and type II cells. Corticosteroid therapy of women in premature labour is currently used to reduce the incidence of infant respiratory distress syndrome (RDS). Treatment of the mother with 12 mg betamethasone causes an approximately four-fold maximal increase in unbound glucocorticoid activity in fetal plasma which is calculated to cause 80% nuclear occupancy by receptor–steroid complex. It is likely that endogenous corticoids influence normal lung development; possible sources of cortisol include the fetal adrenal, maternal adrenal, and conversion of cortisone to cortisol by amniotic membranes and lung fibroblasts.

Thyroid hormones have effects similar to corticosteroids, but appear to influence different biochemical steps. Synthetic analogues of triiodothyronine (T_3) are available which readily cross the placenta, in contrast to T_3 and thyroxine, and accelerate surfactant synthesis and release. Thyroid hormones probably act through nuclear receptors which are present in lung of both animals and the human. Thyroid treatment *in utero* also appears to accelerate lung maturation and prevent RDS in premature infants.

It is now recognized that the fetal lung, like many other differentiating tissues, is subject to hormonal regulation. Research on this topic has proceeded at an increasing pace over the past ten years since the first suggestion that glucocorticoids stimulate lung maturation. There is now experimental evidence that many different hormones or drugs may stimulate or delay fetal lung development (Table 1). This paper will discuss glucocorticoid and thyroid hormones,

Metabolic activities of the lung
(Ciba Foundation symposium 78) p 251-274

TABLE 1

Agents reported to affect fetal lung development

Accelerated maturation	*Delayed maturation*
Glucocorticoids	Metyrapone (Metopirone)
ACTH	Insulin
Thyroid hormones	Phenobarbitone
β-Sympathomimetics	Indomethacin[a]
Thyrotropin-releasing hormone	
Oestradiol	
Cyclic AMP and aminophylline	
Biosolvon metabolite VIII	
Heroin	
Epidermal growth factor	
Fibroblast/pneumonocyte factor	
Prolactin[a]	

[a]Effect disputed.

the two agents that we have investigated most extensively in my laboratory.

In the first section I shall review (1) the effects of glucocorticoids in fetal lung, (2) the properties of glucocorticoid receptors, (3) the use of glucocorticoid treatment to prevent respiratory distress syndrome (RDS), and (4) the possible role of endogenous corticosteroids in normal pulmonary development. The second section considers similar questions regarding thyroid hormones. The methods used in studies from my laboratory have been described in previous publications which are referenced in the text.

GLUCOCORTICOID EFFECTS

Buckingham et al first proposed in 1968 that glucocorticoids might stimulate lung differentiation in a manner analogous to effects in the intestine. The following year, Liggins (1969) reported that lambs which delivered prematurely after glucocorticoid treatment *in utero* were unexpectedly viable. He postulated that corticosteroid treatment accelerated lung differentiation, and a number of subsequent studies have supported this conclusion.

Corticosteroid treatment of the fetus accelerates normal events of pulmonary development, including (1) flattening of epithelial cells and thinning of alveolar septae to increase potential air space and gas exchange, (2) deposition of glycogen in epithelial cells and its depletion later in gestation, (3) development of the rough endoplasmic reticulum and appearance of lamellar bodies and their precursors in type II cells, and (4) release of surfactant from lamellar bodies into the alveoli. Physiologically, there is an increase in total lung volume and stability on deflation, as well as enhanced survival of prematurely born animals (for reviews see Avery 1975 and Ballard et al 1977).

The major action of glucocorticoids on the surfactant system of type II cells is at the level of phospholipid synthesis, which occurs by the CDP-choline incorporation pathway, rather than on release of surfactant *per se* (Brehier et al 1977, Rooney et al 1979, Corbet et al 1978). The characteristics of corticosteroid effects in the lung are consistent with *de novo* induction of enzymes. Studies in my laboratory (Brehier et al 1977) and by others (Rooney et al 1979, Possmayer et al 1979) indicate that corticosteroid treatment increases the activity of microsomal phosphatidic acid phosphatase (PAPase), the enzyme which hydrolyses phosphatidic acid to provide diglycerides for the final step in phosphatidylcholine synthesis. It is likely that additional enzymes are affected by treatment, but there is disagreement at present about which enzymes are involved. Glucocorticoids may also stimulate phospholipid synthesis through increased glycogenolysis and availability of substrate. The generalized morphological maturation in fetal lung after corticosteroid treatment suggests that many different cell types are affected, including both mesenchymal and epithelial elements.

GLUCOCORTICOID RECEPTORS

I proposed several years ago that the effects of glucocorticoids in fetal lung are mediated by specific glucocorticoid receptors (Ballard & Ballard 1972). Our studies (Ballard & Ballard 1972, 1974, Granberg & Ballard 1977, Ballard et al 1978a) and those by Giannopoulos (1973, Giannopoulos et al 1972, 1973) established that fetal rabbit lung contains specific cytoplasmic proteins which bind glucocorticoids with high affinity and specificity. Protein-bound [^{3}H]dexamethasone appears as a single peak on both sucrose gradient sedimentation and gel filtration, and binding data are consistent with a single class of receptor sites. During late fetal life, rabbit lung contains an average of 12 000 binding sites per cell and the apparent equilibrium dissociation constant (K_d) for binding of [^{3}H]dexamethasone at 2°C is about 3 nM. Glucocorticoid receptor is detected as early as 18 days of gestation in the rabbit (term is 31 days), and there is no apparent change in the properties of the cytoplasmic binding reaction during the last trimester.

Receptor is present in both fetal and adult lung of all species examined so far. This includes the rabbit, rat, mouse, sheep, dog, monkey and human. Compared with other fetal tissues, the lung contains a relatively high concentration of binding sites. Recent experiments demonstrated glucocorticoid receptor in both lung fibroblasts and type II cells (Ballard et al 1978a). The concentration of receptor in these isolated cells is similar to that in whole lung tissue, suggesting that most if not all pulmonary cell types contain receptors and are therefore potentially capable of responding to glucocorticoids.

The relative affinity of lung receptor for various steroids has been studied in some detail. Cortisol and corticosterone, the major endogenous steroids with glucocorticoid activity, are bound by receptor with similar affinity. Synthetic corticosteroids such as methylprednisolone, dexamethasone, betamethasone, fluorocortisol, prednisolone and triamcinolone exhibit a higher affinity for binding (from 2- to 12-fold that of cortisol), as would be expected from their greater potency *in vivo*. Cortisone, androgens, oestrogens and other steroids without glucocorticoid activity have little affinity for lung receptor. These results probably reflect the potency of various glucocorticoids at the cellular level *in vivo,* since there is a close correlation in other systems between binding of steroid to receptor and the extent of the physiological response. The unique specificity of receptor binding allowed us to develop a radioreceptor assay which measures plasma glucocorticoid activity due to both endogenous and exogenous steroids (Ballard et al 1975b).

When binding experiments are carried out in intact lung cells, most of the glucocorticoid–receptor complex localizes in the cell nucleus where it binds tightly to chromatin. The nuclear binding presumably initiates the effects of glucocorticoid on *de novo* RNA and protein synthesis.

GLUCOCORTICOID TREATMENT FOR PREVENTION OF RDS

The early studies on lung maturation in fetal animals quickly led to the suggestion that corticosteroid therapy might benefit the human fetus at risk for RDS, a disease of surfactant deficiency. In 1972, Liggins and Howie reported the results of a double-blind clinical trial of prenatal betamethasone therapy for prevention of RDS. They found a significant decrease in the incidence of RDS and increased survival of premature infants less than 34 weeks' gestation who were exposed to maternal steroid therapy. Since then a number of other studies have supported the effectiveness of this preventive therapy. The established benefits of prenatal therapy now include decreased incidence of RDS in infants of 26–34 weeks' gestation, decreased severity of RDS when it does occur, decreased occurrence of intraventricular haemorrhage, and increased survival (reviewed by Ballard & Ballard 1979).

My colleagues and I have assayed betamethasone and cortisol concentrations in cord plasma of treated infants (Ballard et al 1975b). The mean level of betamethasone one hour after the first dose was 14.3 μg cortisol equivalents/dl. This level decreased to 3 μg/dl at 24 hours and increased to a maximal value of 15 μg/dl after the second dose; betamethasone was undetectable in cord blood during the third day after initiation of therapy. In six matched maternal and cord blood samples the mean maternal–fetal gradient of betamethasone was 3:1. Cortisol levels in cord blood of treated infants were suppressed maximally to 45% of the level in untreated infants, and values returned to the normal range by seven days after the last treatment (Ballard et al 1980a).

The sum of unbound (physiologically active fraction) betamethasone and cortisol concentrations, both expressed in terms of cortisol equivalents, should reflect the total amount of glucocorticoid activity in fetal plasma. Fig. 1 shows the calculated levels of glucocorticoid activity occurring in fetal plasma after maternal betamethasone treatment. Maximal concentrations are approximately four-fold higher than in untreated infants. As betamethasone is cleared from the circulation after the second dose, glucocorticoid levels transiently fall below the untreated value because of the suppression of endogenous cortisol. The peak levels of glucocorticoid activity represent an increase into the physiological stress range. For example, untreated newborn infants with RDS develop similar plasma concentrations of unbound cortisol (7.8 μg/dl) in response to the stress of the illness. Thus, prenatal betamethasone therapy at the 12 mg dose used by Liggins & Howie (1972) produces physiological, not pharmacological, concentrations of circulating glucocorticoid activity. This is an important consideration in evaluating possible mechanisms of glucocorticoid therapy.

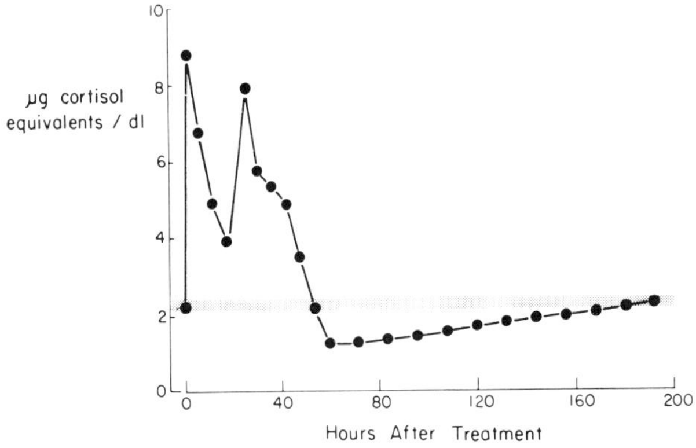

FIG. 1. Time course of unbound glucocorticoid activity in cord plasma after prenatal betamethasone treatment. Results for plasma glucocorticoids (cortisol plus betamethasone) are calculated for intervals after maternal therapy with 12 mg betamethasone. The untreated level is shown by the stippled bar. (Results taken from Ballard et al 1980a.)

We have estimated the amount of receptor–glucocorticoid complex present in nuclei of human lung cells under various conditions. Fig. 2 shows an idealized dose–response curve for nuclear binding of glucocorticoid at 37°C, based on our studies with intact lung cells (Ballard et al 1978a). The vertical bars indicate the level of nuclear receptor–steroid complex that would be expected to occur at the concentrations of plasma glucocorticoids before, during and after betamethasone treatment. In untreated premature infants the mean plasma concentration of unbound corticoids is approximately 40 nM, resulting in 40% nuclear occupancy. Even lower occupancy levels would occur in those untreated infants with lower plasma cortisol. The maximal plasma levels after betamethasone are about 220 nM, which increases nuclear binding to 80%. After the last dose of betamethasone, plasma glucocorticoid decreases to a minimum of 16 nM and nuclear occupancy falls to approximately 20% because of the suppression of the fetal hypothalamic–pituitary–adrenal axis. Thus, prenatal betamethasone therapy results in at least a twofold increase in the amount of receptor–steroid complex in nuclei. Since the binding curve reaches a plateau, this analysis indicates that higher doses of betamethasone would not substantially increase nuclear binding. In other glucocorticoid target tissues there is a close correlation between nuclear binding and biological response. If this is also true in the fetal lung, these calculations suggest that the currently used dose of 12 mg betamethasone should produce a nearly optimal effect on lung maturation. This proposal is

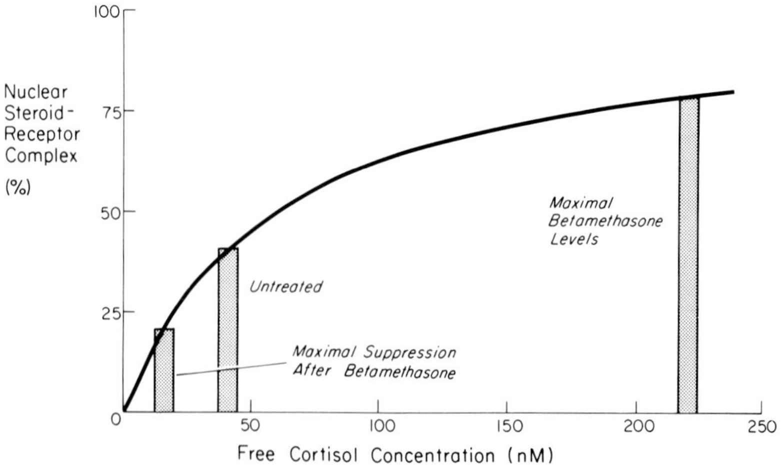

FIG. 2. Calculated nuclear binding of receptor–glucocorticoid complex in human fetal lung as a function of unbound cortisol concentration. The calculations are discussed in the text.

supported by the finding that doubling the dose of betamethasone (24 mg daily) did not improve the efficacy of this therapy in preventing RDS (Liggins & Howie 1974).

The receptor mechanism also predicts that all steroids with glucocorticoid activity should be effective in preventing RDS. The relative activities of various synthetic corticosteroids at the same plasma concentration should be equivalent to the relative affinities, as discussed earlier. However, it is known that different glucocorticoids do not achieve the same distribution between maternal and fetal plasma. Maternal levels of betamethasone, cortisol and prednisolone are about 3, 5 and 10 times higher, respectively, than the levels achieved in the fetal circulation. The clinical effectiveness of various steroids would also be determined by their binding to plasma corticosteroid-binding globulin and by the rate of metabolic clearance. Clinically, maternal treatment with betamethasone, dexamethasone and hydrocortisone appears to be equally efficacious in preventing RDS (Ballard & Ballard 1979). Methylprednisolone therapy was not effective in one study, probably because of limited transfer to the fetus (Block et al 1977).

DO ENDOGENOUS CORTICOIDS REGULATE NORMAL LUNG DEVELOPMENT?

This question has interested a number of investigators and is important both in terms of basic biology and in regard to the mechanism of action of exogenous corticoids. In certain other mammalian tissues there is convincing evidence for the regulatory role of corticosteroids in the process of terminal differentiation (Ballard 1979). The maturation of intestinal enzymes and function, for example, is associated with increasing levels of unbound plasma corticoids, is induced precociously by administration of glucocorticoid, and is delayed by adrenalectomy in the absence of replacement hormone. As reviewed below, the first two conditions are also well documented for lung differentiation; however, the effects of hormone ablation and replacement have not been conclusively demonstrated. Nevertheless, all available data are consistent with a role of endogenous corticoids in influencing the rate of pulmonary development.

Experimental evidence

A variety of experimental approaches have been used to examine the role of endogenous corticosteroids in lung maturation. Blackburn and colleagues (1972, 1973) decapitated fetal rats *in utero,* and Chiswick et al (1973) and Meyrick et al (1975) did this experiment in fetal rabbits. Results were similar in the two species. Compared with control animals, alveolar septae were thicker and more cellular, type II cells contained fewer lamellar bodies and more glycogen, and, in two studies, there was evidence of decreased surface-active material. When decapitated fetuses were exposed to ACTH (Chiswick et al 1973) or dexamethasone (Farrell et al 1977) there was an increase in lamellar bodies and in the rate of incorporation of choline into phospholipid. Although these results support the proposed role of endogenous corticoids, decapitation by neck (and tracheal) ligature may affect lung development by causing the retention of lung fluid in addition to ablation of the hypothalamus and pituitary.

Recent studies in fetal sheep have used hydranencephaly, produced by ligation of both carotid arteries (Platzker et al 1976), and hypophysectomy (Kitterman et al 1979) to remove pituitary hormones. These procedures caused a delay in lung maturation as judged by surfactant levels in tracheal fluid, histology, and lung pressure–volume studies. Preliminary results indicate that replacement therapy with corticosteroid does not prevent the delay in development. This finding suggests that glucocorticoids may act in conjunction with other hormones to regulate fetal lung development. Thyroid hormones are likely candidates for this role in view of their effects in both the fetal lung (discussed later) and other developing tissues.

Metyrapone (Metopirone), an inhibitor of adrenal steroid 11β-hydroxylase activity, has been used as a potentially more selective means of reducing fetal corticosteroid levels. These studies (Vidyasagur & Chernick 1975, Nelson et al 1976) indicated some reduction in lung tissue surface-active material but not in other parameters of lung development. Interpretation of these results is difficult because of the apparently rapid clearance of metyrapone, the absence of data on plasma corticoids after treatment, and the possibility of effects of metyrapone unrelated to steroid production.

Stressful situations in experimental animals can stimulate phospholipid synthesis in fetal lung. Kotas (1973) injected *Staphylococcus aureus* into fetal rabbits and found more stable lungs in pressure–volume studies, presumably as a consequence of stress-induced hormonal changes. After sham surgery of fetal rabbits the rate of incorporation of choline into phospholipid increases and fetal corticoid levels are higher two days later (Ballard et al 1978b) (Table 2). In addition, there is a correlation between fetal plasma corticoid concentration and the activity of lung PAPase (Ballard et al 1980a). These findings suggest that the level of PAPase and the rate of phospholipid synthesis in fetal lung are regulated by physiological levels of endogenous corticoids.

TABLE 2

Effect of surgery on plasma corticoids and choline incorporation into lung phospholipid in the fetal rabbit

Procedure	*Choline incorporation into lecithin (pmol/mg protein per h)*	*Plasma corticoids (μg/dl)*
Unoperated	33.2 ± 1.2 (47)	0.86 ± 0.06 (36)
Sham surgery	52.2 ± 5.1* (22)	1.15 ± 0.07* (20)
Surgery plus diluent injection	45.6 ± 2.3* (21)	1.46 ± 0.07* (21)

*$P < 0.05$ compared with unoperated control.
Mean ± SE values are shown with number of determinations in parentheses. (Data from Ballard et al 1978b.)

Temporal associations

The increase in fetal plasma corticoids (total or unbound fraction) during gestation correlates with the major terminal events in lung maturation. Fig. 3 shows this relationship for the fetal rabbit, with the rise in unbound corticoids preceding accumulation of lamellar bodies and release of surfactant into alveoli. A similar pattern occurs in the fetal rat where unbound corticoid concentrations increase as a result of a decrease in levels of corticosteroid-binding globulin (CBG) before birth (Ballard 1979). Mescher et al (1975) found that corticoid levels in plasma of fetal sheep increase dramatically in late gestation,

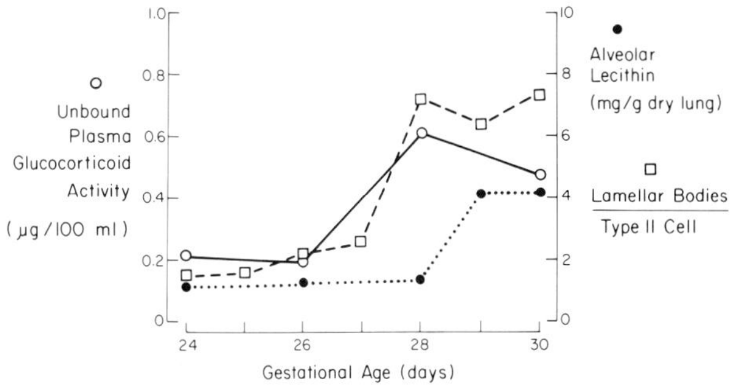

FIG. 3. Developmental patterns of unbound plasma corticoids, lamellar bodies and alveolar surfactant in the fetal rabbit. (From Ballard et al 1977, by permission.)

coincidentally with increasing surfactant levels in tracheal fluid. No change in plasma cortisol was observed earlier in gestation when surfactant was first detected, suggesting that only the later events in lung maturation are normally regulated by endogenous corticosteroids. In the human, cortisol levels in fetal plasma and amniotic fluid begin a major increase about 32 weeks of gestation when the lecithin/sphingomyelin (L/S) ratio increases and the incidence of RDS decreases (Murphy 1978a). These observations are consistent with the regulation of normal lung maturation by increasing levels of endogenous glucocorticoid, but they do not prove this relationship.

Clinical evidence

Gluck et al (1974) find several conditions of pregnancy that are associated with accelerated maturation, and it is proposed that these stresses affect the fetal lung through increased production of fetal cortisol. A similar mechanism may account for the protective effect of labour on the occurrence of RDS (Fedrick & Butler 1972). There is one report that low cortisol levels at birth are associated with RDS in premature infants (Murphy 1974). Similarly, RDS is associated with a reduced production of cortisol by human amniotic membranes (Tanswell & Smith 1978), and possibly with reduced concentrations of cortisol in amniotic fluid. RDS occurs more frequently in males, and cortisol concentrations in amniotic fluid may rise more slowly during gestation in this sex (Nielsen et al 1979). Infants with RDS have larger thymuses at birth (Fletcher et al 1979) and smaller adrenals at *post mortem* (Naeye et al 1971), consistent with less adrenocorticoid production in these infants. As discussed, exogenous betamethasone accelerates lung maturation at plasma glucocorticoid concentrations within the physiological range, suggesting that endogenous corticoids can have the same effect. It is possible that endogenous cortisol, which increases several fold after birth in infants with RDS (Ballard et al 1975a), is responsible in part for the improvement in this disease which often occurs at 48–72 hours.

Sources of fetal corticoids

At least four mechanisms may contribute to the accumulation of cortisol in the fetal lung. The adult zone of the *fetal adrenal* produces cortisol and cortisone as early as 18 weeks of human gestation (Murphy 1973), and adrenal size and steroid production increase through gestation. The autonomy of fetal adrenal function is well documented in the sheep, where fetal levels of cortisol increase many fold in late gestation without any change in maternal levels. In contrast to the sheep, steroids can cross the placenta to some extent in the human, and *maternal corticosteroids* may contribute to fetal levels. Both unbound and total levels of cortisol increase in women during pregnancy, and presumably transfer increases proportionally. However, most of the maternal cortisol is converted to inactive cortisone by the enzyme 11β-hydroxysteroid dehydrogenase in the placenta.

A third source of fetal cortisol, therefore, may involve conversion from cortisone of either fetal or maternal origin. *Amniotic membranes* have a large capacity for metabolizing corticosteroids, and the direction of conversion becomes predominantly cortisone → cortisol after 20 weeks of gestation (Tanswell et al 1977). This activity probably accounts for the increasing concentration of unconjugated cortisol in amniotic fluid during gestation. Amniotic fluid cortisol could be obtained by the fetus through swallowing or transcutaneous absorption.

A fourth interesting possibility is that metabolism of cortisone by *fetal lung fibroblasts* provides cortisol for lung cells. Dehydrogenase activity is present in fetal lung of the rat (Nicholas & Kim 1975), rabbit (Nicholas et al 1978) and human (Smith et al 1973). In the fetal rabbit there is a several-fold increase in the rate of reduction of cortisone to cortisol between Days 22 and 30 of gestation, paralleling the increase in rate of choline incorporation (Nicholas et al 1978). Human fetal lung cells demonstrate an increasing ability to reduce cortisone with time in culture (Smith et al 1973). Furthermore, cells previously exposed to cortisol had a greater rate of conversion. In studies with human fetal specimens, Murphy (1978b) found a change from inactivation of cortisol to cortisone in early fetal life to a slight net production of cortisol at term. The mechanisms of the changes in corticosteroid metabolism during development are not understood. The direction and rate of the reaction may be controlled by the relative concentrations of the cofactors NADP and NADPH and/or by the presence of different enzymes for the oxidative and reductive reactions.

The demonstration of 11β-hydroxysteroid dehydrogenase activity in fetal lung, and its possible regulation by glucocorticoids, suggest that the lung may play a significant role in determining its own tissue levels of glucocorticoid. In assessing the endogenous glucocorticoid influence in lung development one should therefore probably consider the plasma concentrations of both cortisol and cortisone, as well as the activity of 11β-dehydrogenase in the lung.

THYROID HORMONES

Recent studies indicate that thyroid hormones also influence fetal lung maturation. In 1973 Wu et al found more mature lung morphology and greater bubble stability of lung wash after treatment of rabbit fetuses with thyroxine (T_4). Rooney and co-workers (1975) also noted accelerated morphological development with T_4 treatment, and Smith & Torday (1974) reported that T_4 enhanced choline incorporation into phospholipid by cultured fetal lung cells. Clinically, low levels of plasma triiodothyronine (T_3) and T_4 at birth are associated with RDS (Redding & Pereira 1974, Cuestas et al 1976), and there is one report that intraamniotic T_4 treatment stimulates human lung maturation (Mashiach et al 1979).

In vivo studies in fetuses involve surgery and fetal injection (through the exposed uterus) of hormone since neither T_3 nor T_4 readily crosses the placenta. This experimental approach is known to increase corticoids and possibly other stress-related factors (as discussed above) which also affect the fetal lung. Recent studies of the effects of thyroid hormones in the fetus have used a synthetic non-iodinated analogue of T_3, 3,5-dimethyl-3′-isopropyl-L-thyronine (DIMIT), which is more lipophilic than T_3 and binds poorly to plasma thyroxine-binding proteins. Administration of DIMIT to pregnant rats prevents fetal goitre and precociously induces enzymic and morphological changes in fetal liver, suggesting free placental passage (Kriz et al 1978, Comite et al 1978). Experiments in my laboratory with ^{3}H-labelled DIMIT have confirmed that this compound freely passes across the placenta (Ballard et al 1980b).

We have treated pregnant rabbits for 1–2 days with DIMIT in doses of 0.5–3 mg/kg per day and examined the fetuses at 26 and 27 days (Ballard et al 1980b). Treatment did not affect fetal growth or viability. In fetal lung tissue, DIMIT decreased the glycogen content by 38%, but had no effect on DNA, protein or phospholipid levels. As shown in Fig. 4, DIMIT produces a dose-dependent increase (maximum 104%) in the rate of incorporation of choline into phospholipid. There is also an increase in microsomal PAPase activity, but the maximal effect is small (38%) and occurs only with two days of treatment at the higher doses of DIMIT. The limited effect of DIMIT on PAPase compared with the stimulation of choline incorporation contrasts with the effect of glucocorticoid treatment. This suggests that thyroid hormone may act through biochemical mechanisms different from those of glucocorticoids. In addition, DIMIT treatment increased total phospholipid by 163% and saturated phosphatidylcholine by 330% in lung lavage fluid whereas an optimal dose of betamethasone enhanced lavage phospholipid by 50%. These results support those of earlier studies indicating that thyroid hormone accelerates lung maturation. Analogues such as DIMIT will be useful in exploring further the mechanism of thyroid hormone effects and

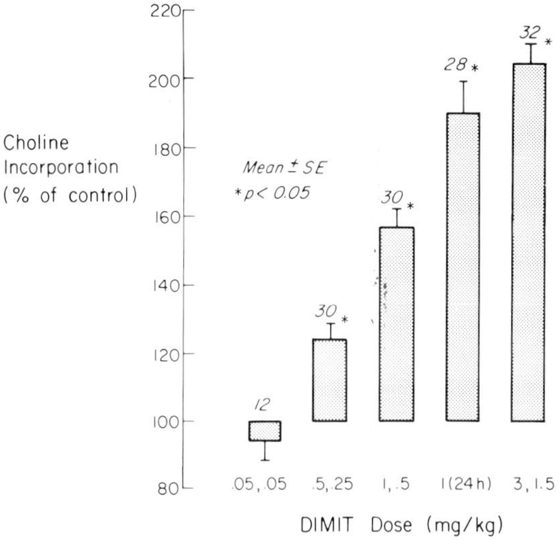

FIG. 4. Rate of choline incorporation into phospholipid by minced fetal rabbit lung after various doses of DIMIT. Pregnant rabbits received diluent or 0.05–3 mg/kg DIMIT on Days 24 and/or 25, and choline incorporation was determined on Day 26 by the method described in Brehier et al (1977).

they may eventually find application in prenatal prevention of RDS in infants.

It is likely that the effects of thyroid hormones in fetal lung are mediated through binding to nuclear receptors and subsequent enzyme induction, analogous to the mechanism which appears to operate for T_3 in adult target tissues. Nuclear T_3 receptors have been described in adult rat lung (Morishige & Guernsey 1978), in both adult and fetal rabbit lung (Lindenberg et al 1978), in human fetal lung, and in two cell lines (A549 and L-2) which apparently originated from type II cells (Lindenberg et al 1978). The concentration and affinity of binding sites is similar among these tissues (Table 3). Properties of the binding reaction in lung nuclei closely resemble those described for other T_4-responsive tissues such as adult liver. T_4 is approximately 7% as active as T_3 for binding to lung nuclear receptor, consistent with the relative *in vivo* potencies. DIMIT is only 0.15% as active as T_3 but, like other analogues, it can completely displace T_3 from receptor at sufficiently high concentrations (Lindenberg et al 1978). This suggests that DIMIT at appropriate doses can optimally induce thyroid hormone-responsive functions in fetal lung. In addition to nuclear receptors, fetal rabbit lung contains cytoplasmic binding sites for T_3 and T_4. The role of these sites in thyroid hormone action is uncertain at present.

TABLE 3

Nuclear receptor for triiodothyronine in lung and cell lines derived from lung

Tissue	*Nuclear binding of [^{125}I]T_3*	
	Sites/cell	*K_d (pM)*
Adult rat lung[a]	900	250
Adult rabbit lung	800	70
Fetal rabbit lung (28 days)	1360	120
Fetal human lung (16–19 wk)	1350	70
L-2 cells[b]	2280	280
A549 cells[b]	1580	200

[a]Data from Morishige & Guernsey (1978).
[b]Data from Lindenberg et al (1978).
The results are mean values obtained from Scatchard analyses of dose–response experiments performed at 37°C (fetal rabbit) or 25°C (adult rabbit and fetal human). L-2 cells were cloned from adult rat lung as presumptive type II cells and A549 cells were cultured from a human alveolar carcinoma.

The role of endogenous T_3 and T_4 in the normal course of lung development is still uncertain. In both sheep and humans there is a temporal association between increasing concentrations of plasma thyroid hormones and maturation of the surfactant system (Fisher et al 1977). Erenberg (1979) found that thyroidectomy of fetal sheep resulted in lower lecithin/sphingomyelin ratios in tracheal fluid, without affecting plasma cortisol levels. Additional studies of this type are needed to fully define the influence of endogenous thyroid hormones.

In view of the extensive list of agents reported to accelerate pulmonary maturation (Table 1) it seems likely that normal lung development is influenced by several agents. The development and metabolic function of other organs are known to be under multi-hormonal regulation. Future experiments should further define the various mechanisms of hormone action, and possible interactions between hormones, in lung differentiation. This knowledge may eventually lead to a better therapeutic means of preventing RDS in premature infants.

ACKNOWLEDGEMENTS

Portions of this work were supported by Grant HL-24075-01 from the National Heart, Lung and Blood Institute. Recent studies on thyroid hormone binding were done in collaboration with L. Gonzales.

References

Avery ME 1975 Pharmacologic approaches to the acceleration of fetal lung maturation. Br Med Bull 31:13

Ballard PL 1979 Glucocorticoids and differentiation. In: Baxter JD, Rousseau GG (eds) Monographs on endocrinology, vol 12. Springer-Verlag, Berlin, p 493

Ballard PL, Ballard RA 1972 Glucocorticoid receptor and the role of glucocorticoids in fetal lung development. Proc Natl Acad Sci USA 69:2688

Ballard PL, Ballard RA 1974 Cytoplasmic receptor for glucocorticoids in lung of the human fetus and neonate. J Clin Invest 53:477

Ballard PL, Ballard RA 1979 Corticosteroids and respiratory distress syndrome: status 1979. Pediatrics 63:163

Ballard PL, Granberg P, Ballard RA 1975a Glucocorticoid levels in maternal and cord serum after prenatal betamethasone therapy to prevent respiratory distress syndrome. J Clin Invest 56:1548

Ballard PL, Carter JP, Graham BS, Baxter JD 1975b A radioreceptor assay for evaluation of the plasma glucocorticoid activity of natural and synthetic steroids in man. J Clin Endocrinol Metab 41:290

Ballard PL, Benson BJ, Brehier A 1977 Glucocorticoid effects in fetal lung. Am Rev Respir Dis 115:29

Ballard PL, Mason RJ, Douglas WHJ 1978a Glucocorticoid binding by isolated lung cells. Endocrinology 102:1570

Ballard PL, Gluckman PD, Brehier A, Kitterman JA, Kaplan SL, Rudolph AM, Grumbach MM 1978b Failure to detect an effect of prolactin on pulmonary surfactant and adrenal steroids in fetal sheep and rabbits. J Clin Invest 62:879

Ballard PL, Gluckman PD, Liggins GC, Kaplan SL, Grumbach MM 1980a Steroid and growth hormone levels in premature infants after prenatal betamethasone therapy to prevent respiratory distress syndrome. Pediatr Res 14:122

Ballard PL, Benson BJ, Brehier A, Carter JP, Kriz BM, Jorgensen EC 1980b Transplacental stimulation of lung development in the fetal rabbit by 3,5-dimethyl-3′-isopropyl-L-thyronine. J Clin Invest 65:1407

Blackburn WR, Travers H, Potter DM 1972 The role of the pituitary–adrenal–thyroid axes in lung differentiation. I. Studies of the cytology and physical properties of anencephalic fetal rat lung. Lab Invest 26:306

Blackburn WR, Kelly JS, Dickman PS, Travers H, Lopata MA, Rhodes RA 1973 The role of the pituitary–adrenal–thyroid axes in lung differentiation. II. Biochemical studies of developing lung in anencephalic fetal rats. Lab Invest 28:352

Block M, Kling O, Crosby W 1977 Antenatal glucocorticoid therapy for the prevention of RDS in the premature infant. Obstet Gynecol 50:186

Brehier A, Benson BJ, Williams MC, Mason RJ, Ballard PL 1977 Corticosteroid induction of phosphatidic acid phosphatase in fetal rabbit lung. Biochem Biophys Res Commun 77:883

Buckingham S, McNary WF, Sommers SC, Rothschild J 1968 Is lung an analogue of Moog's developing intestine? I. Phosphatases and pulmonary alveolar differentiation in fetal rabbits. Fed Proc 27:328 (abstr)

Chiswick ML, Ahmed A, Jack PMB, Milner RDG 1973 Control of fetal lung development in the rabbit. Arch Dis Child 48:709

Comite F, Burrow GN, Jorgensen EC 1978 Thyroid hormone analogs and fetal goiter. Endocrinology 102:1670

Corbet AJ, Flax P, Alstan C, Rudolph AJ 1978 Effect of aminophylline and dexamethasone on secretion of pulmonary surfactant in fetal rabbits. Pediatr Res 12:797

Cuestas RA, Lindall A, Engel RR 1976 Low thyroid hormones and respiratory distress syndrome of the newborn. Studies on cord blood. N Engl J Med 295:297

Erenberg A, Rhodes ML, Weinstein MM, Kennedy RL 1979 Effect of fetal thyroidectomy on ovine fetal lung maturation. Pediatr Res 13:230
Farrell PM, Blackburn WR, Adam AJ 1977 Lung phosphatidylcholine synthesis and choline-phosphotransferase activity in anencephalic rat fetuses with corticosteroid deficiency. Pediatr Res 11:770
Fedrick J, Butler NR 1972 Hyaline membrane disease. (Letter). Lancet 2:768
Fisher DA, Dussalt JG, Sack J, Chopra IH 1977 Ontogenesis of hypothalamic–pituitary–thyroid function and metabolism in man, sheep and rat. Recent Prog Horm Res 33:59
Fletcher BD, Masson M, Lisbona A, Riggs T, Papageorgiou AN 1979 Thymic response to endogenous and exogenous steroids in premature newborn infants. J Pediatr 95:111
Giannopoulos G 1973 Glucorticoid receptors in lung. I. Specific binding of glucocorticoids to cytoplasmic components of rabbit fetal lung. J Biol Chem 248:3876
Giannopoulos G, Mulay S, Solomon S 1972 Cortisol receptors in rabbit fetal lung. Biochem Biophys Res Commun 47:411
Giannopoulos G, Mulay S, Solomon S 1973 Glucocorticoid receptors in lung. II. Specific binding of glucocorticoids to nuclear components of rabbit fetal lung. J Biol Chem 248:5016
Gluck L, Kulovich MV 1974 The evaluation of functional maturity in the human fetus. In: Gluck L (ed) Modern perinatal medicine. Chicago Year Book Medical Publishers, Chicago, p 195-207
Granberg PJ, Ballard PL 1977 Role of sulfhydryl groups in the binding of glucocorticoids by cytoplasmic receptors of lung and other mammalian tissues. Endocrinology 100:1160
Kitterman J, Liggins G, Campos G, Forster C, Creasy R 1979 Hormonal factors in lung maturation in fetal lambs. Pediatr Res 13:537 (abstr)
Kotas RV 1973 Accelerated pulmonary surfactant after intrauterine infection in the fetal rabbit. Pediatrics 51:655
Kriz BM, Jones AL, Jorgensen EC 1978 Effects of a thyroid hormone analog on fetal rat hepatocyte ultrastructure and microsomal function. Endocrinology 102:712
Liggins GC 1969 Premature delivery of foetal lambs infused with glucocorticoids. J Endocrinol 45:515
Liggins GC, Howie RN 1972 A controlled trial of antepartum glucocorticoid treatment for prevention of the respiratory distress syndrome in premature infants. Pediatrics 50:515
Liggins GC, Howie RN 1974 The prevention of RDS by maternal steroid therapy. In: Gluck L (ed) Modern perinatal medicine. Chicago Year Book Medical Publishers, Chicago, p 415-424
Lindenberg JA, Brehier A, Ballard PL 1978 Triiodothyronine nuclear binding in fetal and adult rabbit lung and cultured lung cells. Endocrinology 103:1725
Mashiach S, Barkai G, Sack J, Stern E, Bush M, Goldman B, Serr DM 1979 The effect of intraamniotic thyroxine administration on fetal lung maturity in man. J Perinat Med 7:161
Mescher EJ, Platzker ACG, Ballard PL, Kitterman JA, Clements JA, Tooley WH 1975 Ontogeny of tracheal fluid, pulmonary surfactant, and plasma corticoids in the fetal lamb. J Appl Physiol 39:1017
Meyrick B, Bearn JG, Cobb AG, Monkhouse CR, Reid L 1975 The effect of *in utero* decapitation on the morphologic and physiologic development of the fetal rabbit lung. J Anat 119:517
Morishige WK, Guernsey DL 1978 Triiodothyronine receptors in rat lung. Endocrinology 102:1628
Murphy BEP 1973 Does the human fetal adrenal play a role in parturition? Am J Obstet Gynecol 115:521
Murphy BEP 1974 Cortisol and cortisone levels in the cord blood at delivery of infants with and without the respiratory distress syndrome. Am J Obstet Gynecol 119:112
Murphy BEP 1978a Conjugated glucocorticoids in amniotic fluid and fetal lung maturation. J Clin Endocrinol Metab 47:212
Murphy BEP 1978b Cortisol production and inactivation by the human lung during gestation and infancy. J Clin Endocrinol Metab 47:243

Naeye RL, Harcke HT, Blanc WA 1971 Adrenal gland structure and the development of hyaline membrane disease. Pediatrics 47:650
Nielsen HC, Torday JS, Fencl M, Avery ME 1979 Sex differences in human fetal lung maturation. Pediatr Res 13:361 (abstr)
Nelson GH, Eguchi K, McPherson JC 1976 Effect of gestational age, dexamethasone and metopirone on lecithin concentration in fetal lung tissue and amniotic fluid in rats and guinea pigs. Gynecol Invest 7:337
Nicholas TE, Kim PA 1975 The metabolism of ^{3}H-cortisone and ^{3}H-cortisol by isolated perfused rat and guinea pig lungs. Steroids 25:387
Nicholas TE, Johnson RG, Lugg MA, Kim PA 1978 Pulmonary phospholipid biosynthesis and the ability of the fetal rabbit lung to reduce cortisone to cortisol during the final 10 days of gestation. Life Sci 22:1517
Platzker ACG, Lew CD, Ballard PL, Landing B, Freshman K, Lewis A 1976 Delayed secretion of pulmonary surfactant into tracheal fluid in fetal lambs with hydranencephaly. Clin Res 24:198A (abstr)
Possmayer F, Casola P, Chan F, Hill S, Metcalfe IL, Stewart-Dehaan PJ, Wong T, Heras JL, Gammal EB, Harding PGR 1979 Glucocorticoid induction of pulmonary maturation in the rabbit fetus. The effect of maternal injection of betamethasone on the activity of enzymes in fetal lung. Biochim Biophys Acta 574:197
Redding RR, Pereira C 1974 Thyroid function in respiratory distress syndrome (RDS) of the newborn. Pediatrics 54:423
Rooney SA, Gross I, Gassenheimer LN, Motoyama EK 1975 Stimulation of glycerolphosphate phosphatidyltransferase activity in fetal rabbit lung by cortisol administration. Biochim Biophys Acta 398:433
Rooney SA, Gobran LI, Marino PA, Maniscalco WM, Gross I 1979 Effects of betamethasone on phospholipid content, composition and biosynthesis in fetal rabbit lung. Biochim Biophys Acta 572:64
Smith BT, Torday JS, Giroud CJP 1973 The growth promoting effect of cortisol on human fetal lungs. Steroids 22:515
Smith BT, Torday JS 1974 Factors affecting lecithin synthesis by fetal lung cells in culture. Pediatr Res 8:848
Tanswell AK, Smith BT 1978 The relationship of amniotic membrane 11-oxidoreductase activity to lung maturation in the human fetus. Pediatr Res 12:957
Tanswell AK, Worthington D, Smith BT 1977 Human amniotic membrane corticosteroid 11-oxidoreductase activity. J Clin Endocrinol Metab 45:721
Vidyasagur D, Chernick V 1975 Effect of metopirone on the synthesis of lung surfactant in does and fetal rabbits. Biol Neonate 27:1
Wu B, Kikkawa Y, Orzalesi MM, Motoyama EK, Kaibara M, Zigas CJ, Cook CD 1973 The effect of thyroxin on the maturation of fetal rabbit lungs. Biol Neonate 22:161

Discussion

Vane: Is lung surfactant ingested by macrophages?

Ballard: It is to some extent, although Scarpelli et al (1975) reported that fatty acids derived from alveolar surfactant can enter the pulmonary circulation in fetal sheep. This suggests that fatty acids from fetal lung fluid may be re-utilized for synthesis of surfactant.

Vane: You say that glucocorticoids increase phospholipids, and Dr Flower has shown that steroids prevent phospholipase A_2 activity. Is it simply that phospholipids are being protected in your studies?

Ballard: It appears certain that corticosteroids increase the biosynthetic rate of phosphatidylcholine, from the stimulation of specific enzymes and the rate of choline incorporation. So we definitely have a synthetic component to the steroid effect, but it's not known what happens in regard to degradation.

Vane: We have heard two stories about corticosteroid receptors in the lungs. How do we know that your receptors are doing what you think they are, and Dr Flower's are doing what he says they are?

Ballard: Receptors may mediate many different effects, of course. Most tissues are influenced by glucocorticoids and most tissues contain receptors. The receptors appear to be identical in various target tissues, with the apparent exception of guinea-pig tissues, despite the fact that the biological effects of glucocorticoids are different in different tissues. All steroid effects in fetal lung are consistent with mediation by receptor.

Woods: You showed a good agreement in time between the decrease in glycogen and the increase in phospholipid. Is this decrease in glycogen accompanied by an increase in glycolysis? You would need increased glycolysis to provide one of the substrates for lipid synthesis. In other organs it has been suggested that one of the important functions of glycolysis is as a limiting factor in lipid synthesis through the provision of α-glycerophosphate (Woods & Krebs 1971). Our calculations show good agreement between rates of glycolysis in liver and rates of lipid synthesis; it would be interesting to see whether at the time glycogen stores are rapidly falling in the lung there is an increase in glycolysis.

Ballard: The rate of glucose uptake and lactate production is high in fetal lung compared to the postnatal lung (Hamosh et al 1978); however, as far as I know, the developmental pattern during late fetal life has not been examined.

Stubbs: We also wondered about this, and put forward a hypothesis suggesting that substrate provision may limit phospholipid and surfactant production in certain situations (Stubbs & Stubbs 1978). Does, for example, enzyme induction entirely explain the effects of glucocorticoids on surfactant production, or is there an effect on substrate availability and disposal? Have you looked at the effects of steroids in isolated cells when various concentrations of different substrates are used?

Ballard: No, but Gross & Rooney (1977) have used organ culture of fetal lung to look at the effects of various hormones. They used a high glucose level, but have not varied the level nor, to my knowledge, tried other substrates.

Alberti: This is one of the intriguing things about T_3, which alters the handling of glycerol in liver; it could be making a major difference to substrate supply.

Ballard: Thyroid hormone depletes liver glycogen as well, decreasing the content by about 75% in two days. So an influence of these hormones on substrate levels is certainly likely.

Stubbs: There is some suggestion from morphological studies that T_3 and glucocorticoids cooperate in increasing surfactant production (Hitchcock 1979).

Ballard: This is also implied by our studies, which suggest different biochemical sites of action of glucocorticoids and 3,5-dimethyl-3′-isopropyl-L-thyronine. We are now examining the question of possible permissive or additive effects of these hormones.

Collier: Corticosteroids benefit the respiratory distress syndrome and increase surfactant production. Dr Flower has told us that corticosteroids inhibit prostaglandin synthesis in intact cells. I should like to suggest that there is a relationship between these effects of corticosteroids. The blood plasma of the newborn baby has high levels of E and F prostaglandins, which decline rather quickly during the first month (Mitchell et al 1978a). In premature babies a relatively high level of PGE is associated with patent ductus arteriosus and a high level of PGF with hyaline membrane disease (Lucas & Mitchell 1978a, Mitchell et al 1978b, Turnbull et al 1980). Hence, if steroids lowered levels of these prostaglandins in plasma they would be expected to benefit respiratory distress in neonates. We know that indomethacin gives some benefit in such conditions (Lucas & Mitchell 1978b, Turnbull et al 1980).

Ballard: I included indomethacin in the list of compounds reported to delay fetal lung development (Table 1, p 252). Bustos et al (1978) found less phospholipid in lung wash after indomethacin, but fetal corticoid levels were also decreased. Indomethacin did affect surfactant production in experiments with fetal sheep (J. Kitterman, personal communication 1979).

Collier: It is well established that indomethacin benefits some respiratory problems in premature babies (Turnbull et al 1980).

Ballard: Premature babies benefit from indomethacin not because of a direct effect on RDS but because it helps to close the patent ductus arteriosus, apparently by inhibiting formation of PGE_2 (Clyman et al 1980).

Meyrick: In collaboration with Dr L. Pang and Dr S.A. Stalcup we have recently looked at the lung structure of fetal rabbits whose mothers had been given betamethasone. We have found that the areal density of capillaries is increased above that in control, 24-day fetuses.

We have also looked at the lung structure of fetuses from alloxan-diabetic does (I. Sosenko & B. Meyrick, unpublished observations 1980). As one might expect, we find an overall retardation of lung development, but in the type II cells, while we find a normal number of lamellated bodies and these are of normal size, the majority also contain 10 times the amount of glycogen and 2.5 times the amount of rough endoplasmic reticulum as the control fetuses at 27.5 days. There is also a significant increase (30%) in the areal density of the capillary compartment in the 'alloxan' fetuses compared with controls. This is consistent with previous findings of delayed functional maturation without accompanying change in disaturated phosphatidylcholine levels and lecithin/sphingomyelin ratio (Sosenko et al 1980).

The exciting feature here is the anomaly in vessel maturation. One of the important developmental phases with thinning of the alveolar wall is that the capillary migrates to the epithelium, followed by fusion of the basement membrane and a characteristic jutting of the capillary wall into the alveolar space. It seems to be this process that is delayed in the 'alloxan' fetus.

Woods: Is there any pathological information about the relatively rare occurrence of hyperthyroidism or hypothyroidism in the neonate?

Reid: A few cases of hypothyroidism have been reported: I have seen two. In hypothyroidism one does not see the normal thinning of the alveolar septa. In one child, in whom a diagnosis of hypothyroidism was made in the first weeks of life, thyroid hormone treatment led to clinical improvement in the respiratory symptoms. (This case did not have RDS.)

Ballard: One report (D.W. Smith et al 1975) described several cases of RDS among infants with congenital hypothyroidism who were delivered at 36 or more weeks' gestation. RDS is very uncommon among normal infants near term.

Stalcup: We observed that the rabbit in the final third of fetal life has little converting enzyme activity in the lung; in association with the increase in capillary volume density in corticosteroid-treated fetal lung we showed a rapid maturation of converting-enzyme activity. We think this is important, because a variety of vasoactive phenomena, including lower blood pressure, increased coagulation, decreased serum proteins and increased oedema, are associated with RDS and can't be explained by surfactant deficiency alone.

At birth, the lungs become a target organ for many circulating vasoactive substances including catecholamines, probably angiotensin II, and certainly bradykinin, when the pulmonary circulation is established. Can you speculate about the possible role of failure of development of receptors for circulating vasoactive hormones, or failure of the development of the lung as a target organ at the time of birth, in relation to RDS?

Ballard: Are you asking about the aetiology of RDS and whether those vasoactive substances are involved? It is certainly possible that they play a role in development of the disease. However, I am attracted to the concept that the primary cause of RDS is hormonal deficiency. There is evidence that infants with RDS may have reduced cord blood levels of cortisol (Murphy 1974), and lower T_3 and T_4 levels at birth are also associated with RDS (Redding & Pereira 1974, Cuestas et al 1976). It is likely that the interaction of several hormones is involved in normal lung maturation, but certainly, from studies in animals, a deficiency of cortisol would be expected to retard lung maturation.

Said: What is the common thread between all the different agents that accelerate lung maturation (Table 1, p 252)? You listed heroin, corticosteroids, epidermal growth factor and several others. Heroin itself can produce pulmonary oedema and lung damage, yet babies of women who take heroin have a lower incidence of RDS than those of normal women. What does heroin do to the fetal lung?

Ballard: The mechanism by which heroin acts here is not known. It may fall into the category of prenatal stress, perhaps secondary to repeated episodes of withdrawal symptoms *in utero*. Gluck & Kulovich (1974) proposed that a variety of chronically stressful circumstances during pregnancy, such as maternal hypertension, accelerate lung maturation. The L/S ratio (an index of surfactant in amniotic fluid) matures more quickly in these situations. The idea is that, in response to the stress, the fetus produces more cortisol and stimulates its lung development.

Morishige: Insulin has been shown to antagonize glucocorticoids in fetal lung. B.T. Smith et al (1975), using cultured fetal rabbit lung cells in which choline incorporation was stimulated by cortisol, found that insulin at concentrations of 25 and 100 μU/ml abolished the cortisol effects. Insulin alone had no substantial effect on the rate of choline incorporation, so it seemed to be a reversal of the effect of cortisol.

Ballard: This is indeed an interesting possibility for the action of insulin, and further studies are indicated.

Reid: To add to the receptors that could be important before birth, Nielsen et al (1979) have shown that there really is earlier maturation of the female fetal rabbit lung. It had been shown that human male babies are more susceptible to RDS. This difference in maturation rate has also been shown in rabbits, within the same litter (Kotas & Avery 1980).

Ballard: We have looked at the influence of gender on the efficacy of prenatally administered betamethasone in preventing RDS. In small infants (750–1250 g) the incidence of RDS is very high in untreated males (84%) and decreases to 22% ($P < 0.001$) with treatment, while in females the respective values are 59% and 18% ($P < 0.001$). So both sexes in this weight group benefit from treatment. In older infants (1250–1750 g) the incidence of RDS was 35% in untreated males as against 41% (not significant) in treated males, indicating no apparent benefit; betamethasone remained effective in female infants (35% versus 7%, $P = 0.04$). A similar sex difference has been observed by Taeusch & Tulchinsky (1979). The mechanism of the apparent male disadvantage with treatment is unclear. We have determined that cord serum levels of betamethasone are similar in treated male and female infants, suggesting that there are no sex differences in either the placental transfer or metabolism of betamethasone.

Aiken: When you talk about accelerated maturation of cells, tissues or capillaries, is this the same as cell differentiation?

Ballard: Certainly. We are talking about the normal developmental pattern, or differentiation if you like, of lung cells during fetal life. As part of that pattern the epithelial cells lose glycogen, make more phospholipids, develop lamellar bodies and secrete surfactant. Steroids accelerate this differentiation in epithelial cells and probably affect maturation of other lung cells as well.

Aiken: So the rate of differentiation has changed.

Ballard: Yes: with glucocorticoid treatment there is an increased rate of differentiation which results in more mature cells at any given time.

Reid: If you are looking at biochemical measures such as surfactant activity or L/S ratio you can think of a programme that is delayed, but when you look at structure the picture is more complex. There is a dysmaturity, with an uneven pattern of change. In alloxan diabetes, for example, the number of lamellar bodies within the type II cells gives a normal count, but the pattern of the capillaries is not normal. In another model pattern that we looked at there was the normal number of lamellar bodies but half of them were 'immature', being too small (Meyrick et al 1975). The more closely you analyse the morphological picture the more necessary it is to make a fairly sophisticated list of criteria for maturation.

Burri: Even if you see the usual number of granules or lamellar bodies you don't know from the static picture whether they are actually secreted or not.

Mellins: Administration of corticosteroids may have profound effects on cell growth postnatally. Corticosteroid treatment before birth may enhance maturation of the type II cells with the production of enough surfactant to avoid neonatal RDS, but do we know what effect prenatal administration of corticosteroids has on ultimate cell growth and maturation of the lung and brain? Is the price paid for accelerated lung cell maturation, fewer cells in the lung and in the brain?

Reid: In normal lung development there is a stage of maximum growth or cell division but then a stage of slowing of cell multiplication with a switch to differentiation or maturation. Some clinical cases, and some experimental studies, support the idea that one is at the expense of the other. If lung matures before its complement of cells is complete the lung may be small but, in terms of surfactant production, functionally mature. The babies of heroin addicts tend to be very small, but they have 'mature' lungs in that they do not develop RDS. There are an increasing number of cases where growth in the sense of size and weight has been hindered but a functional maturation exists which seems to protect from some problems, although perhaps not from others (Rendas et al 1980).

Bakhle: Do corticosteroids have any effect on surfactant production and phospholipid turnover in the adult lung?

Ballard: Abe & Tierney (1977) showed that treatment of adult rats with hydrocortisone for seven days increased both the rate of synthesis and tissue content of saturated phosphatidylcholine. Whether there is a physiological role for cortisol in the adult lung is unknown, but it seems unlikely.

Herbaczyńska-Cedro: You mentioned the decreased incidence of intracranial haemorrhage in infants treated with corticosteroids. Some time ago we investigated the effect of hydrocortisone on the release of prostaglandins from the brain, induced by various injurious agents in dogs. It suppressed PG release (Herbaczyńska-Cedro et al 1978). Is there any link between this finding and your observation of a decreased incidence of intracranial haemorrhage?

Ballard: It has been postulated that the stress of RDS *per se* causes haemorrhage, or that therapy for RDS (the application of positive pressure, mechanical ventilation, infusion of fluids, perhaps hypovolaemia) predisposes to intracranial bleeding, or both; so there is an association between bleeding and RDS. Apparently by reducing the incidence of RDS with steroids we have also lowered the incidence of intracranial bleeding. So I don't think a prostaglandin mechanism needs to be invoked.

References

Abe M, Tierney DF 1977 Lung lipid metabolism after 7 days of hydrocortisone administration to adult rats. J Appl Physiol Respirat Exercise Physiol 42:202-205

Bustos R, Ballejo G, Giussi G, Rosas R, Isa JC 1978 Inhibition of fetal lung maturation by indomethacin in pregnant rabbits. J Perinat Med 6:240-245

Clyman RI, Mauray F, Rudolph AM, Heymann MA 1980 Age-dependent sensitivity of the lamb ductus arteriosus to indomethacin and prostaglandins. J Pediatr Res 96:94-98

Cuestas RA, Lindall A, Engel RR 1976 Low thyroid hormones and respiratory distress syndrome of the newborn. Studies on cord blood. N Engl J Med 295:297

Gluck L, Kulovich MV 1974 The evaluation of functional maturity in the human fetus. In: Gluck L (ed) Modern perinatal medicine. Chicago Year Book Medical Publishers, Chicago, p 195-207

Gross I, Rooney SA 1977 Aminophylline stimulates the incorporation of choline into phospholipid in explants of fetal rat lung in organ culture. Biochim Biophys Acta 488:263-269

Hamosh M, Schechter Y, Hamosh P 1978 Metabolic activity of developing rabbit lung. Pediatr Res 12:95-100

Herbaczyńska-Cedro K, Truskolaski P, Ruszczewski P 1978 Inhibitory effect of hydrocortisone on the release of prostaglandins from dog's brain in hypoxia and cerebral embolism. Acta Physiol Pol (Engl Transl) 29:501-507

Hitchcock KR 1979 Hormones and the lung. I. Thyroid hormones and glucocorticoids in lung development. Anat Rec 194:15-40

Kotas RV, Avery ME 1980 The influence of sex on fetal rabbit lung maturation and on the response to glucocorticoid. Am Rev Respir Dis 121:377-380

Lucas A, Mitchell MD 1978a Prostaglandins in patent ductus arteriosus. Lancet 2:937-938

Lucas A, Mitchell MD 1978b Plasma prostaglandins in pre-term neonates before and after treatment for patent ductus arteriosus. Lancet 2:130-132

Meyrick B, Bearn JG, Cobb AG, Monkhouse CR, Reid L 1975 The effect of *in utero* decapitation on the morphological development of the fetal rabbit lung. J Anat 119:517-535

Mitchell MD, Lucas A, Etches P, Brunt J, Turnbull AC 1978a Plasma prostaglandin levels during early neonatal life following term and preterm delivery. Prostaglandins 16:319-326

Mitchell MD, Lucas A, Whitfield M, Brunt JD, Turnbull AC 1978b Selective elevation of prostaglandin concentrations in hyaline membrane disease in pre-term infants. Prostaglandins & Med 1:207-212

Murphy BEP 1974 Cortisol and cortisone levels in the cord blood at delivery of infants with and without the respiratory distress syndrome. Am J Obstet Gynecol 119:112

Nielsen HC, Torday JS, Fencl M, Avery ME 1979 Sex differences in human fetal lung maturation. Pediatr Res 13:361

Redding RR, Pereira C 1974 Thyroid function in respiratory distress syndrome (RDS) of the newborn. Pediatrics 54:423

Rendas A, Brown E, Avery ME, Reid LM 1980 Prematurity, hypoplasia of the pulmonary vascular bed and hypertension: its fatal outcome in a ten month old infant. Am Rev Respir Dis 121:873

Scarpelli EM, Condorelli S, Colacicco G, Cosni EV 1975 Lamb fetal pulmonary fluid. II. Fate of phosphatidylcholine. Pediatr Res 9:195-201

Smith BT, Giroud CJP, Robert M, Avery ME 1975 Insulin antagonism of cortisol action on lecithin synthesis by cultured fetal lung cells. J Pediatr 87:953-955

Smith DW, Klein AM, Henderson JR, Myrianthopoulos NC 1975 Congenital hypothyroidism—signs and symptoms in the newborn period. J Pediatr 87:958-962

Sosenko IRS, Lawson EE, Demottaz V, Frantz ID III 1980 Functional delay in lung maturation in fetuses of diabetic mothers. J Appl Physiol 48:643

Stubbs WA, Stubbs SM 1978 Hyperinsulinism, diabetes mellitus, and respiratory distress syndrome of the newborn: a common link? Lancet 1:308-309

Taeusch HW Jr, Tulchinsky D 1979 Obstetric factors affecting risk of respiratory distress syndrome. In: Premature labor. Mead Johnson Symposium on Perinatal and Developmental Medicine no. 15. Vail, Colorado, June 3-7

Turnbull AC, Lucas A, Mitchell MD 1980 Prostaglandins in the perinatal period. Rev Perinat Med 4, in press

Woods HF, Krebs HA 1971 Lactate production in the perfused rat liver. Biochem J 125:129-139

Pulmonary angiotensin-converting enzyme and its inhibition: a historical survey

Y.S. BAKHLE

Department of Pharmacology, Institute of Basic Medical Sciences, Royal College of Surgeons of England, Lincoln's Inn Fields, London WC2A 3PN, UK

Abstract Angiotensin-converting enzyme, the peptidase hydrolysing angiotensin I to angiotensin II and first discovered in plasma, has been demonstrated in lung tissue on the luminal surface of endothelial cells lining pulmonary blood vessels. Because converting enzyme is the final activating step in the renin–angiotensin system its inhibition prevents the pressor and other effects of increased renin secretion. Lung converting enzyme activity is inhibited specifically by a nonapeptide (BPP_{9a}:SQ 20 881) contained in *Bothrops jararaca* venom. This peptide inhibits the pressor effects of injected angiotensin I in humans and lowers blood pressure in patients with high-renin hypertension. Recently a synthetic inhibitor, captopril, was devised which is effective, given orally, in reducing the blood pressure of high-renin hypertensives and of a proportion of hypertensives with normal renin levels. The latter finding suggests that blood pressure may be maintained by renin-dependent mechanisms without increased renin secretion.

Angiotensin-converting enzyme, or dipeptidyl carboxypeptidase (peptidyldipeptide hydrolase, EC 3.4.15.1), a peptidase hydrolysing the decapeptide angiotensin I to the octapeptide angiotensin II, was first found by Skeggs and his colleagues in horse blood (Skeggs et al 1954). Because angiotensin I and angiotensin II were equipotent as pressor agents *in vivo,* the action of converting enzyme was understandably described as leaving that portion of the peptides responsible for their pressor effect unchanged. Thus this was a biochemically interesting enzyme but not one of direct physiological significance. This conclusion was almost immediately challenged by Hellmer (1955) who showed that angiotensin I was inactive *in vitro* until incubated with plasma, when it became equipotent with angiotensin II. Confirmation of this finding by Skeggs' group followed (Skeggs et al 1956) and it was soon realized that converting enzyme was indeed the final activating step in the renin–angiotensin system (Fig. 1). Even if the more recent suggestion of a physiological role for the heptapeptide angiotensin III (see Goodfriend &

© Excerpta Medica 1980
Metabolic activities of the lung
(Ciba Foundation symposium 78) p 275-292

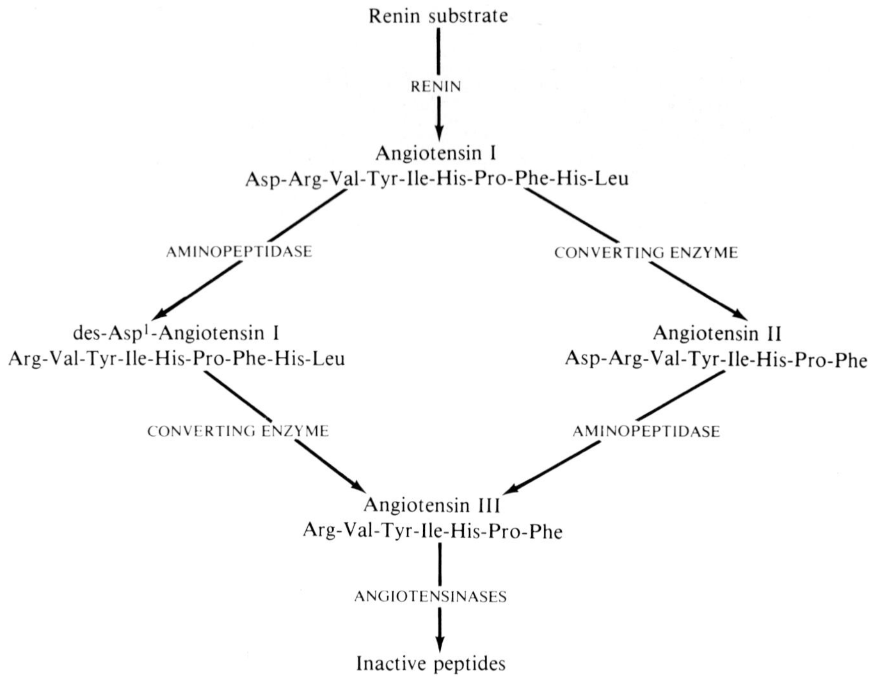

FIG. 1. The renin–angiotensin system. Significant biological activity (vasoconstriction, aldosterone release, etc.) is shown only by angiotensins II and III.

Peach 1975) is finally substantiated, converting enzyme will still play an essential role in the formation of this peptide.

The next chapter in the story of this enzyme concerned its location. The enzyme had been found in the blood of many species and this circulating enzyme was considered to be the physiologically important angiotensin-converting activity. However, in 1967, Ng and Vane found, in the pulmonary circulation, angiotensin-converting activity well in excess of the plasma activity (Fig. 2). They concluded that either some factor had activated the blood converting enzyme while in the pulmonary circulation or, a more likely alternative, cells in the lung had particularly high converting-enzyme activity of their own. Earlier, Ferreira & Vane (1967) had observed a particularly high degree of inactivation of bradykinin, another peptide hormone, in the pulmonary circulation, so the idea of highly active peptidases in the lung was not without precedent.

The conversion of angiotensin I to angiotensin II in the pulmonary circulation has since been amply confirmed by a number of different techniques in

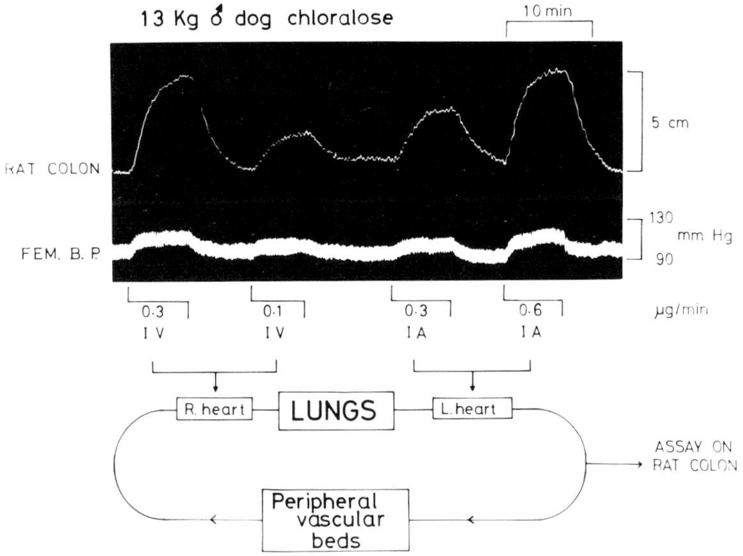

FIG. 2. Increase in activity of angiotensin I on passage through the pulmonary circulation *in vivo*. This tracing shows the responses of a rat isolated colon superfused with femoral arterial blood from a dog and the dog's blood pressure. Angiotensin I was infused as shown either into the right ventricle (i.v.) or the ascending aorta (i.a.). Comparing the first and third responses, an infusion of 0.3 μg/min given i.v. was more effective than the same amount infused i.a. The effects of the angiotensin I that had passed through the pulmonary circulation (0.3 μg/min i.v.) were equivalent to those of twice the infusion (0.6 μg/min) given i.a. (From Ng & Vane 1967 with permission.)

many species including man (for references see Vane 1974). Because the pulmonary enzyme activity was higher than that of blood, the lung became the most physiologically important site of angiotensin I conversion in the body. This is not to say that the pulmonary circulation is the only site of conversion: later work showed conversion in other vascular beds, for instance, arm (Collier & Robinson 1974) and mesentery (Di Salvo & Montefusco 1971), but it still is the only vascular bed to 'export' angiotensin II – that is, to show a net increase in biological activity. In other vascular beds angiotensin II is largely inactivated, so any angiotensin I converted to angiotensin II in these beds is inactivated before it can emerge in the venous effluent, thus leading to an overall inactivation of angiotensin I (Hodge et al 1967, Aiken & Vane 1972).

The conclusions of Ng & Vane (1967) on the intrinsic activity of the cells in the lung were also soon confirmed. Isolated lungs perfused with physiological salt solutions (thus eliminating the blood converting activity) converted angiotensin I to angiotensin II (Fig. 3) and also inactivated bradykinin (Bakhle et al 1969, Ryan et al 1968).

The high levels of converting enzyme activity in lung and the physiological importance of this enzyme combined to encourage several groups to investigate the biochemistry of the pulmonary enzyme. The first rather simple experiments (Bakhle 1968) showed the activity in lung homogenates to be concentrated in a particulate fraction. Several groups have now solubilized and purified this activity to homogeneity (see Soffer 1976). Many of the biochemical properties – K_m, V_{max}, pH optima, ionic requirements – are now known for pulmonary converting enzyme from a number of species. One finding of particular importance was that the purified enzyme also hydrolysed bradykinin (Dorer et al 1974). Thus, the simultaneous activation of angiotensin I and inactivation of bradykinin, already observed in the pulmonary circulation *in vivo,* was most probably due to the action of the same enzyme on the two substrates. This meant that the lung was adding a pressor agent and at the same time removing a depressor agent, acting, on balance, to increase systemic arterial blood pressure – a quasi-endocrine function of lung.

The important question of the location of converting enzyme within the

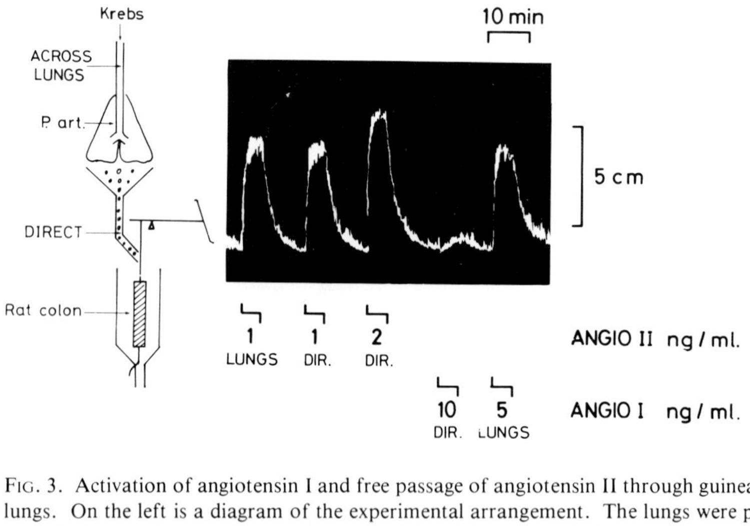

FIG. 3. Activation of angiotensin I and free passage of angiotensin II through guinea-pig isolated lungs. On the left is a diagram of the experimental arrangement. The lungs were perfused with Krebs' solution via the pulmonary artery and the effluent from the lungs superfused a rat isolated colon. The angiotensins were infused either below the lung (direct), or into the cannula in the pulmonary artery so that they passed through the pulmonary circulation before superfusing the assay tissue. The first two responses show that the activity of angiotensin II is unaffected by passage through the pulmonary circulation; that of angiotensin I (last two responses) greatly increased (5 ng/ml through the lungs causes a much greater response than twice that infusion, 10 ng/ml, made directly). (From Bakhle et al 1969 with permission.)

lung was answered soon after purification of the enzyme. Early suggestions that the enzyme was membrane bound, with ready access to blood-borne substrates (Bakhle 1968), had received indirect support; the matter was finally settled by the elegant work of the Ryans, using antibodies to the purified enzyme to locate it immunohistochemically, clearly and unequivocally on the luminal surface of the plasma membrane of endothelial cells in the pulmonary circulation (Ryan et al 1976; Fig. 4a). One of the corollaries of this locus is that Soffer's analysis of the composition of converting enzyme is in fact an analysis of a portion of a cell membrane (Soffer 1976).

Another corollary is that the amount of this enzyme in the pulmonary circulation is as vast as the area of the pulmonary capillaries. However, there is evidence (Ryan & Ryan 1977; Fig. 4b) that the endothelial cells do not form a flat smooth lining of the capillaries but that their surface is covered with projections of the membrane reminiscent of the microvilli of the intestinal epithelium. If this is so, clearly the surface area available for the enzyme may be much greater than that already estimated.

Angiotensin-converting activity is associated not only with pulmonary endothelial cells but with the endothelium of many other vascular beds (see Caldwell et al 1976, Ody & Junod 1977). However, the biological effects of angiotensin I conversion do appear to be greater in strips of pulmonary artery than in strips from any other arterial bed (Aiken & Vane 1970).

INHIBITION OF CONVERTING ENZYME

Another finding first described with the original crude dog lung preparation of converting enzyme (Bakhle 1968) and confirmed with the highly purified enzyme was its inhibition by peptides extracted from *Bothrops jararaca* venom (bradykinin-potentiating factor, BPF; Ferreira 1965). This report was followed by the purification, isolation and synthesis of the component peptides of BPF (Ferreira et al 1970, Ondetti et al 1971). Much of the subsequent work used the penta- and nonapeptides from this source, designated BPP_{5a} or SQ 20 475 and BPP_{9a} or SQ 20 881 respectively (Fig. 5). The results of all the experimental work confirmed the inhibition of angiotensin I conversion by these peptides in very low doses *in vitro,* in perfused lung and *in vivo.*

Furthermore, in animals with high blood pressure resulting from experimentally elevated concentrations of renin in blood, the administration of the nonapeptide BPP_{9a} reduced the blood pressure to normal levels (Krieger et al 1971, Miller et al 1972, Engel et al 1973). This is exactly what would be expected if the conversion of angiotensin I to angiotensin II were blocked by inhibition of converting enzyme.

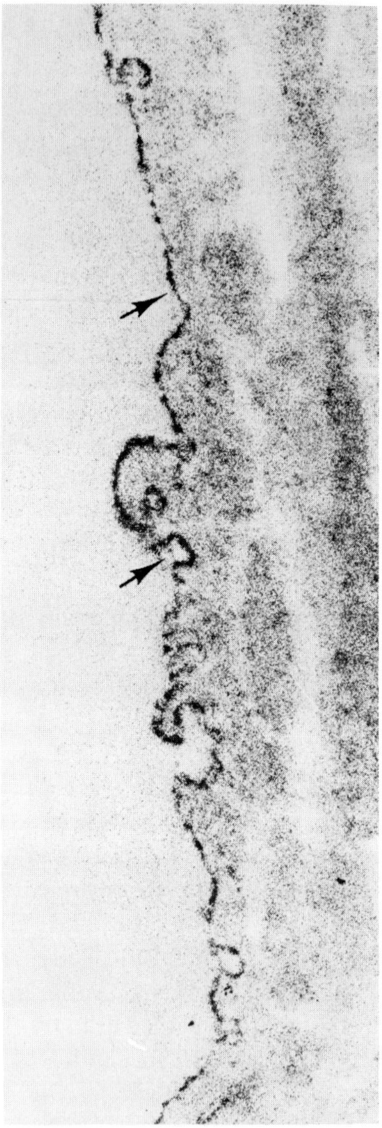

FIG. 4(a) Localization of converting enzyme on membrane of capillary endothelium of rat lung. The section of rat lung was incubated with antibody to converting enzyme coupled to microperoxidase and the immune complex was made electron-dense by reaction with diaminobenzidine and H_2O_2. The reaction product is located on the plasma membrane and caveolae facing the vascular lumen (arrows). × 116 280. (From Ryan et al 1976 with permission.)

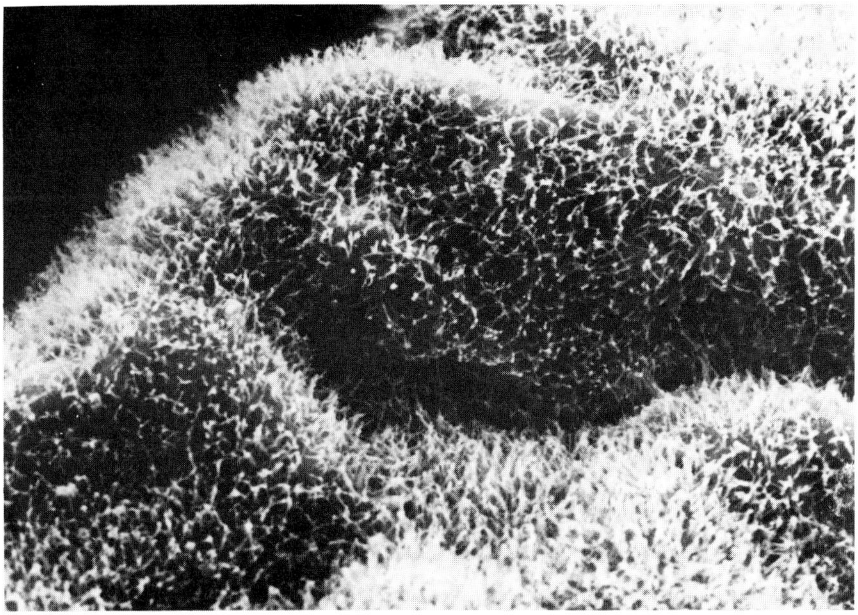

FIG. 4(b) Scanning electron micrograph of the luminal surface of endothelial cells of rat pulmonary artery. The cell surface is covered with a profuse array of finger-like projections. × 2870. (From Ryan & Ryan 1979 with permission.)

In man the nonapeptide was able to prevent increases in blood pressure consequent on the intravenous injection of angiotensin I in healthy volunteers (Collier et al 1973) without altering the pressor effects of injected angiotensin II – effects compatible with inhibition of converting activity without antagonism at the receptor for angiotensin II. This peptide did not affect resting blood pressure; that is, it lacked agonist activity at the angiotensin II receptor. This, coupled with its greater duration of action *in vivo,* favoured it over the angiotensin II antagonist, saralasin, as a method of blocking the effects of the renin–angiotensin system (see Gavras et al 1974, Williams 1977).

Although the efficacy of the nonapeptide in lowering blood pressure in high-renin hypertensives was demonstrated in a number of clinical studies the wider use of this inhibitor seemed unlikely, since it had to be given by injection and the cost of synthesizing a nonapeptide even by the newer methods available was clearly too high. What was needed was a chemically simpler inhibitor that was also effective after oral administration.

This need was met in 1977 with the report that a mercaptopropionic acid derivative of proline – captopril, SQ 14 225 (Fig. 5) – was a potent inhibitor

pyro-Glu-Lys-Trp-Ala-Pro
BPP_{5a} (SQ 20 475)

pyro-Glu-Trp-Pro-Arg-Pro-Gln-Ile-Pro-Pro
BPP_{9a} (SQ 20 881)

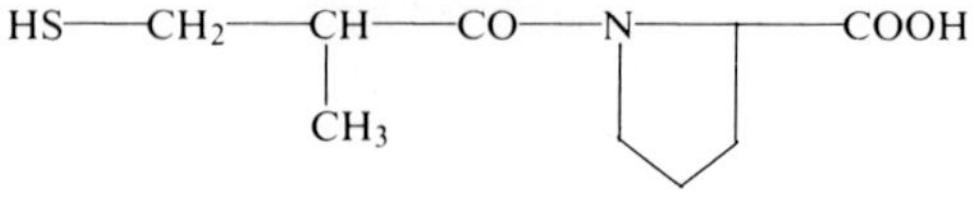

Captopril (SQ 14 225)

FIG. 5. Peptide inhibitors of converting enzyme. The upper two peptides are two of the naturally occurring peptides isolated from *B. jararaca* venom by Ferreira (1965) and later synthesized. The last (captopril) is an entirely synthetic compound. Pyro-Glu, pyroglutamic acid (pyrrolid-2-one-5-carboxylic acid).

of angiotensin I conversion in animals (Ondetti et al 1977) and in man (Ferguson et al 1977), after oral administration. It is important – not only for Cushman and Ondetti's sake, but for the sake of all those who endeavour to *design* drugs rather than to discover them by chance – to realize that this inhibitor of converting enzyme was the product of logical thought. Bearing in mind the probable mode of action of this enzyme (it is a carboxydipeptidase), its inability to hydrolyse peptide bonds involving the imino group of proline, and the structure of a known inhibitor of carboxypeptidase A, Cushman et al (1977) synthesized some simple carboxylic acid derivatives of proline, which, though less potent than captopril, were clearly inhibitors of converting enzyme. Logical development of the structure soon led to the synthesis of captopril and the vindication of their application of basic scientific principles to drug design.

This drug has since been investigated clinically in several countries as a treatment for renal hypertension and has generally been found to be as effective as the nonapeptide and more convenient to use. A recent survey (Atkinson & Robertson 1979) of the use of captopril has commented on the widespread interest in the drug and has welcomed its addition to the therapeutic repertoire.

Captopril is also useful, as was the nonapeptide (Case et al 1977), in treating a proportion of patients with essential hypertension and normal renin levels (see Atkinson & Robertson 1979). The early observation that the hypotensive effect of inhibiting converting enzyme was potentiated by diuretics (Gavras et al 1974) has been confirmed in a longer-term (eight months) treatment of essential hypertension with captopril and hydrochlorothiazide (Johnston et al 1979). This interaction between sodium depletion and the inhibitor can, if disregarded, lead to excessive falls in blood pressure (Atkinson et al 1979). A particularly interesting extension of this interaction has been the demonstration that, in sodium-depleted normotensive subjects, inhibition of converting enzyme impairs the homeostatic mechanisms maintaining blood pressure during tilting (Sancho et al 1976). Thus, although in normal, sodium-replete subjects the renin–angiotensin system seems not to be involved in the maintenance of blood pressure, the loss of sodium insufficient to alter resting blood pressure seems to call into use a renin-dependent mechanism to maintain pressure.

Two intriguing questions arise from this finding: first, how much sodium or volume depletion is needed for this switch to renin dependence? Is the depletion caused by sweating during exercise or heavy manual labour sufficient? The second, related question applies to those being treated with captopril: will they suffer excessive falls in blood pressure if they lose salt and water by sweating?

A further application of the use of converting enzyme inhibitors has been in congestive cardiac failure. The experimental work of Watkins et al (1976) using the nonapeptide in animals has been extended to patients with congestive heart failure treated conventionally (Gavras et al 1978). The results so far are encouraging though the mechanism of the beneficial action is not yet clear.

Since this enzyme also hydrolyses bradykinin, its inhibition implies an increase in circulating bradykinin levels as well as the demonstrable decrease in angiotensin II in blood. Such a change in bradykinin levels would be expected to contribute to the hypotensive effect of converting enzyme inhibition. This possibility has been suggested several times but, in the one study in which blood bradykinin concentrations were measured (Johnston et al 1979), no change was observed at a time when angiotensin II levels fell and angiotensin I levels rose after treatment with captopril. Although the original premise sounds reasonable, there are at least two reasons why it may not be so. Firstly, bradykinin is a better substrate for converting enzyme than is angiotensin I (K_m values of 4 μM and 30 μM respectively; Dorer et al 1974). This means that hydrolysis of angiotensin I would be inhibited more than that of bradykinin by a given amount of inhibitor. Thus extensive inhibition of angiotensin I conversion does not necessarily imply extensive inhibition of bradykinin. Secondly, and perhaps more importantly, whereas only converting enzyme will produce angiotensin II from angiotensin I, there are at least two other peptidases capable of hydrolysing bradykinin in the blood and in the lung and these peptidases are not affected by the inhibitors we have discussed (see Ferreira & Bakhle 1977). Thus, even with total inhibition of the bradykininase activity of converting enzyme there is a large reservoir of uninhibited alternative bradykininase activity. These theoretical modifications to the original simple premise coupled with the one practical result so far obtained make it less likely that inhibition of converting enzyme in these circumstances increases circulating bradykinin enough to contribute to the general hypotensive effect.

Whatever the mechanism of the antihypertensive effect of inhibiting this enzyme may be, this mode of treatment is quite clearly different from established treatments and, as such, is useful as an additional antihypertensive therapy. Furthermore, when side-effects are discovered, they should at least be different from those already known for established antihypertensive drugs.

The story of pulmonary angiotensin-converting enzyme and its inhibition illustrates vividly for me – perhaps because of my own involvement – the way in which biological research should work. In a little over 10 years we have gone from a chance discovery of a physiological event, via a careful investigation of each of the components of that event as an end in itself, to the extrapolation of basic biochemical properties for the treatment of human disease. However, it is more than the story of how a therapeutically useful drug was discovered; inhibition of converting enzyme has allowed us to realize that the renin–angiotensin system may after all be involved in the maintenance of normal blood pressure. We have thus illuminated a physiological problem through a pharmacological approach.

Dr Stalcup is to tell us about what happens to pulmonary converting enzyme during alveolar hypoxia (p 293-307). Perhaps his work with this enzyme will illuminate yet another physiological problem: what causes hypoxic vasoconstriction in lung?

References

Aiken JW, Vane JR 1970 The renin–angiotensin system: inhibition of converting enzyme in isolated tissues. Nature (Lond) 228:30-34

Aiken JW, Vane JR 1972 Inhibition of converting enzyme of the renin–angiotensin system in kidneys and hindlegs of dogs. Circ Res 30:263-273

Atkinson AB, Robertson JIS 1979 Captopril in the treatment of clinical hypertension and cardiac failure. Lancet 2:836-839

Atkinson AB, Brown JJ, Leckie B, Lever AF, Fraser R, Robertson JIS 1979 Captopril in a hypo-natraemic hypertensive: need for caution in initiating therapy. Lancet 2:557-558

Bakhle YS 1968 Conversion of angiotensin I to angiotensin II by cell-free extracts of dog lung. Nature (Lond) 220:919-921

Bakhle YS, Reynard AM, Vane JR 1969 Metabolism of the angiotensins in isolated perfused tissues. Nature (Lond) 222:956-959

Caldwell PRB, Seegal BC, Hsu KC, Das M, Soffer RL 1976 Angiotensin converting enzyme: vascular endothelial localization. Science (Wash DC) 191:1050-1051

Case DB, Wallace JM, Keim HJ, Weber MA, Sealey JE, Laragh JH 1977 Possible role of renin in hypertension as suggested by renin-sodium profiling and inhibition of converting enzyme. N Engl J Med 296:641-646

Collier JG, Robinson BF 1974 Comparison of effects of locally infused angiotensin I and II on hand veins and forearm arteries in man; evidence for converting enzyme activity in limb vessels. Clin Sci Mol Med 47:189-192

Collier JG, Robinson BF, Vane JR 1973 Reduction of pressor effects of angiotensin I in man by synthetic nonapeptide (B.P.P.$_{9a}$ or SQ 20,881) which inhibits converting enzyme. Lancet 1:72-74

Cushman DW, Cheung HS, Sabo EF, Ondetti MA 1977 Design of potent competitive inhibitors of angiotensin-converting enzyme. Carboxyalkanoyl and mercaptoalkanoyl amino acids. Biochemistry 16:5484-5491

Di Salvo J, Montefusco CB 1971 Conversion of angiotensin I to angiotensin II in the canine mesenteric circulation. Am J Physiol 221:1576-1579

Dorer FE, Kahn JR, Lentz KE, Levine M, Skeggs LT 1974 Hydrolysis of bradykinin by angiotensin converting enzyme. Circ Res 34:824-827

Engel SL, Schaeffer TR, Waugh MH, Rubin B 1973 Effects of the nonapeptide SQ 20881 on blood pressure of rats with experimental renovascular hypertension. Proc Soc Exp Biol Med 143:483-487

Ferguson RK, Brunner HR, Turini GA, Gavras H, McKinistry DN 1977 A specific orally active inhibitor of angiotensin-converting enzyme in man. Lancet 1:775-778

Ferreira SH 1965 A bradykinin-potentiating factor (BPF) present in the venom of *Bothrops jararaca*. Br J Pharmacol 24:163-169

Ferreira SH, Vane JR 1967 The disappearance of bradykinin and eledoisin in the circulation and vascular beds of the cat. Br J Pharmacol Chemother 30:417-424

Ferreira SH, Bakhle YS 1977 Inactivation of bradykinin and related peptides in lung. In: Bakhle YS, Vane JR (eds) Metabolic functions of the lung (Lung biology in health and disease, vol 4). Dekker, New York, p 33-53

Ferreira SH, Bartelt DC, Greene LJ 1970 Isolation of bradykinin potentiating peptides from *Bothrops jararaca* venom. Biochemistry 9:2583-2593

Gavras H, Brunner HR, Laragh JH, Sealey JE, Gavras I, Vukovich RA 1974 An angiotensin converting-enzyme inhibitor to identify and treat vasoconstrictor and volume factors in hypertensive patients. N Engl J Med 291:817-821

Gavras H, Faxon DP, Berkoben J, Brunner HR, Ryan TJ 1978 Angiotensin converting enzyme inhibition in patients with congestive heart failure. Circulation 58:770-776

Goodfriend TL, Peach MJ 1975 Angiotensin III: (des-aspartic acid^1)-angiotensin II. Circ Res (Suppl I) 36:38-48

Hellmer OM 1955 A factor in plasma that enhances contraction produced by angiotonin on rabbit aortic strips. Fed Proc 14:728

Hodge RL, Ng KKF, Vane JR 1967 Disappearance of angiotensin from the circulation of the dog. Nature (Lond) 215:138-141

Johnston CI, McGrath BP, Millar JA, Matthews PG 1979 Long-term effects of captopril (SQ 14 225) on blood-pressure and hormone levels in essential hypertension. Lancet 2:493-495

Krieger EM, Salgado HC, Assan CJ, Greene LLJ, Ferreira SH 1971 Potential screening test for detection of overactivity of renin-angiotensin system. Lancet 1:269-271

Miller ED Jr, Samuels AI, Haber E, Barger AC 1972 Inhibition of angiotensin conversion in experimental renovascular hypertension. Science (Wash DC) 117:1108-1109

Ng KKF, Vane JR 1967 The conversion of angiotensin I to angiotensin II. Nature (Lond) 216:762-766

Ody C, Junod AF 1977 Converting enzyme activity in endothelial cells isolated from pig pulmonary artery and aorta. Am J Physiol 232:C95-98

Ondetti MA, Williams NJ, Sabo EF, Pluscec J, Weaver ER, Kocy O 1971 Angiotensin converting enzyme inhibitors from the venom of *Bothrops jararaca*. Isolation, elucidation of structure and synthesis. Biochemistry 10:4033-4039

Ondetti MA, Rubin B, Cushman DW 1977 Design of specific inhibitors of angiotensin converting enzyme: a new class of orally active antihypertensive agents. Science (Wash DC) 196:441-444
Ryan JW, Ryan US 1977 Pulmonary endothelial cells. Fed Proc 36:2683-2691
Ryan US, Ryan JW 1979 Vasoactive substances and the lungs: cellular mechanisms. In: Saldeen T (ed) The microembolism syndrome. Almqvist & Wiksell, Stockholm, p 223-232
Ryan JW, Roblero J, Stewart JM 1968 Inactivation of bradykinin in the pulmonary circulation. Biochem J 110:795-797
Ryan US, Ryan JW, Whitaker C, Chiu A 1976 Localization of angiotensin converting enzyme (kininase II). II. Immunocytochemistry and immunofluorescence. Tissue & Cell 8:125-145
Sancho J, Re R, Burton J, Barger AC, Haber E 1976 The role of the renin-angiotensin-aldosterone system in cardiovascular homeostasis in normal human subjects. Circulation 53:400-405
Skeggs LT, Marsh WH, Kahn JR, Shumway NP 1954 The existence of two forms of hypertensin. J Exp Med 99:275-282
Skeggs LT, Kahn JR, Shumway NP 1956 The preparation and function of the hypertensin converting enzyme. J Exp Med 103:295-299
Soffer RL 1976 Angiotensin converting enzyme. Annu Rev Biochem 45:73-94
Vane JR 1974 The fate of angiotensin I. In: Page IH, Bumpus FM (eds) Angiotensin (Handbook of experimental pharmacology, vol 50). Springer-Verlag, Berlin, p 17-40

Discussion

Reid: I understand Una Ryan to say that if antibody to converting enzyme is injected into the bloodstream the converting enzyme is found only in the caveolae on the luminal endothelial surface, whereas if the antibody is applied to a block of tissue the enzyme can be shown in any of the caveolae of the endothelium. It is a question of whether the polarity of the caveolae is maintained in cell or tissue culture.

Bakhle: When a section of rat lung is incubated with antibody the antibody is fixed on the luminal surface of the endothelial cell; only when Dr Ryan grows endothelial cells in culture does she find the enzyme on both faces of the cells, so the endothelial polarity is lost during culture (Ryan et al 1976).

Burri: What happens to the enzyme if the caveolae move to the abluminal side, as they are thought to do by the process known as micropinocytosis? Is the enzyme lost?

Reid: The angiotensin II produced by this enzyme, whatever its location, has still to reach the extravascular space for its effect, so if the enzyme doesn't cross the cell, the AII *must.* What has been done to look systematically for the receptors or targets for these drugs?

Bakhle: Measurements of the transit time of AI in the pulmonary circulation show that neither AI nor its metabolites leave the vascular space on a single pass (Ryan et al 1970, Fanburg & Glazier 1973), so maybe the AII gets through the endothelium on the second time around the circulation. It is also possible that a small proportion (about 10%) of the AII formed could leave the vascular space without being detected in the experiments I have quoted.

Said: Converting enzyme activity has been found in vascular beds outside the lung but the pulmonary circulation seems to be physiologically the most important. Is it, however, true that where you compare equal lengths, or equal areas, of pulmonary vessels and systemic vessels, the capacity for converting AI is still greater for the pulmonary circulation?

Aiken: Our evidence for converting enzyme activity here was based on the response of the tissue (Aiken & Vane 1970). The aortic strips we used were the same size as the pulmonary artery strips; I would say the surface area of endothelium was about the same. The pulmonary artery was more efficient than the aorta in producing a response to angiotensin I. The dose–response curves for angiotensin II were roughly the same; so it isn't that one arterial strip is much more sensitive than the other.

Burri: We have seen that the pulmonary *artery* is active in converting activity, but we also often refer to the pulmonary circulation; I wouldn't equate these. The major part of the pulmonary circulation is the capillary bed.

Bakhle: Yes. The point I was making is that although all endothelial cells in all capillaries seem to have converting ability, there seems to be a difference in the biological effect.

Junod: We measured converting enzyme activity in freshly isolated cells from the pulmonary artery and aorta of the pig, and obtained identical values, so there might be species differences (Ody & Junod 1977). However, I don't think many people have made the comparison using freshly isolated lung cells. Relating enzyme activity to the pharmacological response of a tissue can cause problems since many other factors could play a role in the tissue response; the contraction of a smooth muscle may not be the best way of measuring converting enzyme. Contraction depends on the presence and number of specific receptors, the diffusion characteristics of the substrate, and so on. This might explain why the pulmonary artery and aorta do not behave the same way in these studies where converting enzyme activity was not assessed directly.

Bakhle: If one is interested in the biological effect of converting enzyme, however, the contractile response to a given amount of AII is a valid assay.

Junod: But how much angiotensin II is there in the pulmonary artery? Probably little, and certainly less than on the venous side. It appears to be generated where it is not supposed to act, namely at the capillary level. In the pulmonary artery there might not be enough time for the generation of AII.

Aiken: In our experiments (Aiken & Vane 1970), one aspect of Dr Junod's criticism is valid. That is that we don't know the angiotensinase activity of the different tissues. It is possible that angiotensinase activity was much higher in the other tissues than in the pulmonary artery and may have been breaking down angiotensin II as fast as it was being produced, to give less apparent conversion in the systemic vessels.

Vane: There is one clear difference between the pulmonary and peripheral vascular beds: the intact pulmonary circulation lacks angiotensinase activity. If angiotensinase is also located in the endothelial cells, that would be a clear difference.

Junod: You can find angiotensinase activity in endothelial cells and if you break them down, angiotensin is degraded (unpublished observation).

Bakhle: In a crude, uncentrifuged homogenate of lung there is an enormous amount of angiotensinase, I agree (Bakhle 1968).

Alberti: What is the physiological importance of angiotensin III? How much of it is present in the blood?

Bakhle: It is as good a stimulator of aldosterone as angiotensin II, but it has only 50% of its pressor effect (see Freeman et al 1977). Semple says that in the rat angiotensin III may constitute up to 20% of the angiotensin II-like immunoreactive material in blood, but in man it is difficult to detect (Semple & Morton 1976). I don't know if anything is known about its ability to interfere with catecholamine uptake, which is another site of angiotensin II action.

IMMUNOBIOLOGY OF PULMONARY ANGIOTENSIN-CONVERTING ENZYME

Soffer: Dr Bakhle has summarized the development of chemical inhibitors of converting enzyme, which was initiated by his discovery (Bakhle 1968) that bradykinin-potentiating factor suppressed angiotensin conversion in a cell-free system. I have used an immunological approach to the inhibition of this enzyme.

Early evidence that pulmonary converting enzyme was directly accessible to the bloodstream (Ryan et al 1972) and that it represented a therapeutic target in experimental renin-dependent hypertension (Krieger et al 1971) suggested to us that the introduction of inhibitory anti-enzyme antibodies into the circulation might be a useful way of controlling blood pressure. To examine this possibility we developed a procedure for isolating rabbit pulmonary converting enzyme. The pure enzyme had bradykininase activity and was characterized as a single glycopolypeptide chain of molecular weight ~ 130 000 which contains a molar equivalent of zinc (Soffer et al 1974, Das & Soffer 1975). Anti-enzyme antibodies were raised in goats.

Our initial immunological investigations focused on the enzyme–antibody interaction *in vitro* (Das & Soffer 1976). Specific anti-holoenzyme antibodies were prepared by immunoadsorbent chromatography and it was established that each molecule could bind two enzyme molecules and that at least 18% of the specific antibody population reacted with determinants of the enzyme which influenced catalysis. The antibodies apparently recognize only the polypeptide part of the enzyme molecule, since the isolated oligosaccharide component did not displace the intact glycoprotein from an immune complex with them, as determined by radioimmunoassay (Hartley & Soffer 1978). This ability to recognize only a part of the molecule – the cognitive property of the antibody – probably accounts for the inability of these antibodies to discriminate between rabbit pulmonary and serum converting enzymes, which differ markedly in the extent to which they are sialylated (Das et al 1977).

The use of these antibodies in inhibition studies and competition radioimmunoassays established that the polypeptide chain responsible for enzyme activity in most rabbit organs and body fluids is closely similar or identical to that in the lung. The seminal fluid enzyme appears to be an exception since, although partially homologous to enzyme elsewhere, it could be distinguished immunologically, specifically in a part of its structure unrelated to catalysis (Das & Soffer 1976). Immunohistochemical studies indicated that, with the exception of epithelial cells containing brush borders, enzyme was localized to vascular endothelial rather than parenchymal cells throughout the body and was therefore probably largely accessible to the circulation (Caldwell et al 1976a).

Enzyme–antibody interaction *in vivo* was first investigated using the goat anti-rabbit enzyme antibodies for passive immunization of homologous recipient animals – that is, rabbits (Caldwell et al 1976b). Unexpectedly, intravenous infusion of the antibodies resulted in an immune-specific lethal reaction and they could not be administered in sufficient quantity to anticipate profound inhibition of enzyme activity. The proximate haemodynamic pathophysiological event was acute pulmonary hypertension, quickly followed by heart failure and death. When lungs from affected rabbits were examined by light microscopy we could not identify a specific pathological process, although there was extensive pulmonary haemorrhage and appropriate histochemical procedures showed antibody fixed to the pulmonary vascular endothelium. The responsible immune mechanism probably does not involve complement or newly synthesized prostaglandins since it occurs after giving Fab fragments and is not prevented by pretreatment with indomethacin (Dickerson & Murthy 1978). The unusual localization of converting enzyme implicates vascular endothelium as the most likely specific cellular determinant of this pathogenicity. If the pathological immune reaction is triggered by association of antibody with a specific binding site on the enzyme molecule, then the lethal and inhibitory properties of anti-holoenzyme antibody preparations may well be dissociated in monoclonal antibodies.

The goat anti-rabbit enzyme antibodies were used to detect immunological homology of rabbit converting enzyme with that in pulmonary extracts of other species (Conroy et al 1976). Such homology was demonstrable with dog, guinea-pig and rat enzymes by anti-catalytic assay, immunodiffusion and competition radioimmunoassay. The effect of passively immunizing the rat with goat anti-rabbit enzyme antibodies was then investigated. In contrast to the rabbit, this heterologous recipient tolerated their administration without deleterious consequences. Infusion of 3–6 times the amount of antibodies required to inhibit the total pulmonary content of rat converting activity *in vitro* suppressed the vasopressor response to angiotensin I and potentiated the vasodepressor action of bradykinin by approximately an order of magnitude, indicating that immunological blockade of the enzyme *in vivo* had been successful. The biological specificity of this immune-dependent blockade was established by failure of the antibodies to modify the vasopressor effect of noradrenaline (norepinephrine). There was, however, a small but unexpected immune-specific inhibition of the vasopressor response to angiotensin II, perhaps mediated by an anatomical proximity of converting enzyme and receptors for the octapeptide. The half-life of the inhibitory antibodies in the circulation was 1–2 days.

After establishing the pharmacological action of the goat anti-rabbit enzyme antibodies on the metabolism of vasoactive peptides in the rat, we investigated these antibodies as antihypertensive agents for the rat renin-dependent model of this disease (Markle et al 1978). Their administration was associated with a striking, immune-specific, relatively long-lived (days) decline in blood pressure to normal values. They produced a smaller but significant immune-dependent vasodepressor effect in normotensive animals, suggesting that the renin–angiotensin system might play a more prominent role in the chronic maintenance of blood pressure than had been discerned in acute experiments with short-lived peptide inhibitors.

Our studies using passive immunization have thus shown that circulating antibodies can inhibit converting activity *in vivo*. However, active immunization against the enzyme might be a more desirable objective, since it would probably preclude the eventual development of serum sickness in recipient animals. We are now examining this possibility by immunizing dogs with the pure rabbit enzyme. This choice of species is based on the extensive immunological homology between canine and rabbit converting enzymes, delineated in reciprocal experiments using the two pure pulmonary glycoproteins and goat antibodies raised against each (Conroy et al 1978). Our rationale is that since these enzymes are so closely related immunologically, the dog may form antibodies against the rabbit enzyme which are capable of inhibiting its own converting activity. Preliminary experiments (unpublished) have already established the feasibility of this concept. Dogs immunized with the pure rabbit enzyme as antigen display no ill-effects. Their sera have an almost comparable, immune-specific inhibitory action on reactions catalysed by thc pure rabbit and dog enzymes. Furthermore, the titre of antibody is sufficient to inhibit almost completely the activity of circulating converting enzyme present in these sera. The effects of these endogenously produced dog anti-rabbit enzyme antibodies on the metabolism of vasoactive peptides in the dog and on the evolution of renovascular hypertension in this species remain to be determined.

References

Aiken JW, Vane JR 1970 The renin–angiotensin system: inhibition of converting enzyme in isolated tissues. Nature (Lond) 228:30-34

Bakhle YS 1968 Conversion of angiotensin I to angiotensin II by cell-free extracts of dog lung. Nature (Lond) 220:919-921

Caldwell PRB, Seegal BC, Hsu KC, Das M, Soffer RL 1976a Angiotensin-converting enzyme. Vascular endothelial localization. Science (Wash DC) 191:1050-1051

Caldwell PRB, Wigger HJ, Das M, Soffer RL 1976b Angiotensin-converting enzyme. Effect of antienzyme antibody *in vivo*. FEBS (Fed Eur Biochem Soc) Lett 63:82-84

Conroy JM, Hoffman H, Kirk ES, Hirzel HO, Sonnenblick EH, Soffer RL 1976 Pulmonary angiotensin-converting enzyme. Interspecies homology and inhibition by heterologous antibody *in vivo*. J Biol Chem 251:4828-4832

Conroy JM, Hartley JL, Soffer RL 1978 Canine pulmonary angiotensin-converting enzyme. Physicochemical, catalytic and immunological properties. Biochim Biophys Acta 524:403-412

Das M, Soffer RL 1975 Pulmonary angiotensin-converting enzyme: structural and catalytic properties. J Biol Chem 250:6762-6768

Das M, Soffer RL 1976 Pulmonary angiotensin-converting enzyme antienzyme antibody. Biochemistry 15:5088-5094

Das M, Hartley JL, Soffer RL 1977 Serum angiotensin-converting enzyme. Isolation and relationship to the pulmonary enzyme. J Biol Chem 252:1316-1319

Dickerson DD, Murthy VS 1978 Anaphylactoid reaction after intravenous injection of antibodies against angiotensin-converting enzyme in anesthetized rabbits. Fed Proc 37:590A

Fanburg BL, Glazier JB 1973 Conversion of angiotensin I to angiotensin II in the isolated perfused dog lung. J Appl Physiol 35:325-331

Freeman RH, Davis JO, Lohmeier TE, Spielman WS 1977 [Des-Asp^{1}]angiotensin II: mediator of the renin angiotensin system? Fed Proc 36:1766-1770

Hartley JL, Soffer RL 1978 On the oligosaccharide moiety of angiotensin-converting enzyme. Biochem Biophys Res Commun 83:1545-1552

Krieger EM, Salgado HC, Assan CJ, Greene LJ, Ferreira SH 1971 Potential screening test for detection of overactivity of the renin–angiotensin system. Lancet 1:269-271

Markle RA, Sonnenblick EH, Conroy JM, Soffer RL 1978 Reversal of renovascular hypertension by antibodies specific for angiotensin-converting enzyme. Proc Natl Acad Sci USA 75:5702-5705

Ody C, Junod AF 1977 Converting enzyme activity in endothelial cells isolated from pig pulmonary artery and aorta. Am J Physiol 232:C95-C98

Ryan JW, Stewart JM, Leary WP, Ledingham JG 1970 Metabolism of angiotensin I in the pulmonary circulation. Biochem J 120:221-223

Ryan JW, Smith U, Niemeyer RS 1972 Angiotensin I metabolism by plasma membranes of the lung. Science (Wash DC) 176:64-66

Ryan US, Ryan JW, Whitaker C, Chiu A 1976 Localization of angiotensin converting enzyme (kininase II). II. Immunocytochemistry and immunofluorescence. Tissue & Cell 8:125-145

Semple PF, Morton JJ 1976 Angiotensin II and angiotensin III in rat blood. Circ Res 38 suppl 2:122-126

Soffer RL, Reza R, Caldwell PRB 1974 Angiotensin-converting enzyme from rabbit pulmonary particles. Proc Natl Acad Sci USA 71:1720-1724

Modulation of converting enzyme activity by hypoxia and its physiological effects

S. ALEX STALCUP, JOEL S. LIPSET and ROBERT B. MELLINS

Department of Pediatrics (Pulmonary Division), Columbia University College of Physicians & Surgeons, and the Babies Hospital, New York, NY 10032, USA

Abstract To explore the haemodynamic consequences of the reduction in converting enzyme activity by acute alveolar hypoxia we made sequential haemodynamic observations in seven saline-infused and 12 bradykinin-infused anaesthetized, catheterized dogs. They were ventilated initially with room air and then for 50 minutes with hypoxic gas mixtures. Within two minutes after starting hypoxic ventilation, converting enzyme activity decreased, arterial angiotensin II concentrations dropped, and, in the bradykinin-infused dogs, arterial bradykinin concentrations rose. Both groups of dogs experienced a rise in systemic and pulmonary arterial blood pressure in response to hypoxia, but by different mechanisms. In the saline-infused (control) dogs there was increased systemic (+40%) and pulmonary (+90%) vascular resistance while cardiac output was unchanged or slightly reduced. Bradykinin-infused dogs demonstrated reduced systemic vascular resistance (−40%), no increase in pulmonary vascular resistance and a 100% increase in cardiac output. Return to room air breathing restored converting enzyme activity, releasing high concentrations of angiotensin II. Oxygen tension thus regulates converting enzyme activity and hence the circulating levels of angiotensin II and bradykinin.

Bradykinin and angiotensin II (AII) are small peptides with powerful opposing effects on systemic vascular resistance: bradykinin is the most potent endogenously produced hypotensive agent (Colman et al 1971) and AII is correspondingly potent as a vasopressor (Khairalla et al 1966). Converting enzyme (dipeptidyl carboxypeptidase, EC 3.4.15.1), located on the surface of endothelial cells of the lung and systemic vasculature, predominantly regulates the circulating levels of these two peptides by efficiently degrading bradykinin and converting angiotensin I to AII (Ryan & Ryan 1977).

We have previously shown that acute hypoxia in dogs inhibits converting enzyme activity: the inhibition is immediate in onset, is rapidly reversible on return to normal oxygen tension, and the extent of inhibition is closely related

Metabolic activities of the lung
(Ciba Foundation symposium 78) p 293-311

to the oxygen tension (Stalcup et al 1979a). At a Pa_{O_2} of 50 mmHg, enzyme activity is reduced to 50% of the activity at normal Pa_{O_2}, and below 30 mmHg oxygen tension there is minimal detectable bradykinin degradation and angiotensin conversion in either the lung or the systemic vasculature. Similar results are obtained when the converting enzyme activity of endothelial cells in tissue culture is studied at reduced oxygen tensions (Stalcup et al 1979b), and when the conversion of angiotensin I to angiotensin II is assessed by bioassay in intact dogs (Leuenberger et al 1978).

These findings suggested that blockade of converting enzyme activity by hypoxia represented a basic model of disease: since conversion of AI to AII and bradykinin degradation are prevented in hypoxia, profound hypotension should ensue when hypoxia occurs in hyperkininaemic states. Nonetheless, in our previous studies, no hypotension was seen despite widening of pulse pressure in hypoxic dogs receiving bradykinin infusions (Stalcup et al 1979a). Since bradykinin concentrations in plasma have been reported to be elevated in several hypoxic disease states, in the range of 1 to 5 ng/ml (Kellermeyer & Graham 1968), and to reach over 50 ng/ml at the time of birth (Heymann et al 1969, Melmon et al 1968), we compared the changes in cardiac output, systemic and pulmonary arterial blood pressure and systemic and pulmonary vascular resistance in dogs made hypoxic ($Pa_{O_2} < 32$ mmHg) during bradykinin infusion and during saline infusion (controls).

METHODS

Nineteen mongrel dogs weighing 18.4 kg (SD = 3.2) were anaesthetized with sodium pentobarbitone (25 mg/kg) and paralysed with a continuous infusion of 1.2 mg/kg per min succinylcholine. The dogs were ventilated with a Harvard animal respirator and hyperinflated to 20 cm H_2O for 30 seconds at 10-minute intervals. The basic preparation used in these studies has been previously described (Stalcup et al 1979a). In brief, a KMF 7F double-lumen thermistor catheter was placed in the pulmonary artery through a right jugular incision. Under fluoroscopic control catheters were placed into the femoral vein and artery, right atrium and left atrium, and in the thoracic aorta approximately 5 cm above the aortic valve. Vascular pressures were continuously measured with Statham 23 Db strain gauges and recorded (Beckman model R612 polygraph). The cardiac output was determined in duplicate at predetermined time intervals using 5–10 ml injections of room-temperature saline solution and the results were analysed with a KMA model 3500 cardiac output computer. Duplicate values differing by more than 10% were repeated. Pulmonary and systemic vascular resistances were calculated using electronically determined mean vascular pressures. Hence, each reported data point represents the mean of at least two determinations made within two minutes of each other.

Bradykinin (Calbiochem) was prepared in a stock solution of 1 mg/ml in distilled water plus 0.1% lysozyme and frozen at −70°C. Fresh dilutions in normal saline were made on the day of each experiment and continuously infused into 12 of the animals (experimental group) at a rate of 1.0 μg/kg per min (volume 0.4 ml/min).

The dogs were ventilated with room air and with an 8% O_2 : balance N_2 gas mixture to yield a Pa_{O_2} in the range of 30 mmHg. This value was chosen because at this low Pa_{O_2} the activity of converting enzyme is almost completely inhibited (Stalcup et al 1979a,b). Blood gas tensions and pH were measured with a semi-automated analyser (IL 513) whenever blood was drawn for peptide determinations and when vascular resistances were measured.

Bradykinin was extracted from blood using our modifications (Stalcup et al 1979a) of the method of Mashford & Roberts (1972). The blood was drawn into syringes containing kallikrein and kininase inhibitors and the bradykinin immediately extracted into ethanol. Bradykinin was assayed using the radioimmunoassay methods of Goodfriend & Odya (1974) as modified by us (Stalcup et al 1979a). The standard deviation from 10 standard curves was 0.24%, the sensitivity of the assay was 20 pg/ml, and the coefficient of variation of 25 samples assayed in different runs was 7.20% ± 0.95 (SD). When blood was handled in the manner described, the lowest pre-infusion level of bradykinin detectable in either the pulmonary artery or the left atrium of the catheterized dog was 0.11 ± 0.005 ng/ml (SD).

Angiotensin II was extracted into ethanol and was assayed by radioimmunoassay. Antibody to AII was produced in New Zealand white rabbits against angiotensin II coupled to ovalbumin by reaction with *N*-ethyl-*N*-(3-dimethylaminopropyl)carbodiimide (Goodfriend et al 1964). We labelled synthetic AII (Calbiochem) with carrier-free ^{125}I (New England Nuclear) by the chloramine-T method of Hunter and Greenwood as modified by Freedlender et al (1974); with antibody used at a final dilution of 1 : 48 000 the assay sensitivity was 3.5 pg/ml. (Sensitivity was defined as the smallest amount of unlabelled AII that results in a significantly different bound/free ratio from that obtained for the zero standard.) The coefficient of variation for samples run in triplicate was 8.1%. Cross-reactivity of this antibody to angiotensin I is less than 0.01%. The antibody exhibits cross-reactivity with the Val^5, 2–8 heptapeptide (86.4 ± 7.5%) and the Val^5, 3–8 hexapeptide (91.6 ± 10.1%) but less than 0.06% with the Val^5, 1–7 heptapeptide. These studies confirm the importance of the carboxy-terminal phenylalanine in determining antigenic specificity (Ruiz-Maza et al 1977). Angiotensin II was extracted from plasma using the ethanol–ether procedure described above. Recovery of ^{3}H-labelled angiotensin II added to the extractions of 35 samples was 64.7 ± 8.6% (SD). Normal values obtained from right atrial blood of eight dogs were 5.6 ± 1.8 pg/ml (SD). AII levels were measured only in the control dogs, since the administration of exogenous bradykinin could artifactually alter the circulating AII levels in the experimental dogs because these two peptides are interrelated in the circulation (Wong et al 1975).

Pulmonary converting enzyme activity was assessed by calculating the instantaneous clearance of bradykinin using the concentration of bradykinin (BK) in simultaneously drawn samples from the pulmonary artery (PA) and left atrium (LA), as follows:

$$\frac{[BK]_{PA} - [BK]_{LA}}{[BK]_{PA}} \times 100 = \% \text{ instantaneous clearance across the pulmonary circulation}$$

Two groups of dogs were studied: control dogs (n = 7) received a saline infusion (0.4 ml/min) and the experimental dogs (n = 12) received a continuous infusion of 1 μg/kg per minute of bradykinin, also in a volume of 0.4 ml/min. Each dog was prepared as described above, and baseline samples for bradykinin, AII and blood gas determinations were drawn during the period at normal oxygen tension. After 20 minutes of either saline or bradykinin infusion the dog was switched to ventilation with hypoxic gas. Blood samples for peptide and blood gas determinations were drawn 2, 4, 6, 11, 16, 21, 31, 41 and 51 minutes after the start of hypoxic ventilation. Blood samples were also drawn at 2, 4, 6, 11 and 21 minutes after the return to room air breathing. The total volume of blood removed over the course of the experiment was 45 ml from each animal. Blood samples were immediately replaced with an equal volume of Ringer's lactate solution. In addition, both groups of dogs received an intravenous saline infusion adjusted so that fluids from all sources, including catheter flushes and thermodilution boluses, equalled a calculated rate of 100 ml/kg per 24 hours.

Statistical analyses were performed using Student's t-test, on a Wang Series 600 computer. Only values achieving P = 0.01 or less are reported as significant.

RESULTS

The effect of acute hypoxia on the clearance of bradykinin by the lung in the 12 bradykinin-infused dogs is shown in Fig. 1. Baseline bradykinin con-

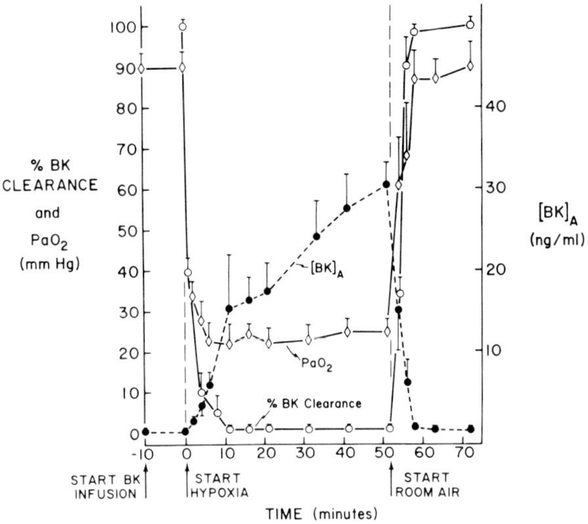

FIG. 1. The effect of acute hypoxia on Pa_{O_2}, the % of bradykinin clearance by the lung, and the arterial bradykinin concentrations ($[BK]_A$) in dogs infused intravenously with bradykinin at 1 μg/kg per minute beginning 10 minutes before the onset of acute hypoxia, during the hypoxic interval and for 20 minutes after return to room air. I, SD.

centrations were not elevated (0.11 ng/ml). After 10 minutes of this infusion the concentration of bradykinin in the pulmonary artery was increased, in the range of 2 ng/ml, but the lung cleared this amount of peptide and the level in the arterial circulation was not elevated. Within two minutes after the onset of hypoxic ventilation the arterial bradykinin concentration rose and its instantaneous clearance (a measure of converting enzyme activity) strikingly decreased. The decline in activity was closely related to the decrease in Pa_{O_2} which in both groups fell below 30 mmHg during the hypoxic interval. There was no significant difference in the Pa_{O_2} values achieved in the control and experimental groups. As a consequence of inhibition of converting enzyme activity the arterial bradykinin concentration continued to rise, reaching about 30 ng/ml by 50 minutes of hypoxia. On return to room air breathing, enzyme activity was rapidly restored and arterial levels of bradykinin returned to baseline values. Pulmonary artery and left atrium bradykinin concentrations were measured simultaneously and at the same time intervals in the saline-infused dogs and were found to remain below 0.11 ng/ml throughout the experiment.

Baseline (pre-hypoxia) systemic and pulmonary haemodynamic data are summarized in Table 1. Fig. 2 compares the effect of hypoxia on systemic

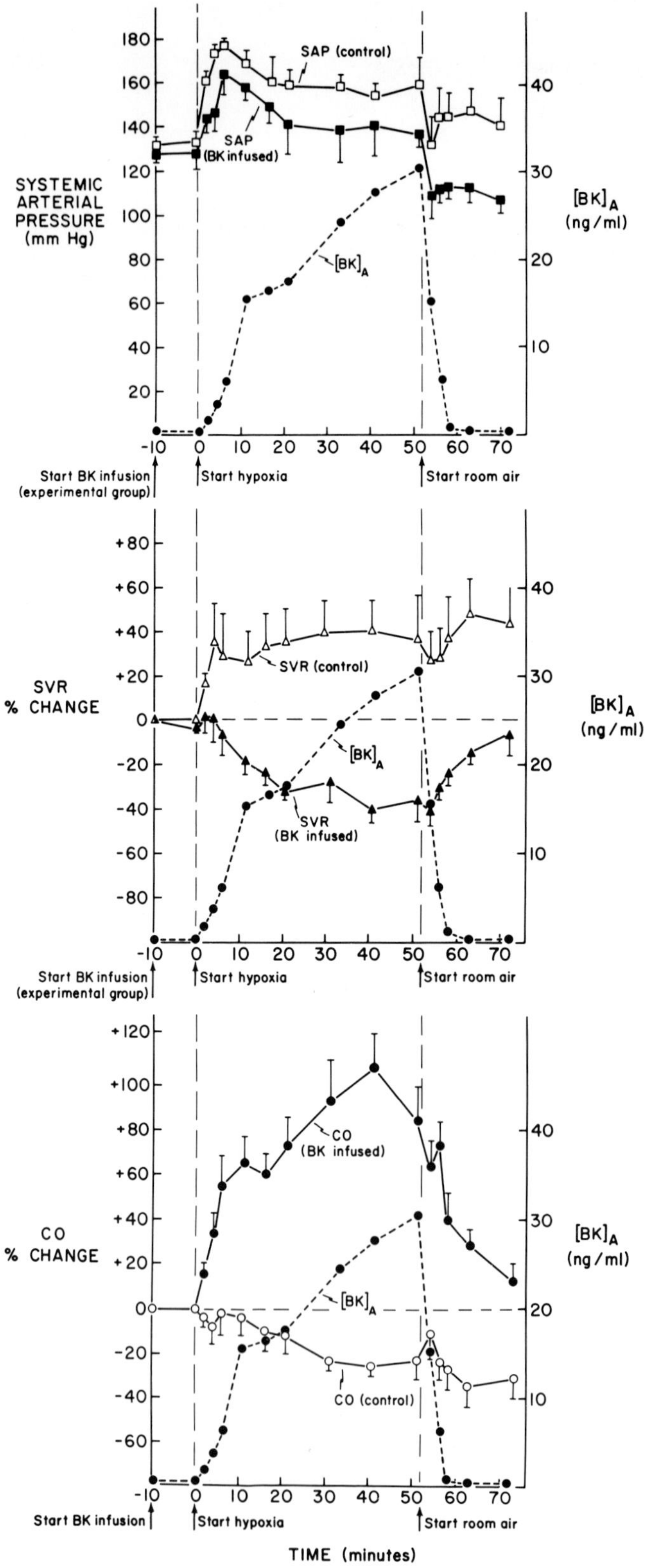

SYSTEMIC ARTERIAL PRESSURE (mm Hg)
SAP (control)
SAP (BK infused)
[BK]A
[BK]A (ng/ml)
Start BK infusion (experimental group)
Start hypoxia
Start room air
SVR % CHANGE
SVR (control)
SVR (BK infused)
CO % CHANGE
CO (BK infused)
CO (control)
Start BK infusion
TIME (minutes)

FIG. 2

TABLE 1

Baseline haemodynamic data in control and bradykinin-infused dogs

	Control (+SD)	*Bradykinin-infused (+SD)*
Cardiac output	2.65 ± 0.78 l min^{-1}	2.52 ± 0.24 l min^{-1}
Systemic arterial pressure	132 ± 19.1 mmHg	129 ± 13.7 mmHg
Systemic vascular resistance	51.32 ± 10.6 mmHg l^{-1} min^{-1}	49.8 ± 30.50 mmHg l^{-1} min^{-1}
Pulmonary arterial pressure	13.5 ± 2.3 mmHg	12.8 ± 0.88 mmHg
Pulmonary vascular resistance	4.23 ± 1.08 mmHg l^{-1} min^{-1}	4.45 ± 2.0 mmHg l^{-1} min^{-1}

arterial pressure, systemic vascular resistance and cardiac output in the control and bradykinin-infused dogs. Although the mean pressures were slightly but consistently lower in the bradykinin-infused group (upper panel), both groups initially experienced a moderate rise in blood pressure, and no hypotension was seen at any time in the experiment. As shown in the middle panel, the control dogs experienced moderate vasoconstriction in response to hypoxia, up to a 40% increase in systemic vascular resistance. As bradykinin levels rose in the bradykinin-infused group, these dogs underwent a 40% decrease in systemic vascular resistance. As expected, since the arterial pressures were similar but the resistances went in opposite directions, there were marked differences in cardiac output: at the low Pa_{O2} achieved in this experiment the control dogs experienced a slight decline in output while the bradykinin-infused dogs showed as much as a 100% increase in cardiac output (Fig. 2, lower panel).

To facilitate comparison of simultaneous changes in systemic vascular resistance, cardiac output and systemic arterial pressure between the two study groups we have summarized these haemodynamic variables in Fig. 3. In the controls (left panel), systemic arterial pressure rose, there was vasoconstriction, and cardiac output was unchanged or slightly reduced. A rise in systemic arterial pressure was also seen in the bradykinin-infused dogs during hypoxia (right panel), but vascular resistance declined while cardiac output increased. Return to room air breathing produced further differences

←

FIG. 2. Effect of acute hypoxia on systemic arterial pressure (SAP), systemic vascular resistance (SVR) and cardiac output (CO) in 12 bradykinin-infused (solid symbols) and seven control, saline-infused dogs (open symbols). Arterial bradykinin ($[BK]_A$) levels rose only in the bradykinin-infused dogs. I, SEM.

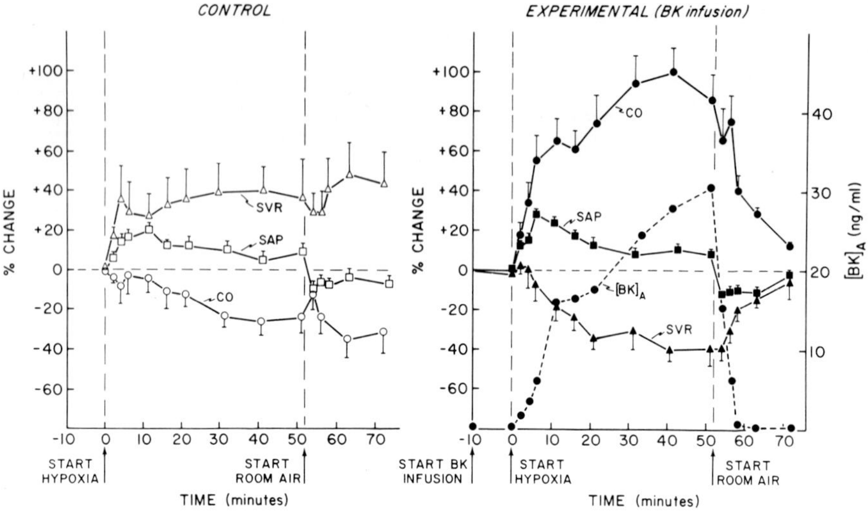

FIG. 3. Simultaneous changes in systemic vascular resistance (SVR), systemic arterial pressure (SAP) and cardiac output (CO) in 12 bradykinin-infused and seven control dogs before, during and after acute hypoxia, expressed as % change from baseline values. I, SEM.

in these haemodynamic variables between the two groups. In control dogs, despite restoration of oxygenation, there was further vasoconstriction and an additional decline in mean cardiac output, with wide swings in systemic arterial pressure and cardiac output. For example, one control dog demonstrated swings in systemic arterial pressure from 114 to 155 mmHg and in cardiac output from 1.04 l/min to 4.34 l/min within two minutes of returning to room air breathing. These findings are contrasted with those in the bradykinin-infused dogs in which these variables returned towards baseline.

Pulmonary haemodynamic alterations in response to hypoxia were also very different in the two groups (Fig. 4). Both groups of dogs demonstrated elevated pulmonary artery pressures during acute hypoxia. However, the control dogs (left panel) showed a rise in pulmonary vascular resistance while there was no change in pulmonary vascular resistance in the bradykinin-infused group (right panel). Thus the rise in cardiac output in the dogs infused with bradykinin was offset by an absence of pulmonary vasoconstriction. Return to room air breathing produced a further increase in pulmonary vascular resistance in the control dogs; the bradykinin-infused dogs showed no change in this value with return of oxygenation.

The levels of angiotensin II measured in the control dogs are shown in Fig. 5. During the hypoxic interval these levels fell to below the limit of detection by our radioimmunoassay method (< 3.5 pg/ml). Within two minutes of

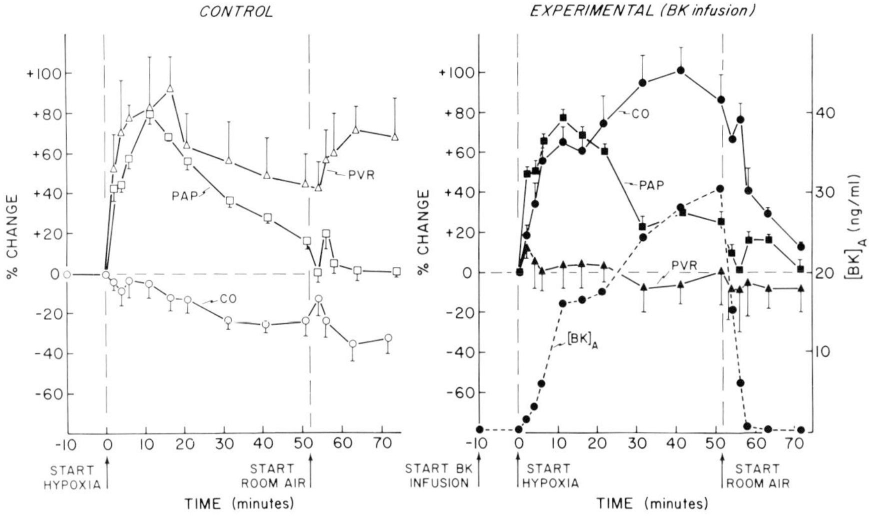

FIG. 4. Simultaneous changes in pulmonary arterial pressure (PAP), pulmonary vascular resistance (PVR) and cardiac output (CO) in 12 bradykinin-infused and seven control dogs in response to acute hypoxia. I, SEM.

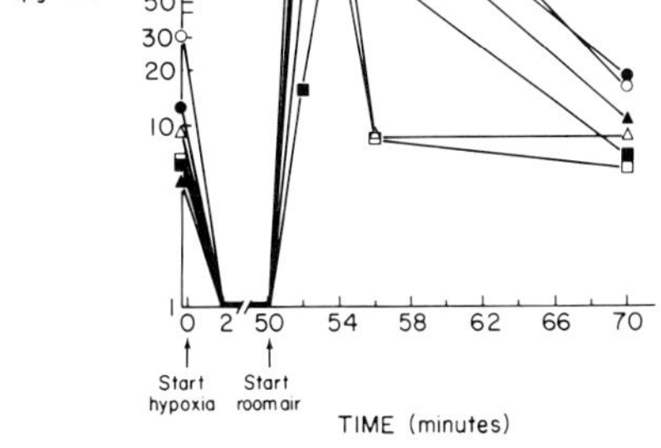

FIG. 5. Effect of acute hypoxia on the concentration of angiotensin II in systemic arterial blood in seven control dogs. Each symbol represents data from a separate dog. Note the logarithmic scale. Peak values from 100 to 3000 pg/ml occurred 2–6 min after returning to room air breathing after a 50-minute period of acute hypoxia.

restoration of room air breathing, peak values of angiotensin II 100- to 300-fold above baseline were seen.

DISCUSSION

It has been speculated that, by virtue of its central location in the circulation and its large surface area, the lung selectively protects the systemic vascular bed from vasoactive agents that are locally released and locally active, such as noradrenaline (norepinephrine), bradykinin and serotonin (Vane 1969). Moreover, by activating or permitting the passage of other agents the lung facilitates the function of systemically active agents such as adrenaline (epinephrine) and angiotensin II. We expected that, with hypoxic inhibition of converting enzyme activity, the loss of the barrier or selective function of the lung with respect to bradykinin and angiotensin II would foster hypotension. Rather, since bradykinin passing through the pulmonary barrier augmented cardiac output, so preventing hypotension, these studies appear to offer further support for the hypothesis that the pulmonary vascular bed actively regulates the arterial levels of systemically active agents. This lung function is in turn modulated by the lung environment – in this instance, altered oxygen tension. In this formulation, infused bradykinin acquires a systemically active role during acute hypoxia. Thus, no untoward effects from hypoxic inhibition of converting enzyme activity were seen, but bradykinin appeared to be protective by enhancing cardiac output.

At normal oxygen tension, in both animals and man, increased arterial concentrations of bradykinin have powerful hypotensive effects because of a decrease in systemic vascular resistance (Nakano 1965). In the present studies, even though the vasodilatory effect of bradykinin persisted during the hypoxic interval, no hypotension was seen despite increases in arterial bradykinin concentration to greater than 30 ng/ml. The amount of the decrease in systemic vascular resistance due to bradykinin was the same as that reported in normoxic dogs (Nakano 1965, 1969), but the decrease seen in vascular resistance was more than offset by increases in cardiac output, so that blood pressure did not fall. Since bradykinin has potent effects on prostaglandin synthesis and metabolism (Needleman et al 1975, Needleman 1976) it is reasonable to suspect that some of the observed effects are mediated locally by kinin-induced release of arachidonic acid metabolites. Additionally, bradykinin stimulates the release of adrenaline from the adrenal medulla (Feldberg & Lewis 1964), which in turn will modify the peripheral effects of bradykinin. The observed changes in pressure and resistance reflect the balance between these constrictor and dilator influences.

The response of cardiac output to acute hypoxia was highly variable in the dogs infused with saline. Initially four dogs had transient slight increases in cardiac output (+2 to +7% of baseline), while three showed no change or slight decreases (0 to −8%). However, by 31 minutes of hypoxic exposure there was a slight but significant decrease in mean cardiac output from baseline in this group of dogs ($P < 0.01$, paired *t*-test). Haemodynamic responses to hypoxia are complex and there is conflicting evidence in the literature on cardiac output responses: Thilenius et al (1964) showed an increase in cardiac output with moderate hypoxia, Borgia & Horvath (1977) found no increase, while Eckenhoff et al (1947) and Rodbard (1959) found depression of output. In conscious, unrestrained animals several studies have shown modest increases in cardiac output, systemic arterial hypertension, and a variable reduction in systemic vascular resistance (Adachi et al 1976, Liang & Gavras 1978, Sylvester et al 1979). Vatner & Braunwald (1975) and Nash et al (1956) suggest that barbiturate anaesthetics can lead both to depressed myocardial function and to relative hypertension, such as we observed in our dogs. We believe this to be the most likely explanation for the modest depression in cardiac output which we observed in this and a previous study (Leuenberger et al 1980). In this regard, the saline-infused and bradykinin-infused dogs received identical doses of the anaesthetic agents; thus it is noteworthy, in the context of possibly impaired myocardial function, that bradykinin enhanced cardiac output in these hypoxic dogs.

The effects of bradykinin on cardiac function during hypoxia were striking. The observed increase in cardiac output may have resulted from coronary vasodilatation with enhancement of myocardial perfusion during hypoxia, from reduced afterload produced by bradykinin-induced systemic vasodilatation, or possibly from enhanced venous return (Nakano 1965) resulting either from the venoconstricting effect of bradykinin (Guth et al 1963, Mason & Melmon 1965) or from increased perfusion to fast-time-constant vascular beds (Caldini et al 1974). A direct inotropic effect cannot be excluded. Several investigators have found bradykinin to be a powerful coronary vasodilator, producing prompt increases in coronary blood flow (Antonio & Rocha e Silva 1962, Maxwell et al 1962, Nakano 1969). The effect of kinin on cardiac function is enhanced and prolonged when converting enzyme activity is inhibited by SQ 20 881 (BPP_{9a}) (Needleman 1976). Several studies suggest that the coronary-vasodilating effects of bradykinin are locally mediated, at least in part by prostaglandin synthesis (Needleman 1976, Needleman et al 1975). A protective role for bradykinin in cardiac function is suggested by the observation that the survival of patients with severely impaired cardiac function secondary to myocardial infarction was greatest in those with elevated circulating levels of bradykinin (Hashimoto et al 1975). Pitt et al (1970) found that acute myocardial ischaemia caused an increase in kallikrein activity and kinin concentration in the blood draining the ischaemic tissue.

The effects of converting enzyme inhibition on peptide concentration and on the circulation have been studied in animals at normal oxygen tensions by giving specific converting enzyme inhibitors. Gavras et al (1978) found that inhibiting converting enzyme activity by administering SQ 20 881 to dogs produced a redistribution of blood flow in favour of the brain, heart and kidneys: flow increased by 64, 76 and 69% respectively. In sodium-deficient dogs, McCaa et al (1978) found that chronic inhibition of angiotensin-converting enzyme with the orally active inhibitor SQ 14 225 (captopril) produced significant increases in blood kinin levels by the second day of enzyme blockade with a corresponding decline in arterial blood pressure. In these experiments, as well as in ours, the observed circulatory effects resulted from simultaneous decreases in angiotensin II levels and increases in bradykinin levels. However, the studies differ in that in ours, converting enzyme activity was inhibited by acute hypoxia rather than by giving exogenous enzyme inhibitors.

Studies on the pulmonary haemodynamic effects of bradykinin have produced conflicting results, with the general consensus that it is, at best, a weak vasodilator (Bishop et al 1962, Hauge et al 1966, Waaler 1961). However, in the transition from fetal to extrauterine life bradykinin exerts profound vasodilating effects, functioning as a principal mediator in the rapid decline in pulmonary vascular resistance occurring with the first breaths (Heymann et al 1969). Also, Segal et al (1970) have previously shown that bradykinin effectively antagonizes hypoxia-induced pulmonary vasoconstriction. Our studies confirm their findings and indicate that the pulmonary vasodilating effects of bradykinin are enhanced when background vascular resistance is high.

The circulatory instability (wide swings in systemic arterial pressure and cardiac output) seen in the control animals on return to room air breathing appears to be in part mediated by angiotensin II. Since converting enzyme activity was found to be close to zero during the hypoxic interval, angiotensin I generated during that time could not be fully converted to AII. On the return to room air and restoration of converting enzyme activity, AII concentrations rose abruptly, reaching extraordinary levels approaching 3000 pg/ml (Fig. 5, p 301). This accounts at least in part for the continued elevation of systemic vascular resistance on return to room air.

These studies suggest that inhibition of converting enzyme activity is a physiological response to hypoxia, acting to adjust the circulating levels of its two peptide substrates, with important secondary effects on vascular resistance and cardiac output. Several studies indicate that the renin–

angiotensin system and autonomic reflex mechanisms are closely interrelated in mediating the net circulatory responses to hypoxia (Hammill et al 1979, Liang & Gavras 1978, Sylvester et al 1979). Moreover, the renin–angiotensin and kallikrein–kinin systems are further interrelated through converting enzyme. In the control dogs the abrupt decline in AII concentrations influences the calculated vascular resistance changes, but these are modified in part by hypoxic stimulation of catecholamine release (Liang & Gavras 1978, Sylvester et al 1979). Thus, net circulatory responses result from interactions between the autonomic nervous system, circulating 'first messengers' (the kallikrein–kinin and renin–angiotensin systems and circulating catecholamines) and tissue-based 'second messengers' (the prostaglandins, cyclic nucleotides, and calcium ion influx).

In order for a physiological role for the kallikrein–kinin system to be invoked in hypoxic states it is necessary that hypoxia bring about the activation of kallikrein, in order for kinin levels to become elevated. The studies in saline-infused dogs indicate that short periods of acute hypoxia do not alone raise endogenous kinin concentrations. In acute severe hypoxia, tissue ischaemia appears to activate the kallikrein–kinin system (Franchi et al 1975, Pitt et al 1970). Our experiments indicate that hypoxic inhibition of converting enzyme activity permits the kinin thereby generated to accumulate. It is not yet known whether converting enzyme activity remains inhibited during *chronic* hypoxia, or whether chronic hypoxia without tissue ischaemia is associated with increased concentrations of bradykinin. In hypoxic animals in which kinin levels do become elevated, we hypothesize that organ blood flow will be inversely related to oxygen tension, in part because in the most hypoxic organs bradykinin levels will rise and angiotensin II levels will fall as a function of decreased converting enzyme activity.

ACKNOWLEDGEMENTS

Supported in part by National Institutes of Health Grants HL 14214 (SCOR), HL 07421 and HL 06012, and grants from the New York Lung Association and the Parker B. Francis Foundation.

References

Adachi H, Strauss HW, Ochi H, Wagner HN 1976 The effect of hypoxia on the regional distribution of cardiac output in the dog. Circ Res 39:314-319

Antonio A, Rocha e Silva M 1962 Coronary vasodilation produced by bradykinin on isolated mammalian heart. Circ Res 11:910-915

Bishop JM, Harris P, Segal N 1962 The effect of synthetic bradykinin on the pulmonary and systemic circulation in man. J Physiol (Lond) 165:37-43

Borgia JF, Horvath SM 1977 Effects of acute prolonged hypoxia on cardiovascular dynamics in dogs. J Appl Physiol:Respirat Environ Exercise Physiol 43:784-789

Caldini P, Permutt S, Waddell JA, Riley RL 1974 Effect of epinephrine on pressure, flow and volume relationships in the systemic circulation of dogs. Circ Res 34:606-623

Colman RW, Girey JD, Zacest R, Talamo RC 1971 The human plasma kallikrein–kinin system. Prog Hematol 8:255-298

Eckenhoff JE, Hafkenschiel JH, Landmesser CM, Harmel M 1947 Cardiac oxygen metabolism and control of the coronary circulation. Am J Physiol 149:634-639

Feldberg W, Lewis GP 1964 The action of peptides on the adrenal medulla. Release of adrenaline by bradykinin and angiotensin. J Physiol (Lond) 171:98-108

Franchi G, Fanciullaci M, Curradi C, Nuzzaci G, Monetti MG, Caternolo M 1975 Kallikreinogen–kallikrein system during muscular work in patients with intermittent claudication: influence of taurine treatment. Adv Exp Med Biol 79:323-327

Freedlender AE, Fyhrquist R, Hollemans HJC 1974 In: Jaffe BM, Behrman HR (eds) Methods in hormone radioimmunoassay. Academic Press, New York, p 455-469

Gavras H, Liang C, Brunner HR 1978 Redistribution of regional blood flow after inhibition of the angiotensin-converting enzyme. Circ Res 43 (Suppl I):59-63

Goodfriend TL, Odya CE 1974 In: Jaffe BM, Behrman HR (eds) Methods in hormone radioimmunoassay. Academic Press, New York, p 439-454

Goodfriend TL, Levine L, Fasman GD 1964 Antibodies to bradykinin and angiotensin: a use of carbodiimides in immunology. Science (Wash DC) 144:1344-1346

Guth PS, Cano G, Jaramillo J 1963 The effect of bradykinin on vascular smooth muscle. Ann NY Acad Sci 104:69-76

Hammill SC, Wagner WW, Latham LP, Frost WW, Weil JV 1979 Autonomic cardiovascular control during hypoxia in the dog. Circ Res 44:569-575

Hashimoto K, Wanka J, Kuhn RN, Wilkens HJ, Steger R, Back N 1975 The vasopeptide kinin system in acute clinical cardiac disease. Adv Exp Med Biol 70:245-263

Hauge A, Launde PKM, Waaler BA 1966 The effect of bradykinin, kallidin, and eledoisin upon the pulmonary vascular bed of an isolated blood-perfused rabbit lung preparation. Acta Physiol Scand 66:269-273

Heymann MA, Rudolph AM, Nies AS, Melmon KL 1969 Bradykinin production associated with oxygenation of the fetal lamb. Circ Res 25:521-534

Kellermeyer RW, Graham RC 1968 Kinins – possible physiologic and pathophysiologic roles in man. N Engl J Med 279:754-759, 802-807, 859-866

Khairallah PA, Page IH, Turker KR 1966 Potentiation of vascular myotropic responses by metanephrine and other noncatecholamines. Circ Res 19:538-543

Leuenberger PJ, Stalcup SA, Mellins RB, Greenbaum LM, Turino GM 1978 Decrease in angiotensin I conversion by acute hypoxia in dogs. Proc Soc Exp Biol Med 158:586-589

Leuenberger PJ, Stalcup SA, Greenbaum LM, Mellins RB, Turino GM 1980 Angiotensin I conversion and vascular reactivity in pathophysiologic states in dogs. J Appl Physiol: Respirat Environ Exercise Physiol 78:308-312

Liang C, Gavras H 1978 Renin–angiotensin inhibition in conscious dogs during acute hypoxemia. J Clin Invest 62:961-970

Mashford ML, Roberts ML 1972 Determination of blood kinin levels by radioimmunoassay. Biochem Pharmacol 21:2727-2735

Mason DT, Melmon KL 1965 Effects of bradykinin on forearm venous tone and vascular resistance in man. Circ Res 17:106-113

Maxwell GM, Elliott RB, Kneebone GM 1962 Effects of bradykinin on the systemic and coronary vascular bed of the intact dog. Circ Res 10:359-363

McCaa RE, Hale JE, McCaa CS 1978 The effects of angiotensin I-converting enzyme inhibitors on arterial blood pressures and urinary sodium excretion; role of the renal renin–angiotensin and kallikrein–kinin systems. Circ Res 43 (Suppl I):32-39

Melmon KL, Cline MJ, Hughes T, Nies AS 1968 Kinins – possible mediators of neonatal circulatory changes in man. J Clin Invest 47:1295–1302
Nakano J 1965 Effects of synthetic bradykinin on the cardiovascular system. Arch Int Pharmacodyn 157:1-13
Nakano J 1969 Effects of bradykinin, eledoisin and physalaemin on cardiovascular dynamics. Adv Exp Med Biol 6:157-170
Nash CB, Davis F, Woodbury RA 1956 Cardiovascular effects of anesthetic doses of pentobarbital sodium. Am J Physiol 185:107-112
Needleman P 1976 The synthesis and function of prostaglandins in the heart. Fed Proc 35:2376-2381
Needleman P, Marshall GR, Sobel BE 1975 Hormone interactions in the isolated rabbit heart; synthesis and coronary vasomotor effects of prostaglandins, angiotensin and bradykinin. Circ Res 37:802-808
Pitt B, Mason J, Conti CR, Colman RW 1970 Observations of the plasma kallikrein system during myocardial ischemia. Adv Exp Med Biol 8:403-412
Rodbard S, Harasawa M 1959 Passivity of the pulmonary vasculature in hypoxia. Am Heart J 57:232-239
Ruiz-Maza R, Teller D, Walker WG 1974 Measurement of angiotensin II in an ultrafiltrate of plasma. Johns Hopkins Med J 135:211-228
Ryan JW, Ryan US 1977 Pulmonary endothelial cells. Fed Proc 36:2683-2691
Segal N, Stanek V, Joshi R, Singhal S 1970 The influence of bradykinin on the pulmonary hypoxic response in normal man. Prog Respir Res 5:119-126
Stalcup SA, Lipset JS, Legant PM, Leuenberger PJ, Mellins RB 1979a Inhibition of converting enzyme activity by acute hypoxia in dogs. J Appl Physiol: Respirat Environ Exercise Physiol 46:227-234
Stalcup SA, Lipset JS, Woan JM, Leuenberger PJ, Turino GM, Mellins RB 1979b Inhibition of angiotensin converting enzyme activity in cultured endothelial cells by hypoxia. J Clin Invest 63:966-976
Sylvester JT, Scharf SM, Gilbert RD, Fitzgerald RS, Traystman RJ 1979 Hypoxic and CO hypoxia in dogs: hemodynamics, carotid reflexes, and catecholamines. Am J Physiol 236:H22-H28
Thilenius OG, Hoffer PB, Fitzgerald RS, Perkins JF 1964 Response of pulmonary circulation of resting, unanesthetized dogs to acute hypoxia. Am J Physiol 206:867-874
Vane JR 1969 The release and fate of vaso-active hormones in the circulation. Br J Pharmacol 35:209-242
Vatner SF, Braunwald E 1975 Cardiovascular control mechanisms in the conscious state. N Engl J Med 293:970-976
Waaler BA 1961 The effect of bradykinin in an isolated perfused dog lung preparation. J Physiol (Lond) 151:475-480
Wong PY, Talamo RL, Williams GH, Colman RW 1975 Response of the kallikrein–kinin and renin–angiotensin systems to saline infusion and upright posture. J Clin Invest 55:691-698

Discussion

Vane: Have you a hypothesis to explain why the intact endothelial cell is sensitive to hypoxia and the enzyme isn't?

Stalcup: The only findings bearing on that question are from some preliminary tissue culture experiments in which we have added captopril to cultured cells previously equilibrated with a hypoxic gas mixture. If we add this inhibitor to normal cells the enzyme activity is inhibited for up to 1½–2 hours; if we add it to hypoxic cells and then wash it off, the enzyme activity is still present. We think this means that the active site with which captopril normally binds is protected in the hypoxic cell, such that the substrate, or in this case the inhibitor, can't gain access to the converting enzyme molecule. As Dr Soffer has indicated (p 142), this suggests an interaction between membrane components of the intact cell and the active site of the enzyme. We probably need to understand converting enzyme in the intact membrane as a functional unit, rather than as an isolated molecule.

Ballard: One implication of your results is that converting enzyme activity might be low during fetal life, since the fetus is quite hypoxic.

Stalcup: We have examined that question. Converting enzyme activity is low in the fetus (as Dr Mellins will discuss, p 313-326).

Vane: You mentioned that renin levels go up during hypoxia and also angiotensin I levels. Is there a dramatic increase in angiotensin I?

Stalcup: For us it was dramatic, but in retrospect it probably wasn't! Using a radioimmunoassay for extracted angiotensin we find normal levels of about 0.1 ng/ml; after several hours of hypoxia these levels increase as much as tenfold.

Vane: So it is probably still being cleared by the aminopeptidase?

Stalcup: Yes. I don't know what is happening to angiotensin III during that time.

Vane: What is the contribution of catecholamine release to the maintenance of the circulation during hypoxia?

Stalcup: With the onset of hypoxic ventilation there is an enormous burst of both noradrenaline and adrenaline. The former rises to a greater extent and is maintained for longer. With the onset of hypoxic ventilation there is also a prompt and significant rise in dopamine level, which stays up for most of the hypoxic period.

Vane: Bradykinin is an active releaser of catecholamines, if it gets to the adrenal medulla.

Gryglewski: Firstly, I don't understand how bradykinin reverses the decrease in cardiac output induced by hypoxia, since it has no stimulating effect on myocardial contractility of its own. Secondly, if hypoxia results in a burst of catecholamines, one ought to see an increase and not a decrease in cardiac output. Does bradykinin cause more adrenaline to be released or does it change the profile of the catecholamines released from the adrenal medulla?

Stalcup: I think converting enzyme is best understood in the circulation in its relations to other vasoactive systems – catecholamines, prostaglandins and prostacyclin. We need to understand the balance between the renin–angiotensin system, where the usual relationships are profoundly disturbed in hypoxic animals, and the 'second messenger' systems. We found that catecholamine levels rise several thousandfold in asphyxia, and Dr Mellins will present our evidence that in newborn animals with hypoxic ventilation catecholamine levels can rise to extreme values (p 313-326). We suspect that this will have secondary effects on prostaglandin and prostacyclin metabolism, and on cyclic AMP and cyclic GMP. It seems that in hypoxia a new balance is achieved and that the net effect on the circulation can't be explained by change in any one mediator, but is best interpreted in the context of a variety of vasoactive systems.

Gryglewski: Perhaps special attention should be paid to the release of prostacyclin by bradykinin. I believe that the prevention by bradykinin of the pulmonary hypertension induced by hypoxia may be explained by the release of prostacyclin by the lungs (Gryglewski et al 1980). Prostacyclin has a selective vasodilatory effect on the pulmonary circulation.

Aiken: Your curve of bradykinin spillover against oxygen tension has a sigmoid shape and a rather steep portion around P_{O_2} of 60 mmHg; the similar plot for angiotensin conversion was a straight line. Is there a real difference or is it just the technique?

Stalcup: There is a striking dissociation in the shape of the two curves which we cannot eliminate by various manipulations. We don't know why this is.

Bakhle: Doesn't the sigmoid shape of the bradykinin spillover curve derive from the fact that you can suddenly measure something where you could measure nothing before, so you will have a break? What disturbs me more about these results is that angiotensin conversion is maintained when bradykinin inactivation has disappeared. I notice that you still call it 'converting enzyme' even when you are measuring bradykinin hydrolysis. I would prefer you to call it 'bradykininase'; that would give a more accurate picture of what is actually measured.

Stalcup: No! Both angiotensin conversion and bradykinin degradation are similarly reduced by hypoxia. We know that the pressor effect of injected angiotensin I (in the linear portion of the dose–response curve) is almost abolished in animals with a P_{O_2} of 30 mmHg, so the biological activity of the renin–angiotensin system is depressed in hypoxic animals. We also know from radioimmunoassay studies that the clearance of AI declines to about 30% in hypoxia from about 95% in normal oxygen tensions. So by biological assay and radioimmunoassay the renin–angiotensin system is affected by hypoxia but to a slightly lesser extent than bradykinin, as has been confirmed by Szidon et al (1980) using tracer doses of injected angiotensin.

Bakhle: To see any conversion of angiotensin I, even as low as 30%, when you find no inactivation of bradykinin at all – that is what puzzles me.

Stalcup: Could it be something to do with the relative preference of the enzyme for bradykinin as a substrate?

Bakhle: But it is the wrong way round; I would expect the better substrate, bradykinin, to be more resistant to inhibition.

Stalcup: Are there heterogeneous regions in the converting enzyme molecule, each with specialized preference for one substrate?

Soffer: No. There *is* something different in the way different substrates fit into converting enzyme, however; some substrates, such as angiotensin I, require chloride ion for their hydrolysis whereas other substrates, such as the bradykinin-potentiating pentapeptide, Pyr-Lys-Trp-Ala-Pro, not only don't require chloride but their cleavage is inhibited by it. However, the substrates all seem to go to the same place on the enzyme.

Stalcup: I would suspect that this has something to do with the fit of the substrate to the active site, and that by some critical interaction of the cell membrane with that site, one substrate is prevented from having access to the active site and the other less so; but this is speculation.

Soffer: It seems possible that you are studying a biological effect of hypoxia that isn't specifically related to converting enzyme but rather to external cellular membranes in general. It might be interesting to look at different types of cells and see whether the external membrane of each, if you can find a test for its function, is particularly sensitive to oxygen concentration.

Stalcup: Yes. We should like to look at 5′-nucleotidase, which appears to be embedded in the surface of the cell membrane, like converting enzyme, at least from the Ryans' studies.

Junod: 5′-Nucleotidase is located on the outer side of the cell membrane, so such measurements would be very interesting. Is the decrease in converting enzyme activity induced by hypoxia calcium dependent?

Stalcup: There are preliminary experiments (unpublished) to suggest that this phenomenon may be calcium dependent.

Junod: If you used compounds that interfere with the action of myofilaments, would you have the same type of effect?

Stalcup: We are about to do those experiments!

Ferreira: Have you exposed hypertensive animals to hypoxia?

Stalcup: Yes, inadvertently. The pentobarbitone-anaesthetized dog is hypertensive, especially if it was anxious before induction, and our experimental animals all had elevated mean blood pressure. With the onset of hypoxia they become more hypertensive still, despite infusions of bradykinin in amounts which are hypotensive in normoxic animals.

References

Gryglewski RJ, Spławiński J, Korbut R 1980 Endogenous mechanisms that regulate prostacyclin release. In: Samuelsson B et al (eds) Advances in prostaglandin and thromboxane research. Raven Press, New York (4th Int Prostaglandin Conference, Washington DC), vol 7:777-787

Szidon P, Bairey N, Oparil S 1980 Effect of acute hypoxia on the pulmonary conversion of angiotensin I to angiotensin II in dogs. Circ Res 46:221-226

Non-respiratory functions of the lung in the perinatal period

ROBERT B. MELLINS, DENNIS DAVIDSON and S. ALEX STALCUP

Department of Pediatrics (Pulmonary Division), Columbia University College of Physicians & Surgeons and the Babies Hospital, New York, NY 10032, USA

Abstract Beginning with the hypothesis that interference with the metabolic function of the lung could lead to perinatal respiratory disease, we explored the role of one of these functions, angiotensin-converting enzyme activity, in the control of the fetal and newborn circulation. Converting enzyme regulates the concentration of two peptides, bradykinin and angiotensin, important in adapting the fetus to extrauterine life. Initial studies demonstrated decreasing amounts of converting enzyme activity and a parallel decrease in vascular surface with decreasing gestational age. Because we had demonstrated that there is little converting enzyme activity at the low P_{O_2} values of the fetus we examined the fetal–placental unit and found that the placenta is the predominant site of converting enzyme activity *in utero* and this activity is modulated by maternal P_{O_2}. We also found that such pathophysiological accompaniments of premature birth as chilling and acidosis can stimulate the kallikrein–kinin system into overactivity. Because the kallikrein–kinin and renin–angiotensin systems are so closely interrelated with other vasoactive substances, an imbalance in production and degradation is likely to produce some of the pathophysiology seen with premature birth, including systemic hypotension, coagulopathy and oedema.

Because vasoactive substances play a prominent role in mediating the circulatory changes that occur at birth (Melmon et al 1968, Stalcup & Mellins 1980) and because the lung is known to play a central role in regulating the arterial concentrations of vasoactive substances, it is reasonable to hypothesize that the non-respiratory functions of the lung are important in the perinatal period. If this is true, a corollary is that disease, such as neonatal respiratory distress syndrome (RDS), could result from interference in the metabolic functions of the lung by perinatal asphyxia or immaturity. Thus we have proposed that the pathogenesis of RDS can best be appreciated if viewed in the context of immature physiological and biochemical control mechanisms

Metabolic activities of the lung
(Ciba Foundation symposium 78) p 313-331

superimposed on the stresses imposed by the transition to extrauterine life (Stalcup & Mellins 1980a). Several lines of evidence indicate that vasoactive substances play an important role in the perinatal period, both in health and in such diseases as respiratory distress syndrome. For the purposes of this discussion we define vasoactive substances as circulating or tissue factors that mediate changes in blood pressure, vascular resistance, cardiac output, blood volume and transvascular exchange of fluid and protein.

We chose to look at the renin–angiotensin and kallikrein–kinin systems because they are believed to be very primitive humoral control systems and because of their demonstrated role at the time of birth and in early life (Mott 1975, Melmon et al 1968, Heymann et al 1969). Thus (1) the immature mammal shows greater activity of the renin–angiotensin system than does the adult and this system appears to play a proportionately greater role in the newborn mammal than in the adult (Mott 1975); (2) the processes of birth lead to activation of the kallikrein–kinin system with very high levels of bradykinin found in umbilical cord blood; bradykinin has been shown to have an important role in adapting the fetal circulation to extrauterine life (Campbell et al 1968, Heymann et al 1969, Assali et al 1971, Gilbert et al 1973).

The concentration of a vasoactive substance depends on the balance of those factors stimulating production and those factors responsible for degradation. In this regard the renin–angiotensin and kallikrein systems are of particular interest since the same enzyme, namely angiotensin–converting enzyme (dipeptidyl carboxypeptidase, EC 3.4.15.1), is responsible for the production of angiotensin II and the inactivation of bradykinin. The interrelationships between the two systems and the pivotal role of converting enzyme are shown in Fig. 1. Because of the known change in vascular oxygen tension

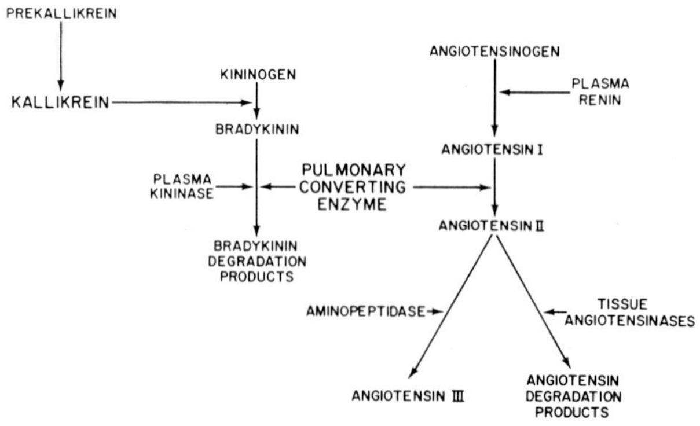

FIG. 1. Interrelationship between the kallikrein–kinin and renin–angiotensin systems.

at the time of birth, our interest in the developmental aspects of this enzyme system was heightened by the observation that converting enzyme activity is modulated by oxygen tension (Leuenberger et al 1978, Stalcup et al 1979a,b, 1980b) with a linear fall in activity as Pa_{O2} decreases.

KALLIKREIN–KININ SYSTEM

The principal components of the kallikrein–kinin system are shown in Fig. 1. The biological activity of this system is terminated by inactivation of bradykinin by converting enzyme. To see how early in gestation this enzyme is present we studied the distribution and development of angiotensin-converting enzyme in fetal and newborn rabbits by immunofluorescence techniques (Wigger & Stalcup 1978). Converting enzyme was noted as early as 17 days of gestation in the lungs, placenta and other organs (term in the rabbit is at 30 days). In parallel with an increase in the number of blood vessels between 17 and 26 days' gestation there was an increase in enzyme localized on the luminal side of the vascular endothelium of the lungs and placenta as well as other organs in the body. These studies also indicated that converting enzyme is a good marker for vascular development during gestational development.

In parallel with these studies we examined the changes in pulmonary converting enzyme activity in the fetal rabbit lung, perfused *in situ* (Stalcup et al 1978). The perfusion pressure used in these studies was approximately 9 mmHg, and the Po_2, 113 mmHg. Thus the oxygen tensions used were those that occur in the postnatal lung. Enzyme activity was assessed by infusing bradykinin in concentrations below those required for enzyme saturation. As demonstrated in the upper panel of Fig. 2 there was a rise in activity over the last third of gestation and the greatest increase did not occur at exactly the same time as the greatest increase in lung or body growth. Much the same findings were obtained when angiotensin I, the other substrate of converting enzyme, was used (lower panel, Fig. 2). Although our studies do not allow precise correlation between vascular growth as indicated by the converting enzyme immunofluorescence studies and these biochemical studies of the enzyme's activity, a close parallel between the two is suggested. The observation that pulmonary converting enzyme activity is lower with decreasing gestation suggests that the prematurely born mammal may be severely handicapped during periods when the kallikrein–kinin system is activated, for example at birth or during episodes of hypotensive stress.

Because these studies were done with perfusates equilibrated with oxygen tensions above 100 mmHg they provide insight into the level of enzyme activity that could be anticipated after premature birth. Since, however, the oxygen

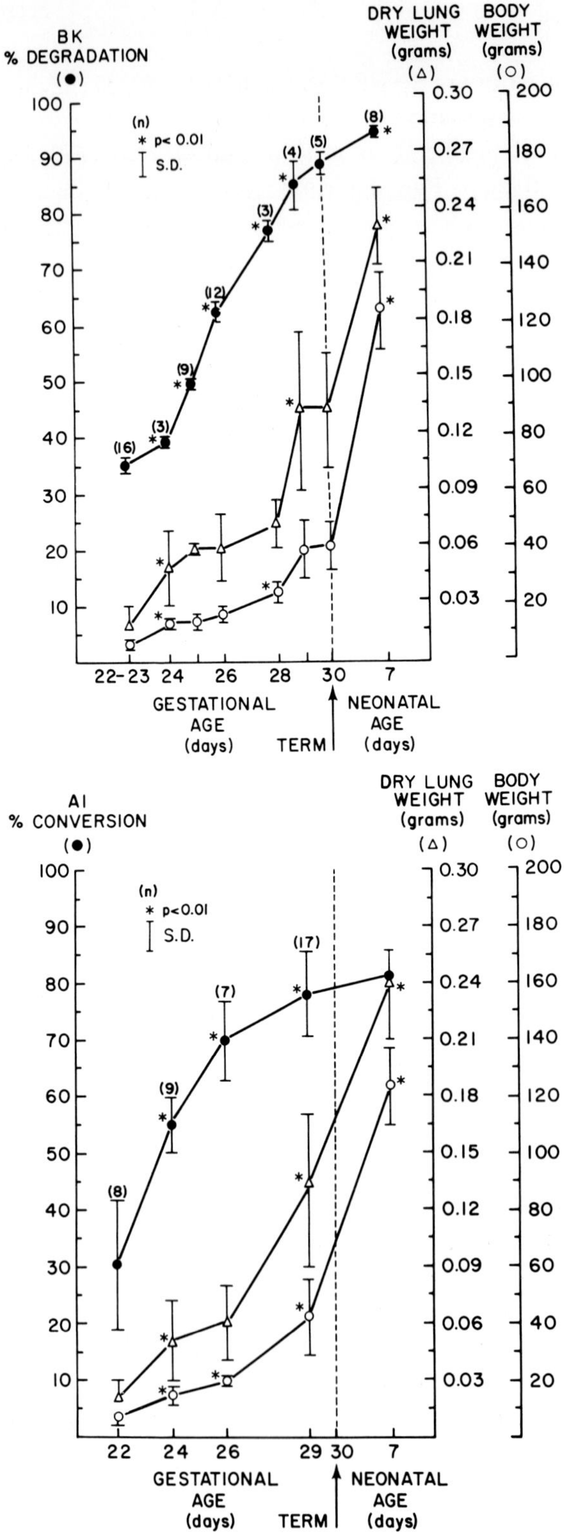
BK
% DEGRADATION
(●)
DRY LUNG WEIGHT (grams) (△)
BODY WEIGHT (grams) (○)
(n)
* p< 0.01
S.D.
GESTATIONAL AGE (days)
TERM
NEONATAL AGE (days)
AI
% CONVERSION
(●)
DRY LUNG WEIGHT (grams) (△)
BODY WEIGHT (grams) (○)
(n)
* p<0.01
S.D.
GESTATIONAL AGE (days)
TERM
NEONATAL AGE (days)

FIG. 2

tension of the fetus is below 30 mmHg and since we have already demonstrated that converting enzyme activity is modulated by P_{O_2} and could be expected to be very low at normal fetal oxygen tensions, we wondered whether the placenta might play an important role in regulating the renin–angiotensin and kallikrein–kinin systems *in utero*. In addition to the fact that converting enzyme is present early in gestational development in the fetal rabbit placenta (Wigger & Stalcup 1978), the mass of the placenta is very large relative to the fetus during gestation and it is exposed to both maternal and fetal oxygen tensions.

In preliminary studies we used the umbilical blood vessels to perfuse separately either the placenta or the fetus *in situ* with angiotensin I and bradykinin, to assess converting enzyme activity (Davidson et al 1980). We showed that at normal fetal and maternal oxygen tensions near term, the converting enzyme previously demonstrated by immunofluorescence to be present in the placenta is biochemically active. Moreover, we found that this activity was modulated by maternal Pa_{O_2}. It will be important to extend these studies since they are likely to have implications for the functioning of both the kallikrein–kinin and renin–angiotensin system at birth.

The kallikrein–kinin system may be stimulated normally at the time of birth by exposure of neonatal granulocytes to increased oxygen tensions and by cooling of the umbilical cord (Melmon et al 1968). We have shown that hypothermia in infants leads to a rise in circulating concentrations of bradykinin (Pang et al 1979); when the lungs (and converting enzyme) were removed from the circulation during cardiopulmonary bypass there was a further rise in the already increased concentrations of bradykinin. As discussed below, severe asphyxia may also lead to increased circulating concentrations of bradykinin. Under these circumstances acidosis activates the kallikrein–kinin system while hypoxia leads to decreased degradation of generated bradykinin. Thus the hypoxic and chilled newborn is especially vulnerable to the effects of excess bradykinin and in the clinical setting these are especially important risk factors for the development of RDS.

Bradykinin has been shown to produce many of the important circulatory changes known to occur at birth (Melmon et al 1968). Bradykinin reduces pulmonary vascular resistance so that blood flows preferentially to the lung (Assali et al 1971, Gilbert et al 1973). It also constricts the ductus arteriosus

---

←

FIG. 2. Change in converting enzyme activity during the last third of gestation in the rabbit, using bradykinin (upper) and angiotensin (lower) as substrates. (Reproduced from Stalcup et al 1978 by permission of The American Heart Association Inc.)

(McMurphy et al 1972). Finally, bradykinin is known to play a role in constriction of the umbilical blood vessels (Eltherington et al 1968). It is clear from all these studies that bradykinin potentiates the effects of oxygen in each of these vascular beds at the time of birth. Hence failure to achieve adequate oxygenation at this time will have an effect not only on converting enzyme activity, as indicated above, but also on the mediation of each of these circulatory adaptations.

RENIN–ANGIOTENSIN SYSTEM

Angiotensin II, the product of converting enzyme's action on angiotensin I, is the potent vasoactive component of the renin–angiotensin system (Fig. 1). Several studies recently reviewed by Mott (1975) indicate the importance of this system in blood pressure homeostasis in the perinatal period. Thus, there is greater sensitivity of the renin–angiotensin system to changes in vascular volume in the fetal lamb than in the adult sheep, with increased renin production in response to haemorrhage and decreased renin and angiotensin II production in response to volume expansion. In neonatal rabbits, less of a drop in blood pressure in response to slow haemorrhage is observed than in adult rabbits. However, after bilateral nephrectomy the neonatal animal becomes more hypotensive than the adult in response to haemorrhage, further emphasizing the importance of the renin–angiotensin system in the defence against hypotensive stress in early life. Other studies demonstrating that umbilical venous levels of angiotensin II are higher than umbilical arterial levels suggest that the placenta may be an important fetal site of converting enzyme activity. These findings cannot be explained by maternal concentrations of renin and angiotensin II because these compounds do not cross the placenta (Symmonds 1979).

Our preliminary studies, described below, suggest that the renin–angiotensin system may also be very important at birth. The increase in Pa_{O2} after the onset of breathing would be expected to increase converting enzyme activity and thus foster production of angiotensin II. Lipset et al (1979) found that in the adult dog the angiotensin II concentration declines rapidly after the onset of hypoxia, despite increased plasma renin activity. The increase in angiotensin I during acute hypoxia results in a bolus production of angiotensin II upon return to normal oxygen tension. Because renin levels are known to be elevated in cord blood (Symmonds 1979) we suspect that similar events are likely at birth. In contrast to the kallikrein–kinin system, the role of the renin–angiotensin system at birth is not yet known. We speculate that angiotensin II could have an important physiological role in maintaining the high systemic resistance required immediately after birth, at a time when its physiological antagonist bradykinin is found in extremely high concentrations. The inability to produce angiotensin II, or its overproduction, could have important effects on blood pressure regulation and the distribution of blood flow in the transitional period.

CIRCULATING VASOACTIVE MEDIATORS AT BIRTH

Because of the relative immaturity of the sympathetic nervous system in the newborn period (Friedman et al 1968, Broughton-Pipkin 1971) and the belief that the newborn relies to a greater extent than the adult on the renin–angiotensin system for defence against hypotensive stress (Mott 1975), we concluded that fresh insights into the role of vasoactive substances at birth could be achieved only by doing serial studies in the unanaesthetized fetus and newborn that interrelate haemodynamic events and simultaneously measured 'first messenger' mediators, namely the kallikrein–kinin, renin–angiotensin and catecholamine systems. To achieve this we placed chronic catheters in the femoral artery of the fetal lamb with the tip below the ductus arteriosus and in the femoral vein with the tip in the right atrium. Blood samples for vasoactive substances were drawn before, during and after delivery by Caesarean section. The results in one preliminary experiment are shown in Fig. 3. Shortly before birth, and coinciding with a modest fall in fetal arterial pH, there is stimulation of the catecholamine, kallikrein–kinin and renin–angiotensin systems. During birth there is an explosive rise in the levels of arterial angiotensin II, bradykinin and total catecholamines in the newborn lamb. These findings confirm previous observations (Melmon et al 1968, Heymann et al 1969) that at birth the arterial concentration of bradykinin is much higher than that in venous blood, indicating a pulmonary origin for bradykinin. Thus in the few moments after birth the systemic circulation is presented with high concentrations of both a vasoconstrictor (angiotensin II) and a vasodilator (bradykinin). Since the persistence of bradykinin and the ongoing generation of angiotensin II depend on oxygen tension (Stalcup et al 1979a,b, 1980b) it is likely that the regional distribution of blood flow will be determined by *local* oxygen tension. The considerable rise in the concentration of catecholamines was unexpected but suggests that it has a physiological role at birth. The observations in Fig. 3 that the rise in catecholamine concentration precedes the rise in plasma renin activity supports previous findings that catecholamines modulate the release of renin through a β-adrenergic mechanism (Ueda et al 1970). Recent studies further suggest an important role for catecholamines in the absorption of fetal lung liquid, and in

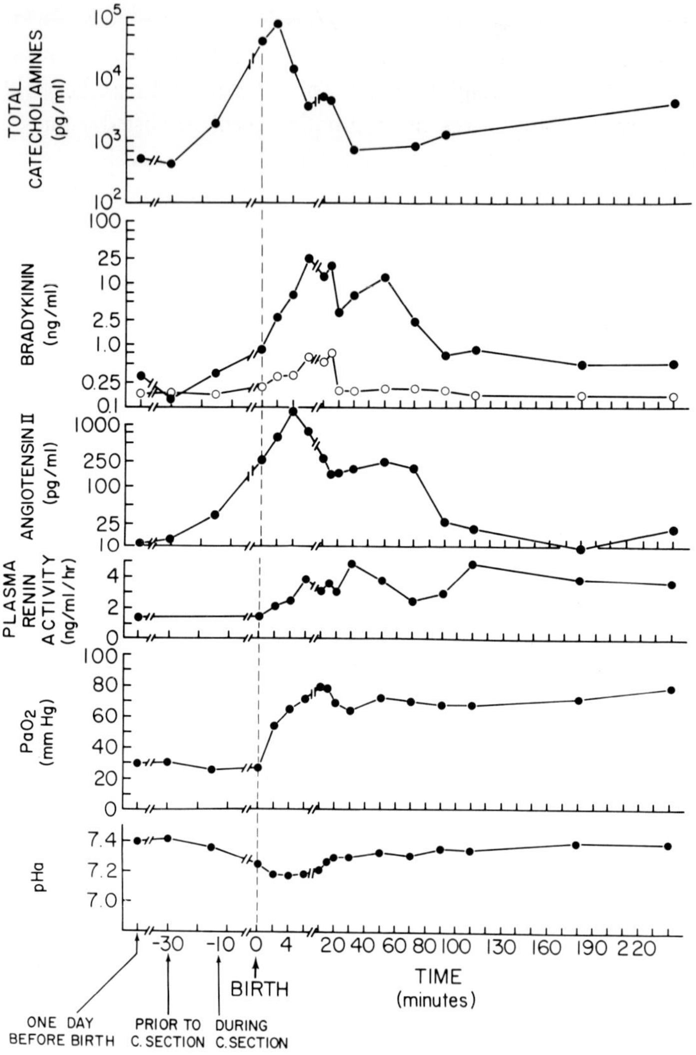

FIG. 3. Sequential changes in circulating vasoactive mediators, Pa_{O2} and pHa before, during and immediately after Caesarean section delivery of the term lamb. •, arterial; ○, venous.

stimulating release of surfactant from type II alveolar cells (Lawson et al 1977, King 1979).

Since acidosis is known to activate the kallikrein–kinin system *in vitro* (Melmon et al 1968) and hypoxia inhibits the degradation of bradykinin, one might anticipate that asphyxia at birth would provoke an extreme disequilibrium between activation and degradation, and this is shown in Fig. 4. The experimental preparation was the same as that in Fig. 3 but this lamb was not allowed to breathe after birth. In contrast to the large amount of bradykinin formed by the lung during normal birth, in this asphyxiated lamb the lung did not make bradykinin. The severe acidosis (pH fell to 6.8 at death) did lead to a rise in the amount of bradykinin leaving systemic tissues, as shown by the higher venous than arterial concentration of bradykinin.

The precise role of the persistent rise in total catecholamines in this asphyxiated lamb is not known but we suspect that it may lead to redistribution of blood flow. The role of circulating catecholamines in the perinatal period has been less extensively studied than the mediator systems already discussed. In the lamb fetus, the infusion of catecholamines has a large effect on the fetal circulation, including pulmonary vasoconstriction (Dawes 1966), and endogenous circulating catecholamines play a prominent role in the redistribution of blood flow to vital fetal organ beds during stress (Rudolph 1969, Jones & Robinson 1975). In the newborn, catecholamines in cord blood samples are increased after a stressful delivery (Cheek et al 1963). This study demonstrated a correlation between cord blood acidosis and raised levels of catecholamines, factors known to cause pulmonary vasoconstriction. The precise relationship between catecholamine excess and the intense pulmonary vasoconstriction in respiratory distress syndrome or persistent pulmonary hypertension of the newborn (Pang & Mellins 1975, Peckham & Fox 1978) remains to be elucidated. Since catecholamines stimulate renin release (Ueda et al 1970) and activate kallikrein (Rothschild et al 1974), clarification of these and other relationships between these mediators is a necessary first step towards developing new therapeutic and preventive approaches.

INTERRELATIONSHIPS BETWEEN 'FIRST' AND 'SECOND' MESSENGER SYSTEMS

There is evidence for widespread intimate interrelationships between mediator systems of all types (Kaplan 1976). As shown in Fig. 5, kallikrein is a major participant in at least two other plasma proteinase cascades, the coagulation and fibrinolysis systems. When kallikrein becomes activated it leads to activation of Hageman factor and plasminogen proactivators; it also feeds back on itself, stimulating further kallikrein activation. The effect of pathophysiological activators of kallikrein such as acidosis and chilling on the ability of kallikrein to activate coagulation and fibrinolysis remains unexplored. Conversely, when tissue injury or shock lead to disseminated intravascular coagulation, the extent to which kallikrein becomes activated is unknown.

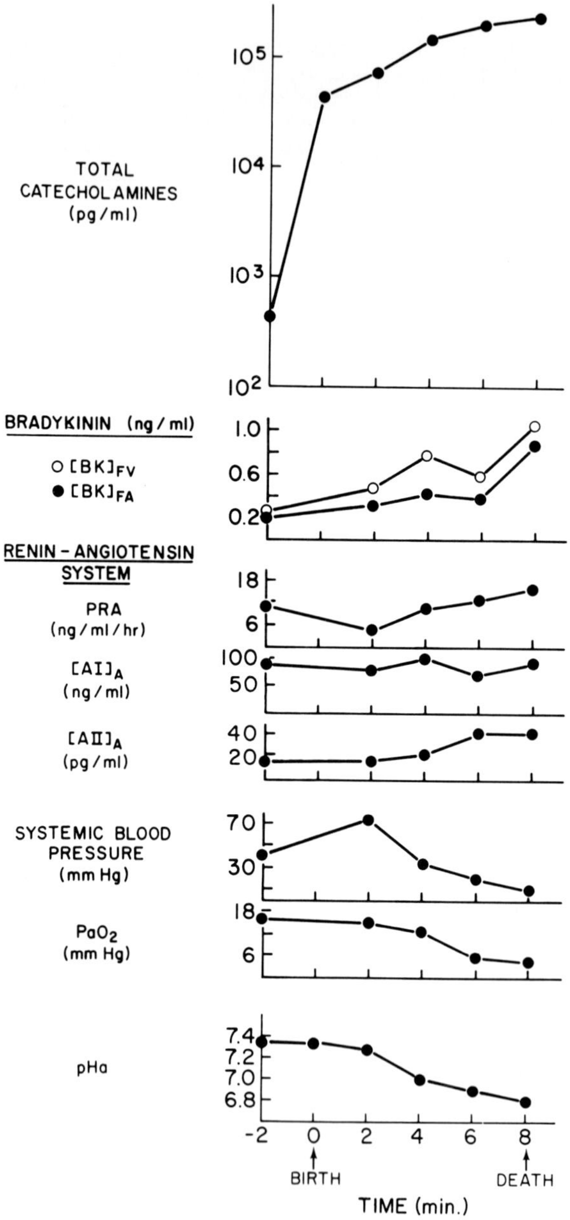

FIG. 4. Sequential changes in circulating vasoactive mediators, systemic blood pressure, Pa_{O2} and pHa during fatal birth asphyxia in the term lamb.

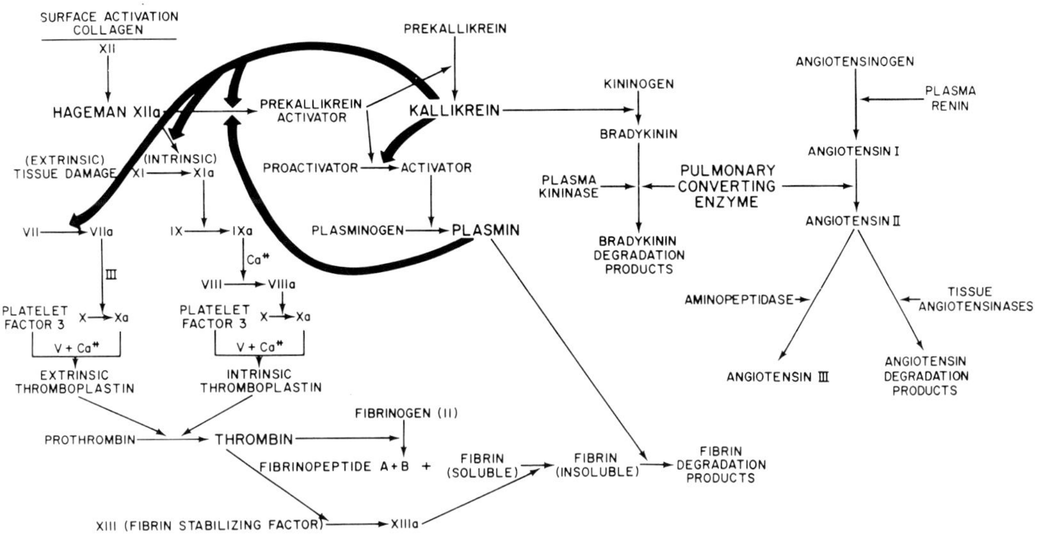

FIG. 5. Interrelationships between the kallikrein–kinin, the coagulation and the fibrinolysis systems and the renin–angiotensin system. (Reproduced from Stalcup & Mellins 1980b, by permission of J.W. Ryan.)

Several aspects of severe neonatal respiratory distress syndrome suggest that control of the activity of these three proteinase pathways is abnormal (Fig. 6) (Stalcup & Mellins 1980a). The coexistence of hypotension, a hypercoagulable state, defective fibrinolysis, systemic tissue oedema, and hypoproteinaemia may relate to vasoactive products of uncontrolled proteinase activity. Hypovolaemia and hypotension are common features of prematurely born high risk infants and have been correlated with the severity of RDS (Chu et al 1967, Neligan et al 1960). Plasma protein concentrations are reduced in premature infants who develop severe RDS and can be used to predict which newborn infants will develop RDS (Bland 1972). Blood pressure regulation in premature infants, especially those with RDS, is markedly unstable; a profound hypotension may be noted within an hour after birth with gradual recovery of blood pressure associated with survival (Chu et al 1967, Neligan et al 1960, Rudolph et al 1961). Pulmonary and peripheral oedema are essential features of RDS and complicate its management (Sutherland 1959). Pulmonary hypotension with right–left shunting of blood (Rudolph et al 1961) and persistence of the transitional circulation (Pang & Mellins 1975) are commonly seen in the course of RDS. These observations, taken together with the gestational immaturity of pulmonary converting enzyme and decreas-

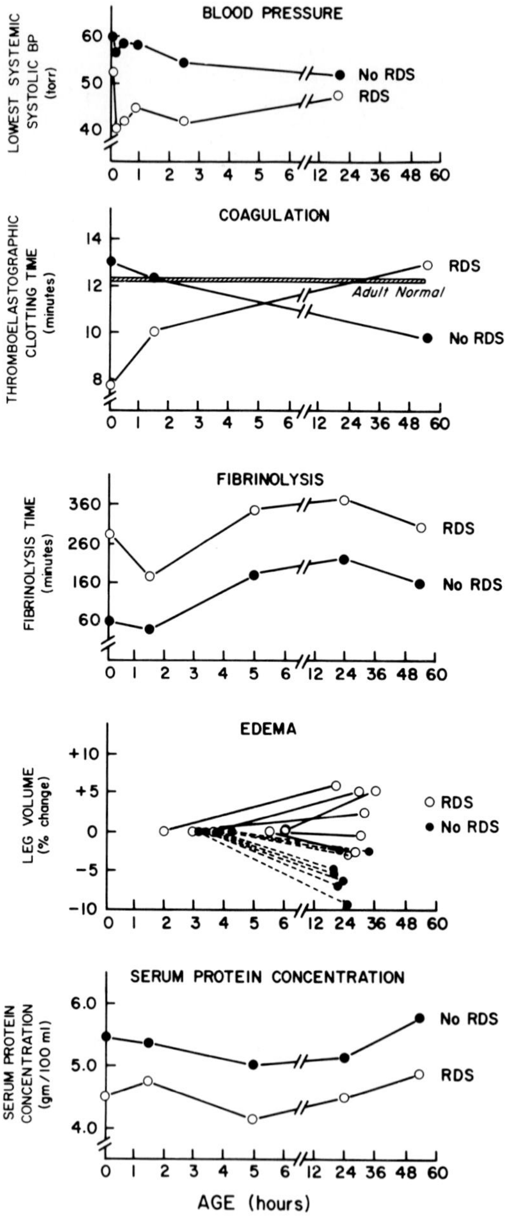

FIG. 6. Sequential changes in neonatal respiratory distress syndrome. (Reproduced from Stalcup & Mellins 1980a. © 1980 A.P. Fishman. Used with the permission of McGraw-Hill Book Company.)

ed converting enzyme activity in hypoxic states, suggest that further investigation of these interrelationships and their control mechanisms is likely to lead to productive insights into neonatal disease.

Circulating 'first messenger' mediators such as catecholamines, bradykinin and angiotensin II exert their effect in part through the production of 'second messenger' mediators such as prostaglandins (Messina et al 1976) and cyclic nucleotides in target organs. We believe that interference with endothelial cell function will result in an imbalance between these interrelated mediator systems and will lead to disease. Finally, modulation of these metabolic functions of the endothelial cell by alterations in physiological state may be important for controlling the activity of these effector systems in health as well as disease.

ACKNOWLEDGEMENTS

Supported by National Institutes of Health Grants HL 06012, HL 07421 and HL 14214 (SCOR), and grants from the Parker B. Francis Foundation and the New York Heart Association.

References

Assali NS, Johnson GH, Brinkman III CR, Huntsman DJ 1971 Effect of bradykinin on the fetal circulation. Am J Physiol 221:1375-1382

Bland RD 1972 Cord-blood total protein level as a screening aid for the idiopathic respiratory distress syndrome. N Engl J Med 287:9-13

Broughton-Pipkin F 1971 Cardiovascular responses in rabbits of different ages to hypertensin and adrenaline. Q J Exp Physiol Cogn Med Sci 56:210-220

Campbell AGM, Dawes GS, Fishman AP, Hyman AL, Perks AM 1968 The release of a bradykinin-like pulmonary vasodilator substance in foetal and newborn lambs. J Physiol (Lond) 195:83-86

Cheek DB, Malinek M, Fraillon JM 1963 Plasma adrenaline and noradrenaline in the neonatal period and in infants with respiratory distress syndrome and placental insufficiency. Pediatrics 31:374-381

Chu J, Clements JA, Cotton EK, Klaus MH, Sweet AY, Tooley WH 1967 Neonatal pulmonary ischemia part I: Clinical and physiologic studies. Pediatrics 40:709-782

Davidson D, Stalcup SA, Mellins RB 1980 Angiotensin converting enzyme activity and its modulation by PO_2 in the guinea pig fetus and placenta. Fed Proc 39:504 (abstr 1250)

Dawes GS 1966 Pulmonary circulation in the foetus and newborn. Br Med Bull 22:61-65

Eltherington LG, Stoff J, Hughes T, Melmon KL 1968 Constriction of human umbilical arteries: interaction between oxygen and bradykinin. Circ Res 22:747-752

Friedman WF, Pool PE, Jacobowitz D, Seagren SC, Braunwald E 1968 Sympathetic innervation of the developing rabbit heart. Circ Res 23:25-32

Gilbert RD, Hessler JR, Eitzman DV, Cassin S 1973 Effect of bradykinin and alterations of blood gases on fetal pulmonary vascular resistance. Am J Physiol 225:1486-1489

Heymann MA, Rudolph AM, Nies AS, Melmon KL 1969 Bradykinin production associated with oxygenation of the fetal lamb. Circ Res 25:521-534

Jones CT, Robinson RO 1975 Plasma catecholamines in fetal and adult sheep. J Physiol (Lond) 248:15-33
Kaplan AP 1976 Activation and control mechanisms of the plasma kinin-forming system and its relationship to coagulation and fibrinolysis. J Invest Dermatol 67:635-637
King RJ 1979 Utilization of alveolar epithelial type II cells for the study of pulmonary surfactant. Fed Proc 38:2637-2643
Lawson EE, Brown EB, Torday JS, Madansky DL, Taeusch Jr HW 1977 Influence of epinephrine on fetal pulmonary fluid production and surfactant release. Physiologist 20:55-65
Leuenberger PJ, Stalcup SA, Mellins RB, Greenbaum LM, Turino GM 1978 Decrease in angiotensin I conversion by acute hypoxia in dogs. Proc Soc Exp Biol Med 158:586-589
Lipset JS, Stalcup SA, Mellins RB 1979 Effect of acute hypoxia on the renin–angiotensin system. Fed Proc 38:689
McMurphy DM, Heymann MA, Rudolph AM, Melmon KL 1972 Developmental changes in constriction of the ductus arteriosus: responses to oxygen and vasoactive agents in the isolated ductus arteriosus of the fetal lamb. Pediatr Res 6:231-238
Melmon KL, Cline MJ, Hughes T, Nies AS 1968 Kinins: possible mediators of neonatal circulatory changes in man. J Clin Invest 47:1295-1302
Messina EJ, Weiner R, Kaley G 1976 Prostaglandins and local circulatory control. Fed Proc 35:2367-2375
Mott JC 1975 The place of the renin–angiotensin system before and after birth. Br Med Bull 31:44-50
Neligan GA, Oxon DM, Smith CA 1960 The blood pressure of newborn infants in asphyxial states and in hyaline membrane disease. Pediatrics 26:735-744
Pang LM, Mellins RB 1975 Neonatal cardiorespiratory physiology. Anesthesiology 43:171-196
Pang LM, Stalcup SA, Lipset JS, Hayes CJ, Bowman Jr FO, Mellins RB 1979 Increased circulating bradykinin during hypothermia and cardiopulmonary bypass in children. Circulation 60:1503-1507
Peckham GL, Fox WW 1978 Physiologic factors affecting pulmonary artery pressure in infants with persistent pulmonary hypertension. J Pediatr 93:1005-1010
Rothschild AM, Cordeiro RSB, Castania A 1974 Lowering of kininogen in rat blood by catecholamines. Arch Pharmacol 282:323-326
Rudolph AM 1969 The course and distribution of the foetal circulation. In: Foetal autonomy. Churchill, London (Ciba Found Symp), p 147
Rudolph AM, Drorbaugh JE, Auld PAM, Rudolph AJ, Nadas AS, Smith CA, Hubbell JP 1961 Studies on the circulation in the neonatal period: the circulation in the respiratory distress syndrome. Pediatrics 27:551-566
Stalcup SA, Mellins RB 1980a Acute respiratory distress in the newborn infant. In: Fishman AP (ed) Pulmonary diseases and disorders. McGraw-Hill, New York, p 1653-1666
Stalcup SA, Mellins RB 1980b Modulation of converting enzyme activity by hypoxia. In: Ryan JW (ed) The lungs, angiotensin converting enzyme and blood pressure control. Plenum Press, New York, in press
Stalcup SA, Pang LM, Lipset JS, Odya CE, Goodfriend TL, Mellins RB 1978 Gestational change in pulmonary converting enzyme activity in the fetal rabbit. Circ Res 43:705-711
Stalcup SA, Lipset JS, Legant PM, Leuenberger PJ, Mellins RB 1979a Inhibition of converting enzyme activity by acute hypoxia in dogs. J Appl Physiol 46:227-234
Stalcup SA, Lipset JS, Woan JM, Leuenberger P, Mellins RB 1979b Inhibition of angiotensin converting enzyme activity in cultured endothelial cells by hypoxia. J Clin Invest 63:966-976
Sutherland JM, Oppe TE, Lucey JF, Smith CA 1959 Leg volume changes observed in hyaline membrane disease. Am J Dis Child 98:24-26
Symmonds ED 1979 The placenta and the renin–angiotensin system. J Reprod Med 23:129-133
Ueda H, Yasuda H, Takabatake Y, Iisuka M, Iizuka T, Ihori M, Sakamoto Y 1970 Observations on the mechanism of renin release by catecholamines. Circ Res 27 (Suppl 2):195-206
Wigger HJ, Stalcup SA 1978 Distribution and development of angiotensin converting enzyme in the fetal and newborn rabbit. Lab Invest 38:581-585

Discussion

Collier: What is the relationship between the respiratory distress syndrome, patent ductus arteriosus and hyaline membrane disease?

Mellins: It is known that the ductus is more likely to stay open in prematurely born infants, probably for reasons connected with muscle development. It is also known that RDS is much more likely to occur in the premature than in the full-term infant. Therefore, the combination of neonatal RDS and patent ductus arteriosus is also more likely to occur in premature infants. As pulmonary vascular resistance falls in these infants postnatally, increased pulmonary vascular blood flow and pressure will lead to increased movement of fluid and protein into the lung and enhanced deposition of fibrin on the alveolar surface, accelerating the course of the hyaline membrane disease (Stalcup & Mellins 1980). I think the patent ductus is a complicating event in RDS but is unlikely to be the cause of the disease.

Collier: It seems that you can have RDS without a patent ductus or hyaline membrane disease, but if you had a patent ductus or hyaline membrane disease you would presumably have RDS? Thinking of prostacyclin here, this may be one of the rarer situations where 'whatever I can do, E can do better', because PGE_2 seems to be more effective than PGI_2 (prostacyclin) in maintaining patency of the ductus (Coceani et al 1979).

Vane: It is true that PGE_2 is more active than prostacyclin in relaxing the ductus, but it could be that the tissue produces much more prostacyclin.

Stalcup: In a few newborns who failed to open up their pulmonary circulation at birth (the persistent fetal circulation syndrome), bolus injections of prostacyclin at birth were effective in opening up the fetal circulation. My working hypothesis is that with the explosive rise in bradykinin at birth there is an augmentation of prostacyclin release and the two have a profound amplifying effect on each other to open up the fetal vascular bed.

Gryglewski: A nice hypothesis can be built on the basis of evidence presented by Dr Stalcup. Let us assume that in the fetal lung arachidonic acid is metabolized mainly to PGE_2; at birth, because of massive activation of the renin–angiotensin and kinin system, instead of PGE_2, prostacyclin starts being produced by the lungs (Gryglewski 1979). Coceani et al (1978) have shown that PGE_2 keeps the ductus arteriosus patent, whereas prostacyclin is not as good as PGE_2 at this job. On the other hand, pulmonary arteries are contracted by PGE_2 and relaxed by prostacyclin (Kadowitz et al 1975). Because of the predominance of PGE_2 produced by the lungs during fetal life the ductus arteriosus remains patent and the pulmonary artery closed. A sudden change in arachidonic acid metabolism at birth along with the development of new mechanical forces is responsible for the reversal of this situation. If this is so, an infusion of prostacyclin into a newborn with patent ductus arteriosus and stenosis of the pulmonary artery will be therapeutically useful.

Professor Markowa in Kraków (our unpublished results) has treated an eight-week-old infant suffering from multiple congenital cardiopulmonary defects (stenosis of the pulmonary artery, an opening between the ventricles and patent ductus arteriosus) with an infusion of prostacyclin (100 ng kg^{-1} min^{-1}, for 48 hours). Serial X-ray photographs clearly demonstrated opening of the pulmonary artery during the infusion of prostacyclin; the blue baby became pink, and this effect persisted for two weeks after the infusion of prostacyclin had been terminated. Unfortunately, three weeks later, the infant's circulation started to deteriorate again. Three other newborns with stenosis of the pulmonary artery were treated with prostacyclin. The opening of the pulmonary artery during the infusion of prostacyclin was seen in all three babies. The aim of this pharmacological treatment is to keep the baby alive until surgery becomes technically possible.

Mellins: Probably in the most severe cases the prostacyclin first reaches the lung in the bronchial circulation, and that is enough to initiate pulmonary vascular dilatation and hence pulmonary perfusion. Once this occurs the prostacyclin may reach the pulmonary vascular bed via the pulmonary arteries.

Gryglewski: Yes, and it is also feasible that as a result of opening up the pulmonary artery, more endogenous prostacyclin is generated by the lung.

Ballard: Studies by Clyman et al (1980) in our institute suggest that PGE_2 is the primary agent maintaining patency of the ductus arteriosus. In fetal sheep the sensitivity of the ductus to PGE_2 decreases during gestation; this would facilitate the effect of oxygen in contracting the vessel with birth at term, as against preterm.

Moncada: PGE_2 seems to be more active *in vitro* than PGI_2.

Vane: One has to be careful in interpreting *in vitro* studies. Terragno et al (1978) showed that slices of fetal vessels in Tris buffer *in vitro* produce five times more prostacyclin than adult vessels, but we don't know what is happening in the fetal circulation. This experiment measures potential rather than actual production.

Mellins: You have also to remember that *in utero* there are vastly different oxygen tensions and that this can be an important modulator of circulating bradykinin. Since, as Dr Moncada has told us (p 165-177), bradykinin itself can be a major stimulus to the prostaglandins, the oxygen tension in these studies is critical.

Junod: If the kinins are important in opening up the pulmonary vessels, why is there such an increase in bradykininase activity at birth?

Stalcup: To maintain the concentration of circulating bradykinin within the range needed for the physiological requirements of the body, especially the pulmonary circulation.

Junod: But why, if you want to keep the vessels open? Is it a good regulatory process? Does it make sense?

Reid: I can't answer that, but perhaps, as Dr Stalcup implies, you need bradykinin only once, to open up the vessels and increase their compliance. The first breaths that the lung takes are the most critical and flow through the arteries once established can maintain itself.

Mellins: It is important to recall that when the bradykinin level is very high the angiotensin II levels are also high; the balance may be critical to the immediate adjustments postnatally. While bradykinin is potent as a pulmonary vasodilator, angiotensin II is most probably responsible for increasing systemic vascular resistance at birth.

Reid: In the first few minutes of life there is a change in function of the pulmonary arteries which leads to a fall in resistance, probably due to a reduction in constriction: there seems to be active vasodilatation. In the first three days of life the distensibility, or compliance, of the smallest, most muscular resistance vessels of the lung increases. The wall thickness of these arteries falls to adult levels although the larger arteries take months (Hislop & Reid 1974, 1977). This must be an important medium- to long-term change being produced by these vasoactive substances. It is not just the fall in blood pressure. The question is whether components of the kinin system or the prostacyclin system are seeping out through the endothelial wall to the basement membrane and smooth muscle and producing changes in the physicochemical behaviour of the muscle and the connective tissue, very selectively, in that part of the vascular bed. At the pressure at which we inject, these vessels achieve an increased external diameter.

Bakhle: To return to Dr Mellins' studies, when both hypoxia and acidosis were present the bradykinin levels in the pulmonary artery were higher than with acidosis alone. Was that due to lack of bradykinin degradation?

Mellins: Yes, combined with the effects of acidosis, which stimulates the formation of kinin.

Stalcup: Hypoxia alone doesn't generate kinin; this occurs only when acidosis is superimposed. Acidosis generates some kinin, but not very much. The greater bradykinin concentration is mainly the effect of absence of degradation.

Bakhle: Have you estimated destruction of angiotensin II in the periphery during hypoxia?

Stalcup: Yes. At normal P_{O_2}, left atrial angiotensin II levels are about 22 pg/ml and right atrial levels, 5.6 pg/ml. In hypoxic animals the levels in left atrial blood fall almost to the limits of the assay, limiting the use of endogenous AII in this experiment.

Bakhle: You could infuse AII into the arterial circulation and see how much survives in the mixed venous blood. If you can reduce one enzyme with hypoxia, you may well affect another, so a part of the fall in AII levels may be not inhibited generation but increased degradation.

Finally, may I repeat my plea that you don't refer to the activity that results in the degradation of bradykinin as 'converting enzyme'? The two activities are not always the same; degradation of bradykinin can result from the action of many enzymes apart from converting enzyme.

Mellins: I accept your point, and we should be careful here. On the other hand, one cannot fail to be impressed by the closeness of the values for angiotensin-converting enzyme activity from both our fetal and our hypoxia studies, whether angiotensin I or bradykinin is used as the substrate.

Vane: Are there likely to be difficulties if captopril is used to treat hypertension in pregnant women?

Stalcup: It could present a problem for the newborn, if captopril crosses the placenta, because the baby needs angiotensin II at birth. The newborn baby also apparently needs a transient rise in bradykinin, and a sustained rise could be detrimental. We have not yet worked with captopril in newborn animals but believe that its use in pregnancy should be evaluated with these considerations in mind. Do you think captopril should be used in exercising individuals?

Vane: You imply that a possible increase in bradykinin followed by the release of prostacyclin might cause a severe fall in blood pressure?

Stalcup: This seems a reasonable hypothesis, and one worth testing.

Mellins: There appears to be a difference in the relative sensitivity of the response of the newborn and the mature individual to stimulation of the renin–angiotensin and catecholamine systems. The nephrectomized newborn rabbit or lamb responds to volume loss with a much greater rise in renin activity than the adult (Mott 1975). In interpreting changes in blood pressure in response to volume loss, one needs to look at both the catecholamine and renin–angiotensin systems. There may be major shifts in the primary control of blood pressure from one system to the other.

Incidentally, there is more than one explanation for the massive catecholamine release at birth. Firstly, it is known to enhance the release of surfactant. Secondly, there are other broad biological effects of catecholamines, such as removal of fetal lung fluid. Thus we don't imagine that catecholamines are there only for circulatory reasons.

Alberti: How much of the catecholamine release was due to Caesarean section?

Mellins: We use a spinal anaesthetic, so the study in the lamb is applicable to newborns delivered by Caesarean section, and not necessarily to normal delivery with concomitant squeezing of the fetus passing through the birth canal. We chose this method to be able to predict the time of birth and be able to make the appropriate measurements.

Stalcup: Cord blood from vaginal delivery at term in the human has levels of catecholamines that are comparable to the ones in Caesarean section in the lamb.

Vane: You are both looking for a reason for the catecholamine release; I am also looking for the cause of that release. This could well be the high angiotensin II levels or bradykinin levels, since both are strong stimulators of catecholamine release from the adrenal medulla.

Bakhle: Is prostacyclin released from the adrenal medulla?

Vane: I don't know. I don't think it has been studied.

References

Clyman RI, Mauray F, Rudolph AM, Heymann MA 1980 Age-dependent sensitivity of the lamb ductus arteriosus to indomethacin and prostaglandins. J Pediatr 96:94-98

Coceani F, Olley PM, Bishai I, Bodach E, White EP 1978 Significance of the prostaglandin system to the control of muscle tone of the ductus arteriosus. In: Coceani F, Olley PM (eds) Advances in prostaglandin and thromboxane research. Raven Press, New York, vol 4:325-333

Coceani F, Bodach E, Dumbrille A, Olley PM 1979 Effect of PGE_2 and PGI_2 on the ductus arteriosus from immature fetal lambs. Abstracts 4th International Prostaglandin Conference, Washington DC, May 1979, p 21

Gryglewski RJ 1979 Is the lung an endocrine organ that secretes prostacyclin? In: Vane JR, Bergström S (eds) Prostacyclin. Raven Press, New York, vol 1:275-288

Hislop A, Reid L 1974 Growth and development of the respiratory system. In: Davis JA, Dobbing J (eds) Scientific foundations of paediatrics. Heinemann, London, p 214-254

Hislop A, Reid L 1977 Formation of the pulmonary vasculature. In: Hodson WA (ed) Development of the lung. (Lung biology in health and disease, vol 6) Dekker, New York, p 37-86

Kadowitz PJ, Joiner PD, Hyman AL 1975 Effect of prostaglandin E_2 on pulmonary vascular resistance in intact dog, swine and lamb. Eur J Pharmacol 31:72-80

Mott JC 1975 The place of the renin–angiotensin system before and after birth. Br Med Bull 31:41-50

Stalcup SA, Mellins RB 1980 Acute respiratory distress in the newborn infant. In: Fishman AP (ed) Pulmonary diseases and disorders. McGraw-Hill, New York, vol 2:1653-1666

Terragno NA, McGiff JC, Smigel M, Terragno A 1978 Prostacyclin (PGI_2): the most abundant prostaglandin (PG) in the fetal vasculature. Fed Proc 37:7321 (abstr)

Prostaglandin receptors in the airways

H.O.J. COLLIER and P.J. GARDINER

Miles Laboratories Ltd, Stoke Poges, Slough, Berkshire, SL2 4LY, UK

Abstract An analysis of the effects of some natural prostaglandins and of synthetic analogues with more selective actions points to the existence of several receptors for prostaglandins in the airways. Three effects have been studied: the contraction and relaxation of bronchial smooth muscle *in vitro* and the cough elicited by inhalation of prostaglandin aerosols by the conscious cat. From the rank orders of potency of a group of prostaglandins and analogues, from tachyphylaxis induced by continued exposure to a single species and from antagonism by indomethacin or mefenamic acid, three prostaglandin receptors have been distinguished: (1) for contraction (χ receptor) and (2) for relaxation (ψ receptor) of bronchial smooth muscle, and (3) for cough (ω receptor). The natural prostaglandins tested stimulated to different extents each of these three receptors; but synthetic analogues with selective actions on only one or two receptors were identified. It seems likely that (1) prostaglandins or thromboxanes not yet tested will interact with these receptors, (2) other receptors for these substances may be distinguished in the airways, (3) the receptors so far distinguished may also be found in other sites, and (4) the receptor categories described may be subdivisible.

The work described here sprang from two paradoxes that were observed during study of the actions of prostaglandins on tracheobronchial smooth muscle. The primary paradox is that any one of the usual prostaglandins, whether PGE_1, PGE_2, $PGF_{2\alpha}$ or PGI_2, if tested over a sufficient range of doses on isolated tracheobronchial muscle, sometimes contracts and sometimes relaxes the preparation. Sweatman and Collier observed this effect in 1967 with prostaglandin E_2 on human isolated bronchial muscle (Sweatman & Collier 1968); recently we have explored it systematically with PGE_1, PGE_2, $PGF_{2\alpha}$, $PGF_{2\beta}$ and PGI_2, and some synthetic derivatives of PGE (Collier & Gardiner 1974, Gardiner 1975, Gardiner & Collier 1980a,b).

The second paradox behind this work is probably related to the first. If a prostaglandin is applied to a strip of tracheobronchial muscle *in vitro* the

Metabolic activities of the lung
(Ciba Foundation symposium 78) p 333-350

resultant response occurs after a long latency, during which a miniature contraction, and/or relaxation, may be seen (Sweatman & Collier 1968).

It has been observed that neither the contractant nor the relaxant actions of prostaglandins on tracheobronchial smooth muscle are modified by propranolol, phentolamine, atropine, mepyramine or methysergide, which antagonize other known bronchoactive endogenous substances (Sheard 1968, Adolphson & Townley 1970, Gardiner & Collier 1980a,b). These observations, and the findings summarized above that the various prostaglandins contract and relax tracheobronchial muscle to different extents, have led us to consider the hypothesis that the responses are due to activation of distinct prostanoid (including thromboxane) receptors subserving contraction or relaxation and that the prostaglandins tested have affinities for both receptors at concentrations within the same range.

When E prostaglandins were first administered by inhalation to man as potential bronchodilators in asthma, cough was found to be their main side-effect (Cuthbert 1969, Herxheimer & Roetscher 1971). Since we observed that the same prostaglandins also elicit cough in the cat, whereas the synthetic bronchodilator derivative, TR4161, was virtually inactive (Gardiner et al 1978, 1980, Gardiner & Collier 1980a,b), it seemed reasonable to postulate that a third prostaglandin receptor, for irritancy, might also exist in the airways. The work we describe here is an exploration of these hypotheses.

METHODS

Theoretical basis

Two principles may be used to distinguish between two receptors for substances of one pharmacological type. One of these principles was used by Ahlquist (1948) to distinguish α and β receptors for adrenaline and by Black et al (1972) to distinguish H_1 and H_2 receptors for histamine. This principle is that, whatever the reaction elicited by the binding of a drug with a receptor at a particular site, the relative potencies of a sufficiently large number of different substances of the same pharmacological group will be comparable if they interact with a single type of receptor and different if they interact with different receptor types.

This principle should apply also to receptor antagonists. Agonists or antagonists specific to a single type of receptor would constitute an extension of this principle from a quantitative to a qualitative form, if the agonist specific to one receptor were supposed to have an affinity for the other receptor too low to elicit a response at practicable doses.

Specific antagonists for prostaglandins are in short supply; but, in tracheobronchial muscle, drugs of the aspirin group can antagonize the contractant action of prostaglandins without antagonizing the relaxant action. Aspirin itself acts in this way, as was first reported in 1968 (Collier & Sweatman 1968); but more impressive activity is shown by the fenamates.

We have used this selective antagonism by non-steroidal anti-inflammatory drugs to help distinguish between prostaglandin receptors for contraction and those for relaxation in tracheobronchial muscle.

A second method, which may be termed 'selective tachyphylaxis', can also be used to distinguish between two receptors present in the same preparation. Tachyphylaxis is a rapidly developing tolerance to a drug. It is known that selective tachyphylaxis applies to prostaglandins (Sweatman & Collier 1968).

To use selective tachyphylaxis effectively it is desirable to find an agonist that binds with only one of the pair of receptors to be distinguished. Fortunately, we have been able to identify, among synthetic prostaglandin derivatives, a compound that fulfils this requirement (TR4752).

Experimental

Test preparations. Three test preparations were used. Two of these were designed to record the contraction or relaxation of the isolated tracheobronchial smooth muscle of man or guinea-pig. The details have been described elsewhere (Gardiner & Collier 1980b). In brief, spirally cut human tertiary bronchiole or guinea-pig trachea cut in a zig-zag fashion was suspended in Krebs' bicarbonate solution at 37°C and movements were recorded with a Harvard isotonic transducer.

The third preparation was designed to record cough in response to inhalation of prostaglandin aerosol by the restrained, conscious cat (Gardiner et al 1978).

Test drugs. In work of this type it is important to use a sufficiently wide range of test drugs of the same pharmacological group. In addition to using the natural prostaglandins E_1, E_2, $F_{2\alpha}$ and I_2, we were fortunate in receiving, from John Wyeth & Brother, $PGF_{2\beta}$, and, from Dr H.C. Kluender of Miles Laboratories Inc., the E prostaglandin derivatives, TR4161, TR4367 and TR4752, which we identified as having marked selectivity in eliciting only one or two of the three effects studied. These derivatives were: 2-decarboxy-2-hydroxymethyl PGE_1 (TR4161); 2-decarboxy-2-hydroxymethyl-15-deoxy-16,20-methano PGE_2 (TR4367); and 2-decarboxy-2-hydroxymethyl-15-deoxy-16,*S*-hydroxy-17,17-dimethyl PGE_1 (TR4752).

SMOOTH MUSCLE CONTRACTION AND RELAXATION

Human bronchial muscle

To determine the relative incidence of contractant and relaxant responses of human bronchial muscle we challenged many preparations with one prostaglandin over a wide range of concentrations. As Table 1 shows, this incidence varied with each prostaglandin. $PGF_{2\alpha}$ and PGE_2 were predominantly contractant on human bronchial muscle; but, on occasions, each produced paradoxical relaxation. PGE_1, $PGF_{2\beta}$ and PGI_2 were predominantly relaxant. Although with PGE_1 paradoxical contractant responses were very rare, with $PGF_{2\beta}$ and PGI_2 they were frequent.

TR4161 and TR4752 had no net contractant effects, although they might have exerted some subliminal contractant action that was masked by the relaxant. TR4161 and TR4752 were tested on 29 and 43 occasions respectively; had they been tested as many times as PGE_1, it is possible that paradoxical contractions might have occurred.

The degree of contractant activity possessed by each prostaglandin was derived from the ratios of total contractant responses to overall total responses in Table 1. From these ratios, the following rank order of contractant activity emerges: $PGF_{2\alpha} > PGE_2 > PGF_{2\beta} > PGI_2 > PGE_1 >$ TR4161 = TR4752. For relaxant activity, these prostaglandins would fall in the reverse order.

In an attempt to handle these paradoxical results further, and to determine in another way the relative activities of the several compounds tested, we derived a mean resultant value from the algebraic sum of the responses to each

TABLE 1

Relative incidence of contractant and relaxant responses to seven prostaglandins by human isolated bronchial muscle

Prostaglandin	*Concn. range at 10-fold dose increments (μg/ml)*	*Total no. of responses observed*	*Total no. of contractions*	*Ratio of contractions to relaxations*
E_1	0.01 –100	626	11	0.018
E_2	0.01 –100	112	84	3.0
$F_{2\alpha}$	0.01 –100	127	121	20
$F_{2\beta}$	0.01 –100	40	18	0.82
I_2	0.001–100	50	11	0.28
TR4161	0.001–100	29	0	0
TR4752	0.01 –100	43	0	0

concentration of each prostaglandin. These means were then plotted against concentration to give a resultant concentration/response line. Fig. 1 gives these lines for some natural prostaglandins, expressed in terms of contraction in response to histamine or relaxation in response to isoprenaline. Fig. 2 gives corresponding lines for $PGF_{2\beta}$, TR4161 and TR4752, expressed in terms of the mean maximal response to PGE_1.

Up to a concentration of 10 μg/ml these concentration/response lines are monophasic and they show a significant slope. An approximate rank order for relaxant activity could be derived from the mean resultant concentration/response lines in Fig. 1 and 2. This order is TR4752 > PGE_1 > TR4161 > PGI_2 > $PGF_{2\beta}$ > PGE_2 > $PGF_{2\alpha}$. This order resembles, but is not identical with, the order for relaxant activity derived from the ratios in Table 1.

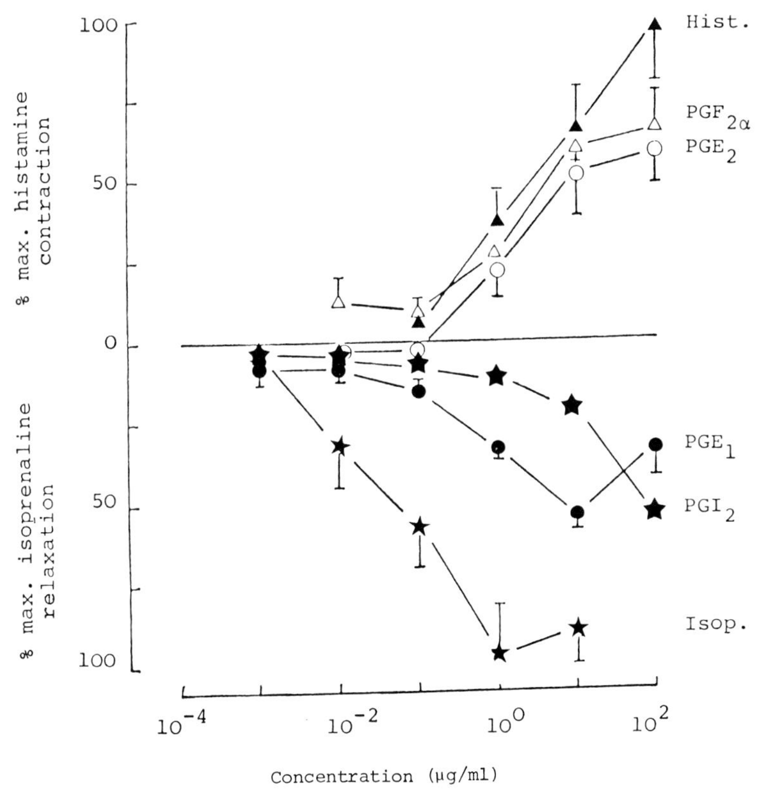

FIG. 1. Mean resultant concentration/response lines of reference prostaglandins on human isolated bronchial muscle. Each point is the mean of at least 4 observations. Vertical lines, SEM. (From Gardiner & Collier 1980b by permission of the publishers.)

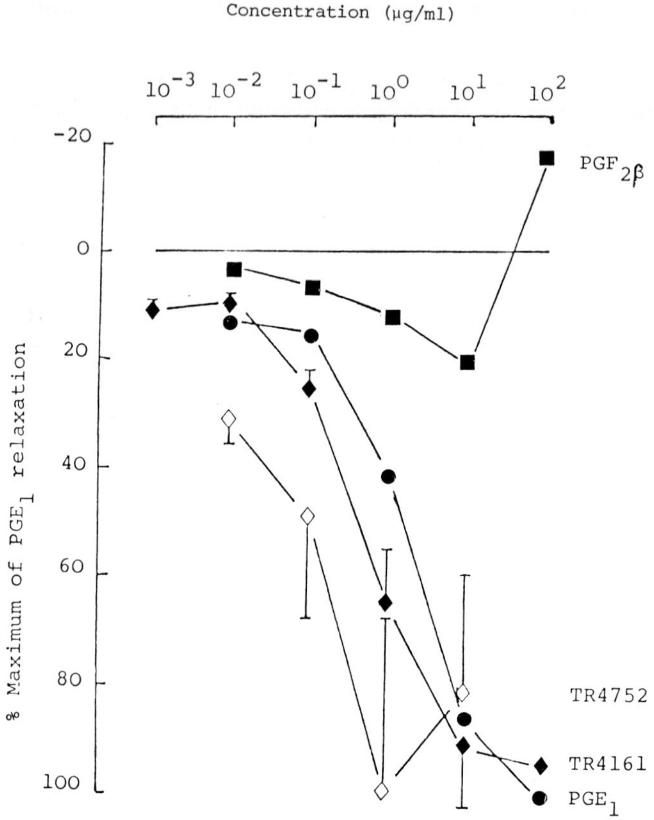

FIG. 2. Mean resultant concentration/response lines of some prostaglandin analogues on human isolated bronchial muscle. Each point represents the mean of at least 4 observations. Vertical lines, SEM. (From Gardiner & Collier 1980b by permission of the publishers.)

Guinea-pig trachea

Contraction and relaxation. Although the paradoxes underlying this study were first met in human bronchial muscle their explanation was more fully investigated in guinea-pig trachea, in which they also occurred, as this tissue was more readily available.

We again determined the activities of test prostaglandins over a wide concentration range. We found that, as with the human muscle, when many tracheal preparations were challenged with a single prostaglandin, some contracted and others relaxed to the same test dose. The relative incidence of contractant and relaxant responses, however, differed somewhat from that in human bronchial muscle, although it also varied with the particular prostaglandin used and its concentration. Table 2 indicates which are the predominant and which the paradoxical actions of each prostaglandin. $PGF_{2\alpha}$ alone was predominantly contractant on the guinea-pig trachea, whereas the remainder were to varying extents predominantly relaxant. PGE_1, $PGF_{2\beta}$, TR4161 and TR4752 had little or no net contractant activity, although they may have had some subliminal contractant action that was masked by the relaxant. In general, guinea-pig trachea more readily relaxed to prostaglandins than did human bronchial muscle.

From the results on which Table 2 was based, mean resultant concentration/response lines were derived, as for human bronchial muscle. Figs. 3 and 4 give these lines. These figures show that, within a wide range of concentrations, the concentration/response lines were monophasic and, except for PGI_2 and TR4367, had significant slopes.

From the data in Table 2 and Figs. 4 and 5 we derived rank orders of activity on guinea-pig trachea, as for human bronchial muscle. A rank order of contractant activity was obtained from the ratios of contractions to relaxations in the last column of Table 2. From these ratios the following rank order of contractant activity emerges: $PGF_{2\alpha} > PGE_2 >$ TR4367 $> PGI_2 > PGE_1 > PGF_{2\beta} =$ TR4161 = TR4752. For relaxant activity, these prostaglandins would fall in the reverse order.

An approximate rank order for relaxant activity was also derived from the mean resultant concentration/response lines in Fig. 4 and 5. This order is: TR4752 > TR4161 > $PGE_1 > PGF_{2\beta} > PGE_2 > PGI_2 >$ TR4367 $> PGF_{2\alpha}$.

TABLE 2

Relative incidence of contractant and relaxant responses to eight prostaglandins by guinea-pig isolated trachea

Prostaglandin	*Concn. range at 10-fold dose increments (μg/ml)*	*Total no. of responses observed*	*Total no. of contractions*	*Ratio of contractions to relaxations*
E_1	0.001 –100	912	3	0.0033
E_2	0.001 –10	168	32	0.24
$F_{2\alpha}$	0.01 –10	374	216	1.4
$F_{2\beta}$	0.01 –10	40	0	0
I_2	0.001 –100	47	5	0.12
TR4161	0.001 –10	51	0	0
TR4367	0.01 –10	16	2	0.14
TR4752	0.000001–10	50	0	0

This order approximates to but is not the same as the rank order for relaxant activity derived from the ratios in Table 2.

Selective antagonism. To extend the evidence that separate prostaglandin receptors subserve contraction and relaxation in tracheobronchial smooth muscle we used indomethacin selectively to antagonize the contractant, without antagonizing the relaxant action of prostaglandins. Since it has been suggested that changes in tone of the muscle explain the paradoxical effects of prostaglandins (Lambley & Smith 1975), histamine was used to restore the tone depressed by indomethacin.

Fig. 5 illustrates experiments on guinea-pig trachea in which a high concentration of indomethacin (100 μg/ml) converted a contractant effect of $PGF_{2\alpha}$ to a relaxant one, without removing the relaxant effects of PGE_1 or PGE_2. In the presence of indomethacin, the latency or the relaxant action was short. These findings support the hypothesis that separate prostaglandin receptors

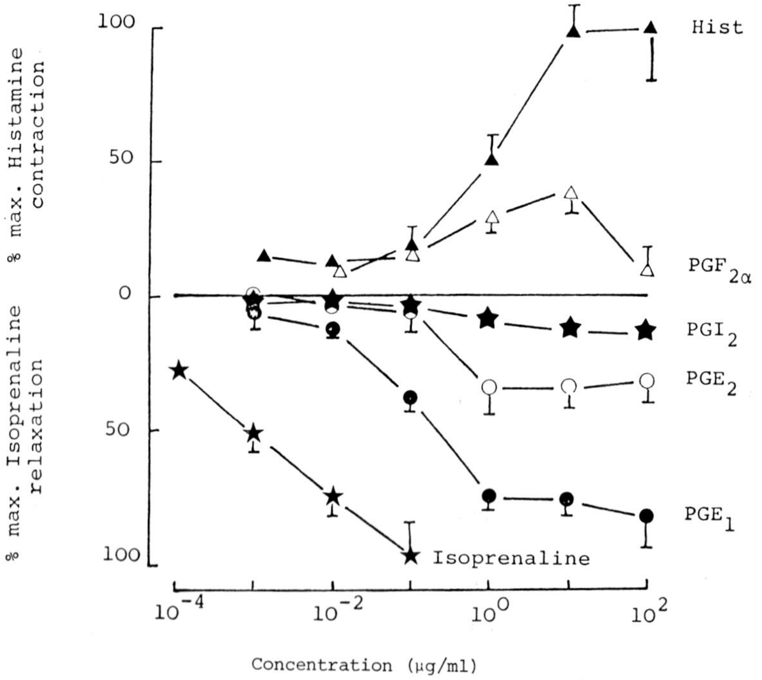

FIG. 3. Mean resultant concentration/response lines of reference prostaglandins on the isolated guinea-pig trachea. Each point represents the mean of at least 6 observations. Vertical lines, SEM. (From Gardiner & Collier 1980b by permission of the publishers.)

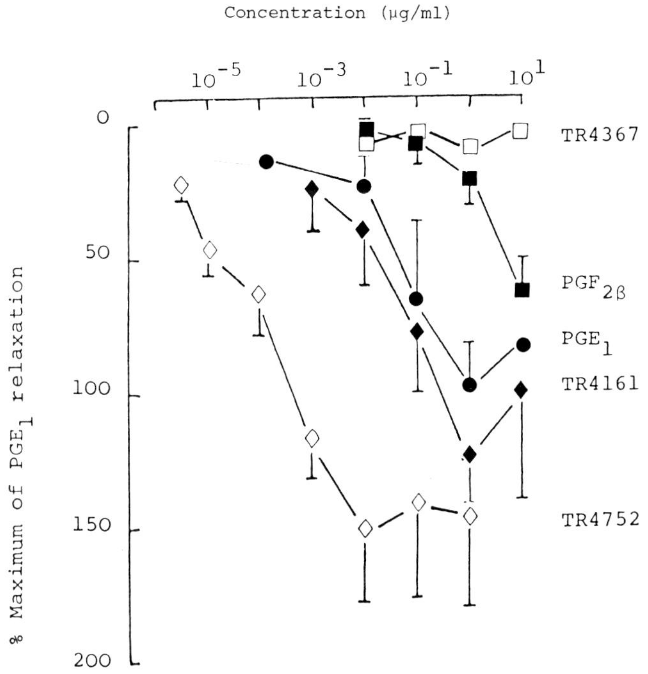

FIG. 4. Mean resultant concentration/response lines of some prostaglandin analogues on the isolated guinea-pig trachea. Each point is the mean of at least 6 observations. Vertical lines, SEM. (From Gardiner & Collier 1980b by permission of the publishers.)

for contraction and relaxation exist in tracheobronchial muscle and that prostaglandins can affect both of them.

Selective tachyphylaxis. Further to distinguish contractant and relaxant receptors in the trachea we induced tachyphylaxis to TR4752, which appeared to be free of contractant effects, by leaving preparations in contact with this prostaglandin derivative at a concentration of 1 μg/ml for 15–30 min. After prolonged exposure to TR4752 the trachea readily contracted in response to PGE_1, but not to TR4752 itself, as Fig. 6 (lower) shows. Similar experiments showed that tachyphylaxis could be induced to the relaxant action of PGE_1 without removing the contractant effect of PGE_2 (Fig. 6, upper). After tachyphylaxis to a relaxant prostaglandin the latency of the contractant responses was short.

These findings indicate that tachyphylaxis can be induced to the relaxant action of prostaglandins without removing their contractant action. They are

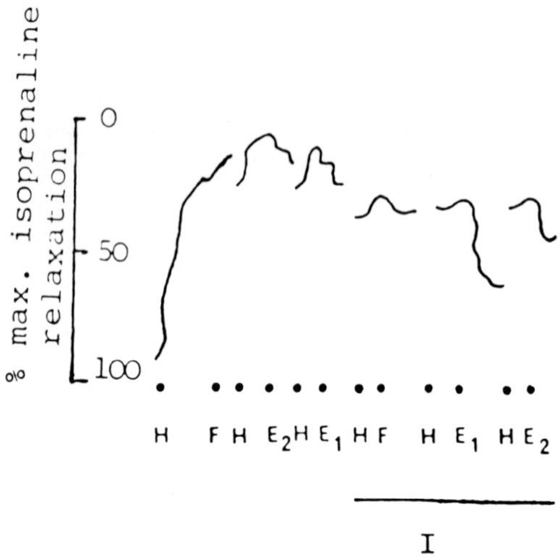

FIG. 5. Blockade by indomethacin of contractant but not relaxant responses of guinea-pig trachea to prostaglandins. H, histamine 1 μg/ml; E_1, PGE_1 0.1 μg/ml; E_2, PGE_2 0.1 μg/ml; F, $PGF_{2\alpha}$ 1 μg/ml; I, indomethacin 100 μg/ml. (From Gardiner & Collier 1980b by permission of the publishers.)

consistent with the hypothesis of separate receptors for relaxation and contraction.

TRACHEOBRONCHIAL IRRITANCY

PGE_1, $PGF_{2\alpha}$, $PGF_{2\beta}$, TR4161, TR4367 and TR4752 were tested for ability to induce cough when inhaled in aerosols by restrained, conscious cats. The irritant activity of each compound was calculated as a percentage of the maximal effect of PGE_1, which was included in the same experiment (Fig. 7). $PGF_{2\beta}$ was tested only at an aerosol concentration of 100 μg/ml. The approximate rank order of irritant activity was $PGF_{2\alpha}$ > TR4367 > TR4752 > PGE_1 > $PGF_{2\beta}$ > TR4161.

DISCUSSION

The same prostaglandin, at the same concentration, relaxes some preparations of tracheobronchial smooth muscle and contracts others. Occasionally the same preparation contracts on one occasion and relaxes on another to the same dose of one prostaglandin. What is the mechanism of this? It has been argued that these paradoxical effects depend on the initial tone of the prepara-

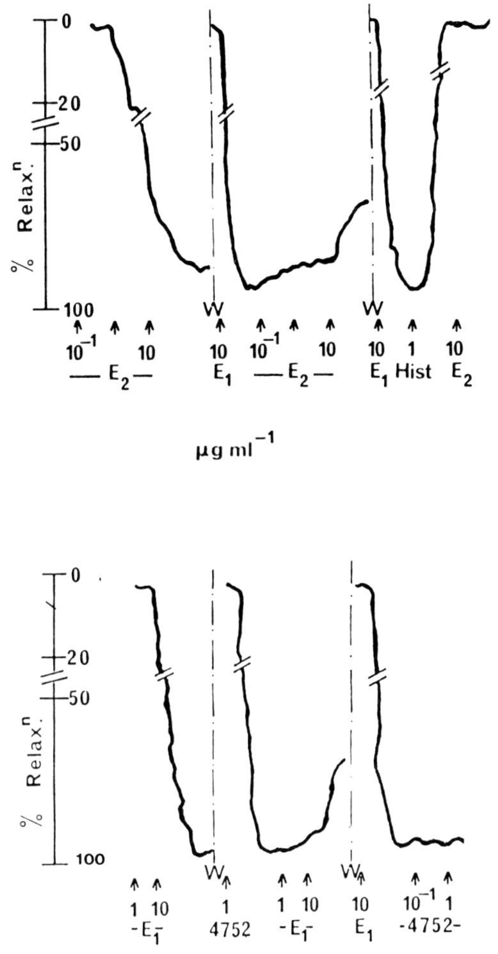

FIG. 6. Tachyphylaxis to the relaxant prostaglandins, TR4752 and PGE_1, unmasks the contractant component of PGE_1 (lower) and PGE_2 (upper) on guinea-pig trachea. To induce tachyphylaxis the prostaglandins were left in contact with the preparation for 30 min. At W it was washed for 1 min. Drug concentrations in μg/ml. (From Gardiner & Collier 1980b by permission of the publishers.)

tion (Lambley & Smith 1975); experiments with theophylline do not fully support this. Although in our hands theophylline greatly reduced tracheal tone, it did not alter the contractant effect of $PGF_{2\alpha}$ or histamine, nor did it convert relaxation induced by PGE_1 or PGE_2 to contraction. The inadequacy of this explanation encouraged us to explore the possibility that two distinct recep-

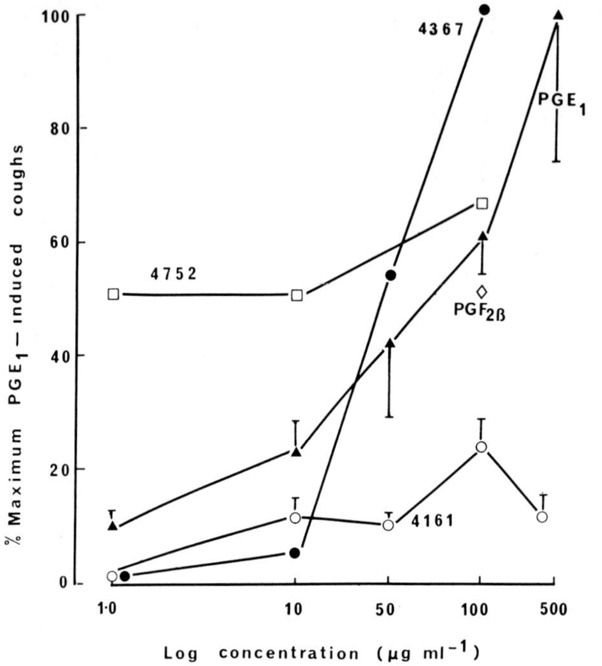

FIG. 7. Tracheobronchial irritant activity of inhaled prostaglandins E_1, $F_{2\beta}$, TR4161, TR4367 and TR4752 in restrained, conscious cats. (From Gardiner et al 1980 by permission of the publishers.)

tors for prostaglandins, one of which subserves contraction and the other relaxation, occur on tracheobronchial muscle.

The hypothesis of two opposed receptors on tracheobronchial muscle, however, raises difficult questions. We shall consider two of these questions below, but the immediately practical question is: how can one obtain evidence for this hypothesis with data on the relative potencies of different prostaglandins? While recognizing the imperfection of our methods, we have obtained approximate rank orders of contractant and relaxant activities of a group of prostaglandins in the ways described. The results are summarized in Table 3, which also gives the approximate rank order of irritant activity in most of these prostaglandins.

Whereas the rank orders for relaxant activity are comparable and not significantly different in human and guinea-pig muscle, the orders for contractant and relaxant activities are obviously different. These rank orders support the hypothesis of two opposed receptors in the muscle; but it will be desirable to confirm the rank orders by determining the contractant and relax-

TABLE 3

Rank orders of activity of prostaglandins on guinea-pig and human tracheobronchial muscle and on cat cough

Action	*Rank order of activity*
(a) Contraction human bronchiole[a]	$F_{2\alpha} > E_2 > F_{2\beta} > I_2 > E_1 >$ TR4161 = 4752
(b) Relaxation human bronchiole[b]	$4752 > E_1 > 4161 > I_2 > F_{2\beta} > E_2 > F_{2\alpha}$
(c) Contraction guinea-pig trachea[a]	$F_{2\alpha} > E_2 > 4367 > I_2 > E_1 > F_{2\beta} = 4161 = 4752$
(d) Relaxation guinea-pig trachea[b]	$4752 > 4161 > E_1 > F_{2\beta} > E_2 > I_2 > 4367 > F_{2\alpha}$
(e) Cat cough	$F_{2\alpha} > 4367 > 4752 > E_1 > F_{2\beta} > 4161$

[a]Based on ratio of total contractions to relaxations recorded for each prostaglandin (Tables 1 and 2).
[b]Based on mean resultant concentration/response lines (Figs. 1–4).

ant potencies of all these prostaglandins in conditions in which one putative receptor has been inactivated. As a step in this direction we have shown that a high concentration of indomethacin blocks the contractant but not the relaxant effect of $PGF_{2\alpha}$ on guinea-pig trachea and that tachyphylaxis to TR4752, which appears to be free of contractant action, unmasks a contractant activity in PGE_1.

A factor that has not been excluded is the spontaneous production of prostanoids by isolated tracheobronchial muscle, indicated by the loss of tone in the presence of non-steroidal anti-inflammatory drugs (Collier & Sweatman 1968, Collier & Gardiner 1974). This may exert a modifying effect that cannot yet be assessed.

The question also arises: is there a distinct, third receptor for the irritant action of prostaglandins? That the rank order for irritancy in Table 3 is different from those obtained for contraction or relaxation of smooth muscle supports this distinction. Further evidence is provided by individual prostaglandin analogues. For example, TR4367 has irritant, but little contractant or relaxant activity. Again, TR4161 has little irritant or contractant, but potent relaxant activity, whereas TR4752 has irritant and relaxant, but no contractant activity. Furthermore, a number of other prostaglandin analogues, which show no obvious contractant but high relaxant activity on guinea-pig trachea and human bronchial muscle, readily induce cough in the cat. Taking into account also that $PGF_{2\alpha}$ has potent irritant and contractant, but little relaxant activity, the argument for a separate cough receptor appears to be strong. Table 4 summarizes these selective actions.

In summary, therefore, our experiments support the hypothesis that at least three types of prostaglandin receptor exist in the airways. We have provisionally termed these the χ (contractant), ψ (relaxant) and ω (irritant) recep-

TABLE 4

Selective actions of prostaglandins on airways, assessed on human and guinea-pig tracheobronchial muscle and on cat cough

Prostaglandin	*Tracheobronchial contraction*		*Tracheobronchial relaxation*		*Cough (cat)*
	Human	*Guinea-pig*	*Human*	*Guinea-pig*	
E_1	±	±	+ + +	+ + +	+ +
E_2	+ +	+	+	+ +	+ +
$F_{2\alpha}$	+ +	+ +	±	±	+ + +
$F_{2\beta}$	+	−	+	+ +	+
I_2	+	−	+ +	+	NT
4161	−	±	+ + +	+ + +	±
4367	NT	±	NT	±	+ +
4752	−	−	+ + + +	+ + + +	+ +
Putative receptors	χ		ψ		ω

+, + +, + + +, + + + + indicate degree of activity; −, inactive; NT, not tested.

tors in airways for prostaglandins and possibly other prostanoids. Until potent and selective antagonists of all three putative receptors are found, however, and the appropriate receptor binding studies have been done, this hypothesis will remain provisional.

It seems possible that further prostanoid receptors will be distinguished in the lungs and equally possible that the three receptors so far distinguished will be found to exist in other sites than the airways. For example, there could be more than one variety of contractant receptor for prostaglandins in the airways. A contractant receptor detected in guinea-pig lung strip by Coleman et al (1980) appears, however, insofar as a comparison can be made, to resemble the χ receptor that we have postulated.

The hypothesis that both contractant and relaxant receptors exist in tracheobronchial muscle and that both are stimulated to different extents by natural prostaglandins resolves one paradox, but raises fresh questions. The paradox resolved is the length of the latency of the response of tracheobronchial muscle to a prostaglandin and the presence, during that period, of miniature contractions, and/or relaxation.

One of the outstanding questions that remains is: what is the mechanism by which one prostaglandin activates one receptor on one occasion and another on another? In answer, one might suppose that each prostaglandin receptor is readily modulated by events such as the presence of another local hormone or the continued presence of one prostaglandin, so that the relative sensitivities of the two receptors can readily be altered.

The second, broader outstanding question is: what is the value to the organism of this paradoxical arrangement? The answer we should like to sketch is in terms of the general functions of prostaglandins recently proposed (Collier 1980). These are two: first, to act as local hormones participating in the defensive, including expulsive, activities of the organism. Second, to control excessive defensive activity arising in the exercise of the first function. In the airways, one might suppose that cough and bronchoconstriction are defensive responses to potentially toxic materials inhaled. Bronchodilatation would be a corrective action, to control a dangerous excess of bronchoconstriction.

ACKNOWLEDGEMENTS

We thank the several chest surgeons and nurses who supplied specimens of human lung, and Miss Julia L. Copas for technical help and Mr S.A. Wilson for useful discussions.

References

Adolphson RL, Town RG 1970 A comparison of the bronchodilator activities of isoproterenol and prostaglandin E_1 aerosols. J Allergy 45:119-120

Ahlquist RP 1948 A study of the adrenotropic receptors. Am J Physiol 153:586-600

Black JW, Duncan WAM, Durant CJ, Ganellin CR, Parsons EM 1972 Definition and antagonism of histamine H_2-receptors. Nature (Lond) 236:385-390

Coleman RA, Humphrey PPA, Kennedy I, Levy GP, Lumley P 1980 Preliminary characterization of three types of prostanoid receptor. Br J Pharmacol 69:265P-266P

Collier HOJ 1980 Prostaglandin synthetase function, pain and drug action. In: Ramwell PW (ed) Prostaglandin synthetase inhibitors in clinical medicine. Alan Liss, New York, p 87-105

Collier HOJ, Gardiner PJ 1974 Pharmacology of airways smooth muscle. In: Burley DM et al (eds) Evaluation of bronchodilator drugs. Trust for Education and Research in Therapeutics, London, p 17-25

Collier HOJ, Sweatman WJF 1968 Antagonism by fenamates of prostaglandin $F_{2\alpha}$ and of slow reacting substance on human bronchial muscle. Nature (Lond) 219:864-865

Cuthbert MF 1969 Effect on airways resistance of prostaglandin E_1 given by aerosol to healthy and asthmatic volunteers. Br Med J 4:723-726

Gardiner PJ 1975 The effects of some natural prostaglandins on isolated human circular bronchial muscle. Prostaglandins 10:607-616

Gardiner PJ, Collier HOJ 1980a Receptors for E and F prostaglandins in airways. In: Samuelsson B et al (eds) Advances in prostaglandins and thromboxane research, vol 7 (4th Int Prostaglandin Conference, Washington DC), Raven Press, New York, p 1003-1008

Gardiner PJ, Collier HOJ 1980b Specific receptors for prostaglandins in airways. Prostaglandins 19:819-843

Gardiner PJ, Copas JL, Elliott RD, Collier HOJ 1978 Tracheobronchial irritancy of inhaled prostaglandins in the conscious cat. Prostaglandins 15:303-315

Gardiner PJ, Copas JL, Schneider C, Collier HOJ 1980 2-Decarboxy-2-hydroxymethyl prostaglandin E_1 (TR4161), a prostaglandin bronchodilator of low tracheobronchial irritancy. Prostaglandins 19:349-370

Herxheimer H, Roetscher I 1971 Effects of prostaglandin E_1 on lung function in bronchial asthma. Eur J Clin Pharmacol 3:123-125
Lambley JE, Smith AP 1975 The effects of arachidonic acid, indomethacin and SC-19220 on guinea-pig tracheal muscle tone. Eur J Pharmacol 30:148-153
Sheard P 1968 The effect of prostaglandin E_1 on isolated bronchial muscle from man. J Pharm Pharmacol 20:232-233
Sweatman WJF, Collier HOJ 1968 Effects of prostaglandins on human bronchial muscle. Nature (Lond) 217:69

Discussion

Vane: You have found some prostaglandin analogues with an increased selectivity towards bronchodilatation. Have you managed to eliminate other side-effects of the prostaglandins, such as diarrhoea and fall in blood pressure?

Collier: Yes; with TR4161 almost all side-effects are reduced to various extents, compared with PGE_1 (Gardiner et al 1980).

Vane: And you lose the anti-aggregating activity as well?

Collier: Yes.

Bakhle: You gave these compounds to cats by inhalation, so enough must get into the systemic circulation to cause diarrhoea?

Collier: Yes, with large doses; but the cat may have swallowed some of it and not inhaled it.

Said: There is a hypothesis that agents that cause bronchial relaxation do so by inducing the accumulation of cyclic AMP in tracheal and bronchial smooth muscle. Have you any measurements of cyclic nucleotides to support or refute this? Secondly, do you think the variability you find in the response of airways to a given prostaglandin could be due in part to the tone of the smooth muscle before the agent is applied?

Collier: We haven't any evidence to contradict the idea that a rise in cyclic AMP is associated with relaxation, and your findings with VIP are consistent with this idea. Changes in tone have been claimed as the reason for the change in responsiveness to prostaglandins, determining whether contraction or relaxation occurs, but our experience using theophylline or histamine to modify tone is that tone is only one of the factors involved.

Mellins: Since you give the drugs to cats by inhalation, how do the receptors that you are looking for relate to the irritant receptors and the likelihood of reflex bronchoconstriction? Could you be stimulating irritant receptors in variable ways, and could some of the variability in response relate to reflex bronchoconstriction?

Collier: Are we using the word 'receptor' ambiguously? The irritant receptors might be considered as sensory receptors as well as pharmacoreceptors. I think that a chemoreceptor could be either sensory or pharmacological or both. Our work on bronchoconstriction was done on isolated smooth muscle; so there is no question of a reflex effect there.

Aiken: The endogenous production of prostaglandins may well be contributing to the responses. To draw firm conclusions about the order of potency it would be necessary to do the experiments on indomethacin-treated tissues, wouldn't it?

Collier: I agree that the endogenous production of prostaglandin is confusing. This applies particularly to the guinea-pig trachea. We are now looking at these responses after indomethacin. We have to repeat the studies in the absence as far as possible of endogenous prostanoids, and with the experiment more fully controlled.

Reid: Do these prostaglandins or their analogues affect mucus secretion? One use of $PGF_{2\alpha}$ is that it helps the normal subject, who does not normally bring up sputum, to produce bronchial secretion for study. We found that the mucus glycoprotein content of secretion induced in this way was similar to that of a mild bronchitic, but it lacked the serum component (Lopez-Vidriero et al 1977). This raised the question whether the drug had stimulated the secretory cells of the gland or surface epithelium or simply squeezed the gland duct to release preformed secretion. The effect on mucus secretion is an important aspect of the properties of these drugs.

Collier: I think it's important too; we haven't yet studied the effect on mucus secretion but we obviously should do so.

Gryglewski: How specific is the antagonism between meclofenamate and $PGF_{2\alpha}$ receptors? Is it found in smooth muscle other than that of the trachea or bronchi?

Collier: Yes. Bennett et al (1980) showed that meclofenamate potently antagonizes PGE_2 on the longitudinal muscle of guinea-pig ileum and $PGF_{2\alpha}$ on that of human intestine. We obtained similar results with rat stomach strip.

Piper: What are the effects of bradykinin on guinea-pig trachea, relative to the fenamates? Did the fenamates antagonize bradykinin? They do so in the whole guinea-pig, but there is a rather complicated story in the isolated trachea.

Collier: I don't recall our testing fenamates against bradykinin in the isolated guinea-pig trachea, although, as you say, they are active against bradykinin in the guinea-pig *in vivo* (Collier et al 1968).

Piper: Does the inhibition of contraction caused by bradykinin suggest that bradykinin was releasing a bronchoconstrictor prostaglandin?

Collier: There is little doubt but that in the guinea-pig *in vivo* bradykinin liberates a bronchoconstrictor of the prostaglandin group.

Moncada: The response of tracheal strips to arachidonic acid is sometimes relaxation and sometimes contraction!

Collier: I agree; but in the guinea-pig *in vivo* the response to intravenous arachidonic acid is usually bronchoconstriction.

Aiken: The response of the isolated guinea-pig trachea to arachidonic acid depends on the tone of the muscle (Aiken & Waddell 1976). When the tone is low it produces contraction; when the tone is higher, arachidonic acid relaxes tracheal muscle. Both responses are blocked by low doses of indomethacin or aspirin.

Vane: And is the tone changed by indomethacin?

Aiken: Yes. It usually relaxes!

Datta: What is the concentration of circulating arachidonic acid?

Moncada: In humans the concentration of arachidonic acid in plasma is low, about 3 μg/ml, which represents no more than 1–2% of the total free fatty acids. In dogs it is much higher, about 30–100 μg/ml (Ramwell et al 1977).

Bakhle: We have perfused guinea-pig lung with [^{14}C]arachidonate using Krebs' solution without albumin: 80% was taken up into the lung lipids and 20% came out as metabolite. When 1% albumin is added to the perfusing medium, uptake of arachidonate into lung is reduced to 50% and the rest comes out in the effluent almost all as unchanged arachidonate (Al-Ubaidi & Bakhle 1979). We feel this shows that the cyclo-oxygenase has less chance to compete for arachidonate in albumin-bound form, but arachidonate is still taken up into lung lipids.

References

Aiken JW, Waddell JE 1976 Relaxation of isolated tracheal smooth muscle produced by prostaglandin precursors and bradykinin: antagonism by aspirin-like drugs. Fed Proc 35:803

Al-Ubaidi F, Bakhle YS 1979 The fate of exogenous arachidonic acid in guinea-pig isolated lungs. J Physiol (Lond) 295:445-455

Bennett A, Pratt D, Sanger GJ 1980 Antagonism by fenamates of prostaglandin action in guinea-pig and human alimentary muscle. Br J Pharmacol 68:357-362

Collier HOJ, James GWL, Piper PJ 1968 Antagonism by fenamates and like-acting drugs of bronchoconstriction induced by bradykinin or antigen in the guinea-pig. Br J Pharmacol 34:76-87

Gardiner PJ, Copas J, Schneider C, Collier HOJ 1980 2-Decarboxy-2-hydroxymethyl prostaglandin E_1 (TR4161), a prostaglandin bronchodilator of low tracheobronchial irritancy. Prostaglandins 19:349-370

Lopez-Vidriero MT, Das I, Smith AP, Picot R, Reid L 1977 Bronchial secretion from normal human airways after inhalation of prostaglandin $F_{2\alpha}$, acetylcholine, histamine and citric acid. Thorax 32:734-739

Ramwell PW, Leovey EMK, Sintetos AL 1977 Regulation of the arachidonic acid cascade. Biol Reprod 16:70-87

The lung, whole-body metabolism and disease

W.A. STUBBS and K.G.M.M. ALBERTI*

*Department of Medicine, St. Bartholomew's Hospital, West Smithfield, London EC1A 7BE, and *Department of Clinical Biochemistry and Metabolic Medicine, Royal Victoria Infirmary, Newcastle upon Tyne, NE1 4LP, UK*

Abstract It is well recognized that the lung has its own hormonally responsive endogenous metabolism. Less well recognized is the potential of the lung to influence and, in turn, be influenced by the homeostatic mechanisms of the body. It is suggested that the lung could modulate concentrations of circulating hormones and thereby play an indirect exogenous metabolic role in whole-body metabolism. Investigations of patients undergoing cardiopulmonary bypass as well as studies with the perfused rat lung suggest that the lung could make an important direct contribution to whole-body lactate and perhaps alanine production.

The control of the endogenous and exogenous metabolism of the lung may be exerted through circulating hormones, substrates, blood gases and lung movement. Disorders of the lung or the whole body may disturb these relationships. In patients with chronic lung disease circulating blood metabolites are affected and conversely in diabetes there are effects on lung metabolism.

The unified concept of lung/whole-body metabolism is discussed in relation to therapeutic approaches for the prevention and investigation of neonatal and adult respiratory distress syndromes.

The lung has received little attention as an organ which may contribute significantly to whole-body metabolism, despite its anatomical siting, which means that it receives the total blood supply of the body.

In this context four proposals will be made and discussed. These are as follows:

(1) The lung has not only its own endogenous metabolism but also an influence on the metabolism of the rest of the body; that is, it has an exogenous role.

(2) Both the endogenous and exogenous metabolic functions of the lung are controlled by the hormonal and metabolic mechanisms of the rest of the body.

(3) Lung disease produces metabolic disturbances in the body and *vice versa*.

Metabolic activities of the lung
(Ciba Foundation symposium 78) p 351-372

(4) The modification of metabolic interactions between the lung and the rest of the body may promise therapeutic benefit.

ENDOGENOUS AND EXOGENOUS LUNG METABOLISM

Many of the endogenous aspects of lung metabolism have been discussed earlier (Datta et al 1980). The exogenous metabolic role could be mediated through effects on either circulating blood metabolites or hormones.

In animal preparations the lung can utilize a variety of substrates including glucose, non-esterified fatty acids (NEFA), lactate, ketone bodies, and certain amino acids (see Datta et al 1980). The uptake of even a major substrate such as glucose, however, probably accounts for only a few per cent of the whole-body turnover (Searle 1976). Similarly, although the lung may oxidize non-esterified fatty acids (NEFA) (Felts 1964), only 2% of a dose of radioactive palmitate injected into animals appears in the lungs (Young & Tierney 1972). Thus the contribution of the substrate uptake by the lungs to whole-body utilization of glucose and NEFA is probably small, although it may be somewhat greater for lactate (Wolfe et al 1979).

These results are derived from animal models. In man, studies have been restricted to measurement of arterio-venous (A-V) differences. The large pulmonary blood flow tends, however, to conceal concentration differences resulting from the uptake or production of substrates by the lung; Tierney (1974) calculated that the A-V concentration difference for glucose would be expected to be only 0.02 mmol/l. It is hardly surprising that consistent A-V differences for substrates across the lung have been difficult to demonstrate, and there is considerable uncertainty about substrate utilization by the lung *in vivo*.

We re-examined this problem by taking simultaneous pulmonary artery and aortic blood samples from six anaesthetized patients immediately before cardiopulmonary bypass for open-heart surgery. The samples were subsequently analysed for blood levels of glucose, lactate, alanine, pyruvate, 3-hydroxybutyrate and glycerol.

Lactate and alanine were consistently produced by the lungs of these patients (Table 1). The other substrates showed no consistent pattern. The mean production by the lung of lactate was 150 μmol/l and of alanine 16 μmol/l. If we assume a cardiac output of 4 l/min, this could account for over 50% of the whole-body turnover of lactate (Krebs et al 1975) and over 20% of that of alanine (Chochinov et al 1978). These figures appear high but it must be remembered that the lungs in this study were exposed to a variety of drugs, anaesthetic agents and mechanical ventilation. Nonetheless the lung in man,

TABLE 1

Mean (± SEM) blood glucose, lactate, pyruvate and alanine concentrations in the pulmonary artery and aorta of six patients before and five patients after cardiopulmonary bypass

	Pulmonary artery (P) (mmol/l)	*Aorta (A) (mmol/l)*	*% extraction*[c]
Glucose	before 5.4 ± 0.2	5.5 ± 0.2	−2 ± 2
	after 8.5 ± 0.4[b]	8.6 ± 0.3[b]	−2 ± 3
Lactate	before 1.2 ± 0.1	1.4 ± 0.1[a]	−13 ± 4
	after 2.1 ± 0.2[b]	2.1 ± 0.3[b]	1 ± 3[b]
Pyruvate	before 0.07 ± 0.01	0.08 ± 0.01	−10 ± 9
	after 0.13 ± 0.01[b]	0.11 ± 0.01[b]	6 ± 3
Alanine	before 0.27 ± 0.02	0.29 ± 0.02[a]	−7 ± 2
	after 0.42 ± 0.05[b]	0.41 ± 0.04[b]	2 ± 1[b]

[a] $P < 0.05$ compared with pulmonary artery concentrations.
[b] $P < 0.05$ compared with values before cardiopulmonary bypass.
[c] % extraction = [(P − A/P] × 100.

as in the rat, may be a lactate-producing organ. It is tempting to speculate that lung could account for the observation by Krebs et al (1975) that the computed lactate production for the individual major organs was about 17% lower than that observed for the whole body.

The direct contribution of the lung to substrate turnover in normal healthy subjects has still to be established. It seems likely, however, that the lung may make, at least in some circumstances, a significant contribution to whole-body lactate and alanine turnover.

In addition to any contribution to substrate turnover, the lung may also have an exogenous metabolic effect, through the modulation and production of circulating hormones.

Normal lungs have long been known to contain neurosecretory or Feyrter cells that may have an endocrine function. Recently, the neuropeptide bombesin has been identified in fetal and neonatal lungs (Wharton et al 1978) and it is probably only a matter of time before other representatives of this family of neuropeptides are discovered in the lung. Thus the lung may be an integral part of a peptidergic nervous system analogous to that of the gastrointestinal tract (Buchanan 1979). It is well known that lung tumours can produce a variety of hormones which have effects throughout the body (Said 1980). Whether this is a reflection of a physiological rather than a purely pathological property remains unclear.

The lung can also concentrate, inactivate, activate, modify or produce a wide range of bioactive substances, often through carrier-mediated processes requiring intact metabolism (Junod 1975). This rapidly increasing list now includes prostaglandins, prostacyclins, thromboxane, serotonin (5-hydroxytryptamine), noradrenaline, angiotensin, bradykinin and vasoactive intestinal polypeptide (VIP), discussed elsewhere in the symposium. The lung also affects the hormones of 'classical' endocrinology, such as cortisol, testosterone, dihydrotestosterone, aldosterone, gastrin, ACTH, thyroxine and, as discussed in the next section, insulin (Junod 1975, Editorial 1974, Hitchcock 1979).

CONTROL OF ENDOGENOUS AND EXOGENOUS METABOLISM

Endogenous metabolism

The metabolic goal of the body is the continuous provision of appropriate energy-yielding substrates for tissue use. Glucose is of overriding importance in that neuronal tissue depends entirely on glucose for metabolism except in chronic starvation. Glucose homeostasis therefore tends to take preference over other metabolic reactions. In starvation, alternative substances such as ketone bodies and NEFA are provided for tissues other than brain so that glucose supplies are preserved for neural use. The whole system is regulated by a fine balance between insulin, the anabolic hormone, and the catabolic hormones, glucocorticoids, catecholamines and glucagon, with growth hormone playing an intermediate role. In the long term, thyroid hormones are also catabolic. In the fed state the balance tilts in favour of insulin with catabolic hormones predominating in starvation and stress states. The catabolic hormones serve to mobilize fuels, the anabolic hormones to conserve them.

In the fed state the liver stores glucose as glycogen or by converting it to fatty acids. Muscle builds up its own stores of glycogen and triglycerides are laid down in adipose tissue. The reverse happens in starvation with additionally amino acids such as alanine being released from muscle and peripheral tissues for gluconeogenesis in the liver. Thus through a series of complex hormonal and metabolic events there is both an alteration in the balance of substrates presented to the tissues and a change in the metabolic pathways of the tissues themselves.

If the lung is an integral part of this homeostatic system there should be similar changes in its substrate uptake and utilization during periods of increased catabolism, such as fasting. In the isolated lung, glucose is the predominant substrate used, even with high concentrations of NEFA available (Rhoades 1974), although the addition of palmitate (Shaw & Rhoades 1977) or lactate (Wolfe et al 1979) does decrease glucose oxidation. Thus glucose can indeed be spared.

The metabolic pathways of the lung can be altered in response to changes in whole-body homeostasis such as fasting. During fasting glucose uptake (Perez-Diaz et al 1977a) and the activity of the glycolytic pathways (Gregorio et al 1976, Chaisson & Massaro 1978) are decreased. There is preferential oxidation of fatty acids and reduced production of both total lipids and phospholipids (Gross 1977, Shaw & Rhoades 1977, Gregorio et al 1976). There is also decreased amino acid incorporation, increased proteolysis and decreased protein synthesis (Gacad et al 1972, Thet et al 1977).

The metabolism of the lung is now known to be under hormonal control. As Morishige (1980) and Ballard (1980) have discussed in this symposium, receptors for glucocorticoids, insulin, thyroxine and androgens have been identified in the lung. The metabolism of the lung has been shown to respond to catecholamines, histamine, thyroxine, glucocorticoids and insulin (Barnett et al 1978, Hitchcock 1979, Datta et al 1980).

The responses of the lung to glucocorticoids and insulin are precisely what one would predict from the metabolic adaptations during starvation. Thus the glucose uptake of *in situ* perfused lungs from fed rats is increased by insulin (Stubbs et al 1977) and decreased by corticosterone (Stubbs 1979). Interestingly, the effect of insulin at physiological concentrations is absent from lungs of fasted animals (Stubbs 1979).

It is therefore evident that the lung is under close hormonal and metabolic control, lung metabolism being modulated through effects on the levels and uptake of circulating substrates, on the activity of the metabolic pathways, and on the degree of response to circulating hormones.

Two additional control mechanisms should also be mentioned: blood gases and ventilatory movements. We were able to examine the effect of respiratory movements and P_{CO_2} independently, since ventilation is not obligatory in the rat lung perfused *in situ* (Stubbs 1979). Ventilation of the lungs at 8 breaths/min decreased the glucose uptake by over 40%. Glucose uptake in the rapidly ventilated lungs (120 breaths/min), however, was similar to control values (unventilated) (Fig. 1). Conversely, lactate production was increased by 28% in response to rapid ventilation but remained unchanged in the slowly ventilated lungs. It is also interesting to note that more lactate was produced than could be accounted for by glucose uptake, suggesting that the lung may have been drawing on substrate reserves.

The effects of P_{CO_2} at low (20 mmHg), medium (40 mmHg) and high (60

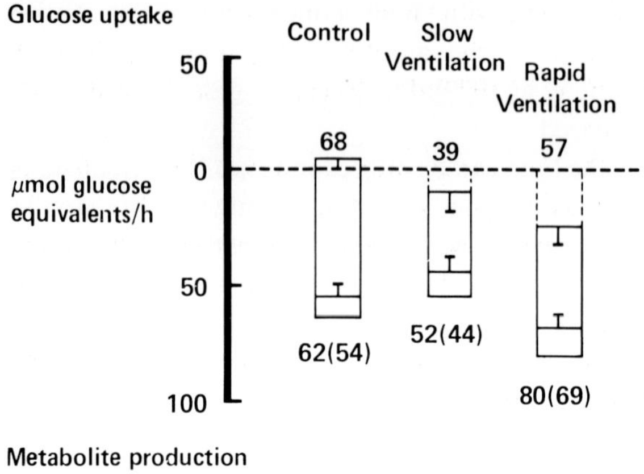

FIG. 1. Glucose uptake and metabolite production at 4 h in the unventilated (control) and ventilated rat lung, perfused *in situ*. The lungs were ventilated at either 8 (slow ventilation) or 120 (rapid ventilation) breaths/min with 95% oxygen and 5% carbon dioxide with a tidal volume of 5 ml. Metabolite production and glucose uptake are plotted as a 'metabolic balance', metabolite production being plotted downwards and glucose uptake upwards. A 'positive balance' lies above and a 'negative balance' below the dotted line.

The upper figures give glucose uptake; the lower figures give total metabolite production (i.e. the sum of lactate, pyruvate, glycerol and alanine production) with lactate production also shown separately in brackets. Results are expressed as mean ± SEM of μmol glucose equivalents/h at 4 h. To obtain the value for the metabolites produced in μmol/h the lower figures should be multiplied by two.

mmHg) values were also examined in the unventilated rat lung perfused *in situ*. Glucose uptake after four hours of perfusion was similar for all values of P_{CO_2}. In the lungs exposed to a high P_{CO_2}, however, lactate production was decreased below that of the other two groups (Stubbs 1979). These results suggest that the effects of a high P_{CO_2} on lung metabolism are selective, since lactate production decreased while glucose uptake remained unchanged. This may represent the diversion of glucose to other metabolic pathways, such as phospholipids, whose production is increased in response to a rise in P_{CO_2} (Longmore & Mourning 1977).

Increased pH (Pérez-Díaz et al 1977b), prolonged hyperoxia (Clark 1971), Fisher 1978) and hypoxia (Bassett et al 1974, Rhoades 1975) also affect lung metabolism. Whether any of these 'respiratory' functions of the lung influence endogenous metabolism *in vivo* is unknown.

In conclusion, the endogenous metabolism of the lung appears to be sensitive to a wide range of hormonal, metabolic and respiratory influences *in vitro*.

Exogenous metabolism

That the lung is a regulator of circulating hormones was initially suggested by Comroe in 1953.

The effect of circulating substrates on the clearance of circulating bioactive substances was demonstrated in the isolated guinea-pig lung by Fisher et al (1979). The clearance of serotonin by the lung was decreased by a metabolic inhibitor, 2-deoxyglucose, and this effect could be reversed by adding substrates such as pyruvate, lactate, acetate, alanine, 3-hydroxybutyrate, palmitate and glycerol. Since the circulating concentrations, uptake and disposal of these substrates are under hormonal control, there is a potential mechanism for one or several hormones to influence the metabolism of another hormone or bioactive substance.

There is also evidence for more direct interactions between hormones; some of these have been discussed elsewhere in the symposium. The uptake or generation of prostaglandins can be affected by thromboxanes (Boura & Murphy 1978), histamine (Berti et al 1979) or glucocorticoids (Gryglewski 1975). It can also be inferred that hormones, either directly or indirectly, may have a role in the alteration of prostaglandin metabolism in thyrotoxic (Moore & Hoult 1978) and pregnant animals (Bedwani 1975). However, while many of these bioactive substances, including the prostacyclins, have metabolic effects (Samuelsson et al 1975, Gryglewski 1980) they are not generally accepted as classical regulators of intermediary metabolism. We therefore looked at the clearance of insulin, one of the 'classic' regulators. There was a slow removal of insulin by perfused lungs from both fed and fasted rats. The half-life of insulin was greater in the fed (5.3 $\pm$ 0.4 h) than the fasted animals (3.6 $\pm$ 0.2 h).

In the isolated perfused rat liver, the half-life of insulin is less than 30 min; it is less than four minutes in intact man. In comparison, therefore, the clearance of insulin by the lung is small. The lungs may however make some contribution to insulin clearance, since in patients with heart disease the serum insulin concentrations in arterial blood were 10–18% lower than in venous blood (Rubenstein et al 1968). The main point nonetheless is that the exposure of the lung to different metabolic environments, such as fasting, produces a change in the clearance of a hormone.

In addition to these hormonal influences ventilation *per se* has long been recognized to release prostaglandins and bioactive substances, including peptides such as VIP (Piper & Vane 1971, Said 1979). Roth & Gillis (1977) also showed that the clearance of drugs was influenced by ventilation, and the same could hold for hormones.

The fact that the endogenous metabolism of the lung is influenced by the metabolic control systems of the rest of the body suggests that this organ should be considered an integral part of whole-body metabolism. In addition, the homeostatic mechanisms of the body influence and, in turn, may be influenced by the exogenous metabolism of the lung. The lung may therefore have an important hormone regulatory role, acting, in effect, as a 'hormonostat'.

LUNG/WHOLE-BODY INTERACTIONS IN DISEASE

The complex series of interactions between the lung and the rest of the body is vulnerable to disease. In the previous section we discussed the various ways in which metabolic stress, such as starvation, produce changes in both endogenous and exogenous metabolism. In prolonged starvation the changes in endogenous metabolism may be accompanied by a decrease in the phospholipid and surfactant production, surface activity and pulmonary compliance of the lung (Gross 1977, Sahebjami et al 1978).

An exaggeration of this whole-body catabolic response might be expected to produce similar changes. One such condition is diabetic ketoacidosis, where there is relative or absolute insulin deficiency and a marked increase in catabolic hormones (see Datta et al 1980, Morishige 1980). Thus glucose uptake in lungs from ketoacidotic rats, perfused *in situ,* was only 68% of that of non-diabetic controls, although lactate production was similar.

When lungs are perfused they are removed from the metabolic environment of the animal. The failure of added insulin to increase the glucose uptake in the lungs from diabetic animals suggests persisting abnormalities of the hormonal response and metabolic pathways of the lungs. Such abnormalities include decreased glucose oxidation, and altered insulin receptors and lipid production (Moxley & Longmore 1977, Morishige 1980).

The effects of severe uncontrolled diabetes on pulmonary function have been little studied. Schuyler et al (1976), however, reported abnormal elastic properties of the lungs in diabetics, although the blood glucose levels of the patients were not stated.

It is apparent that changes in whole-body homeostasis, such as the excessive catabolism accompanying ketoacidosis, may produce disturbances in endogenous lung metabolism in animals and abnormalities of respiratory function in man. In addition, since the generation of prostacyclin may be affected in diabetics (Gryglewski 1980), exogenous lung metabolism may also be disturbed. The possible effects on the lung of excessive catabolism in other situations will be returned to later (p 364). We shall first discuss disturbances of whole-body metabolism resulting from chronic lung disease.

When a metabolically active organ such as the liver is diseased, derangements in whole-body metabolism may be reflected by changes in circulating intermediary metabolites (Johnston & Alberti 1976). We therefore measured fasting venous blood concentrations of hormones and metabolites in 21 patients with chronic lung disease. The metabolic effects of treatment with oral steroids or steroids plus salbutamol were also examined.

In the patients with chronic lung disease not receiving any drugs there was a 100% increase in total blood ketone bodies, a 36% increase in plasma NEFA and a 21% decrease in blood alanine (Table 2). In addition the [lactate]/[pyruvate] and [3-hydroxybutyrate]/[acetoacetate] ratios were elevated.

In the patients treated orally with steroids, only the blood lactate level was raised, but treatment with steroids plus adrenergic agents produced a rise in blood lactate and glycerol concentrations and in [lactate]/[pyruvate] ratio.

The changes in circulating levels of metabolites in patients treated with steroids or steroids plus adrenergic agents was probably a consequence of the drugs used rather than of the lung disease itself. However, in normal subjects

TABLE 2

Circulating venous blood levels of metabolites, hormones, pH, P_{O_2} and P_{CO_2} in control subjects and patients with chronic lung disease without therapy or receiving steroids or steroid plus catecholamines

	Control subjects (12)	*Chronic lung disease*		
		No treatment (9)	*Steroids (6)*	*Steroids + adrenergic agents (6)*
Lactate (mmol/l)	0.76 ± 0.05	0.71 ± 0.04	1.24 ± 0.15***	1.24 ± 0.12***
Pyruvate (mmol/l)	0.07 ± 0.01	0.06 ± 0.01	0.1 ± 0.01	0.09 ± 0.01
Glucose (mmol/l)	5.2 ± 0.2	5.2 ± 0.2	5.1 ± 0.2	5.1 ± 0.03
Alanine (mmol/l)	0.28 ± 0.02	0.22 ± 0.01**	0.25 ± 0.02	0.33 ± 0.04
Glycerol (mmol/l)	0.05 ± 0.01	0.06 ± 0.01	0.10 ± 0.03	0.08 ± 0.01*
Total ketone bodies (mmol/l)	1.12 ± 0.04	0.24 ± 0.05**	0.23 ± 0.09	0.05 ± 0.01
NEFA (mmol/l)	0.50 ± 0.04	0.68 ± 0.07*(6)	–	–
[Lactate]/[pyruvate]	10.5 ± 0.3	12.0 ± 0.3***	12.9 ± 1.5	13.8 ± 0.6****
[3-Hydroxybutyrate]/[acetoacetate]	0.8 ± 0.1	1.9 ± 0.4*	1.2 ± 0.4	2.2 ± 1.0
pH	7.36 ± 0.01	7.37 ± 0.01	7.38 ± 0.03	7.33 ± 0.02
P_{CO_2} (kPa)	5.7 ± 0.1	6.8 ± 0.4*	6.7 ± 0.3***	7.3 ± 0.5***
P_{O_2} (kPa)	4.9 ± 0.4	3.3 ± 0.3***	4.7 ± 0.8	3.6 ± 0.4*
Cortisol (mmol/l)	401 ± 25	486 ± 51(6)	–	–
Insulin (mU/l)	8.3 ± 1.0	5.3 ± 1.1(6)	–	–

Number of subjects in parentheses.
*$P < 0.05$; **$P < 0.02$; ***$P < 0.01$; ****$P < 0.001$.

given salbutamol by aerosol, we were unable to demonstrate an effect on circulating blood metabolites (Holgate et al 1980), so the possibility that lung disease modifies the response to drugs cannot be eliminated.

It seems unlikely that hypoxia, hypercapnia, respiratory work or circulatory changes produced the increases in [lactate]/[pyruvate] ratio seen in the absence of drug treatment, since these are usually accompanied by a rise in blood lactate levels. Could a disturbance of the metabolic functions of the lung be responsible? A direct effect on circulating blood metabolites is unlikely since the diseased lung will probably increase rather than decrease circulating blood lactate levels (Rochester et al 1973). Disturbances in the production or metabolism of hormones such as noradrenaline by the lung could explain the changes in blood metabolites. Ueda (1975) observed a decreased clearance of vasoactive hormones in animals with pneumonitis and in man the clearance of noradrenaline is decreased in patients with pulmonary hypertension (Sole et al 1979). In addition, plasma levels of testosterone, a hormone metabolized by the lung, are decreased in patients with respiratory disease (d'A Semple et al 1979), although the mechanism is unknown.

These results suggest that the lung has a role in maintaining the normal metabolic homeostasis of the body. One can also speculate that these changes in whole-body metabolism may, in turn, influence the lung and thus set up a vicious circle of lung damage, changes in whole-body metabolism, and further lung damage. In the next section this concept of interactions between the whole body and the lung in disease and the implications for treatment will be discussed.

THERAPEUTIC POTENTIAL OF LUNG/WHOLE-BODY INTERACTIONS

One area where a metabolic approach has met with some success is in the treatment of respiratory distress syndrome of the newborn (RDS, hyaline membrane disease). This is now thought to result from either a deficiency or, in some circumstances, a qualitative abnormality of surfactant (Ballard 1980, Gluck 1978).

RDS occurs not only in immature or premature babies but also in certain other groups, for example the infant of the diabetic mother. From our work on the isolated rat lung we suggested that the failure of glycolytic flux to match the activity of pyruvate dehydrogenase might produce a deficiency of the essential glycerol constituents of surfactant (Stubbs & Stubbs 1978) (Fig. 2). The mechanism for RDS that we proposed could also explain the occasional occurrence of RDS in the infants of diabetic mothers with previously normal lysolecithin/sphingomyelin (L/S) ratios, where it has been suggested

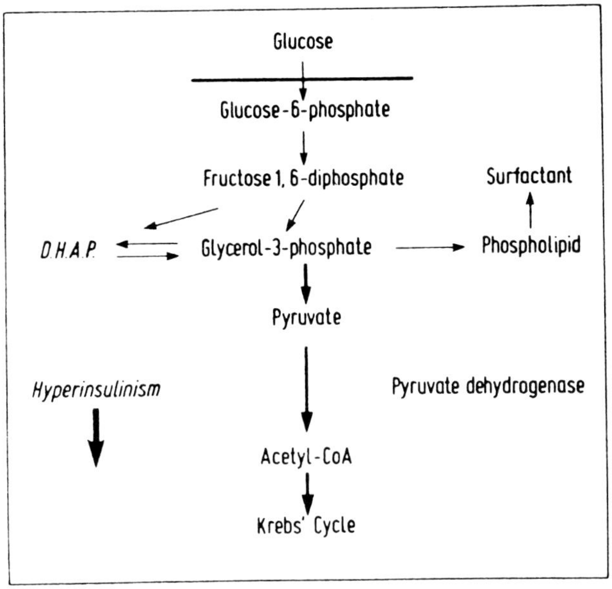

FIG. 2. Glycolysis and the possible effects of hyperinsulinism on the production of surfactant. (Reproduced with kind permission of *The Lancet*.)

that lung phospholipids may be deficient in disphosphatidylglycerol (Gluck 1978). A deficiency of glycerol-3-phosphate would be predicted particularly to limit the production of disphosphatidylglycerol.

Corticosteroids and to a lesser extent adrenergic agents are now widely used to treat RDS (Ballard 1980). These and other drugs, although of considerable value, have met with uneven success. An examination of the metabolic effects of these drugs in relation to whole-body metabolism may provide some clues to their failure to prevent RDS.

This can be illustrated by the responses of the *in situ* adult male rat lung to glucocorticoids (Fig. 3). Markedly different metabolic responses to these hormones can be produced, depending upon the type and duration of glucocorticoid treatment and the degree of whole-body catabolism – that is, whether the animal was fed or fasted.

In fed adult rats, corticosterone added to the perfusate led to a 25–30% fall in the uptake of glucose, and in the production of lactate and pyruvate. Prior treatment of the animals with ACTH produced a fall in glycerol and lactate production. In fasted rats corticosterone still suppressed glucose uptake but lactate and pyruvate production were no longer affected and alanine produc-

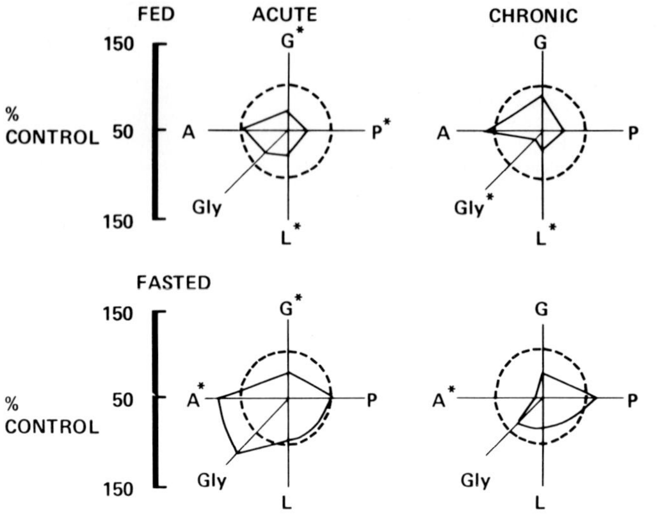

FIG. 3. The uptake of glucose (G) and the production of pyruvate (P), lactate (L), glycerol (Gly) and alanine (A) at 4 h in lungs from fed or 48 h-fasted rats perfused *in situ*. Acute effects of glucocorticoids were examined by adding corticosterone (100 μg/100 ml) to the perfusate. Chronic effects were examined after subcutaneous injection of ACTH (Synacthen Depot, 0.3 mg/kg) 12 h and 36 h before lung perfusion. Results expressed as % of control values (dotted circle).
*$P < 0.05$ compared with control values.

tion was increased. In the fasted animals treated with ACTH the effect on lactate was absent, but alanine production was suppressed.

We do not know what these observations mean in terms of surfactant production, although phospholipid synthesis (Abe & Tierney 1977) and the mechanical characteristics of the lung in adult rats can be influenced by glucocorticoids (Picken et al 1974). Nor do we know whether the differences between the responses of the lung to ACTH and corticosterone are related to the duration of the treatment or merely reflect differences in the circulating concentrations of glucocorticoids.

The treatment of RDS may be further complicated by the need to give these drugs to the mother rather than directly to the fetus. This may produce secondary effects. Stubbs et al (1978), for example, reported that changes in maternal metabolism may be associated with alterations in fetal breathing patterns.

The other group of drugs sometimes used to treat RDS are the adrenergic agents. These can produce marked effects on intermediary metabolism and even precipitate diabetic ketoacidosis (Thomas et al 1977). In addition, metabolic tolerance to these agents may develop (Holgate et al 1980). This suggests that if treatment with adrenergic agents is continued for long periods, the metabolic response may be different from that seen over shorter periods.

It is apparent that the response of the lung to drugs is modified by the metabolic setting and the response of the rest of the body. This investigational mountain of metabolic interactions could prove to be an academic mole-hill if, as some believe, the action of drugs used in the prevention of RDS is only that of non-specific enzyme induction.

Respiratory distress syndromes also develop in the adult. Pulmonary oedema occurs after a variety of insults (Robin et al 1973), including substrate deprivation. In the late 1930s pulmonary oedema was found in 0.3–16% of patients undergoing insulin treatment for psychiatric conditions (Nielsen et al 1938). If insulin hypoglycaemia is continued for several hours in animals pulmonary oedema invariably develops (Mackay & Pecka 1950). The addition of an inhibitor of glycolysis, iodoacetic acid, increased albumin permeability in dog lungs (Goodale et al 1970). There is good evidence, therefore, that substrate deprivation, or the inhibition of glycolysis, can produce pulmonary damage and oedema.

We investigated the possible protective role of substrate in the rat lung perfused *in situ* and found that adding glucose to the perfusate prolonged the time before flow ceased and oedema developed (Fig. 4).

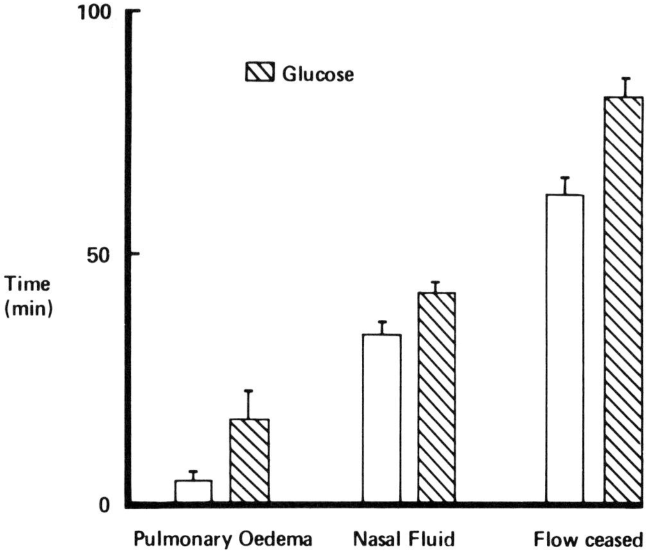

FIG. 4. The protective effect of glucose (4 mmol/l) on pulmonary oedema, judged by the time at which flow ceased, nasal fluid appeared and oedema developed, after the cessation of gassing of the perfusate. (Mean ± SEM.)

In adult respiratory distress syndrome there is marked interstitial oedema and an increase in lung weight. Clinically four phases have been described (Beyer 1979). After the initial event, such as major trauma, there may be hypotension, poor tissue perfusion, hyperventilation, respiratory alkalosis and hypoxaemia. This is followed some hours or days later by respiratory failure. The lung is therefore exposed to a highly catabolic whole-body metabolism and the accompanying disturbances in blood gases and ventilation. In addition, pulmonary oedema may increase the glucose requirements of the lung (Tierney et al 1977). There are therefore several adverse features of the endogenous metabolism of the lung associated with the development of the adult respiratory distress syndrome.

The histological changes in the lung after cardiopulmonary bypass are similar to those described for adult RDS (Pennock et al 1977). We examined circulating levels of glucose and intermediary metabolites in the pulmonary artery and aorta in five patients after cardiopulmonary bypass and compared them with the levels in six patients studied before cardiopulmonary bypass (see Table 1, p 353). After bypass the blood glucose, alanine, lactate and pyruvate levels were much higher than in the patients examined before cardiopulmonary bypass. Some of these effects on carbohydrate metabolism are well recognized and are accompanied by changes in circulating levels of insulin, growth hormone and catecholamines (see Nuutinen et al 1977).

There was also a marked difference in the effects of the lung on circulating substrates. For example, the consistent production of lactate and alanine by the lung before cardiopulmonary bypass (Table 1) was absent after bypass.

It is not clear whether these changes reflect damage to the lungs or the response of the lung to the changes in whole-body metabolism, nor do we know the effects of these changes on the exogenous functions of the lung; but it seems likely that the combination of so many features unfavourable to endogenous metabolism will interfere with its exogenous metabolism.

In animals, prostaglandin clearance is decreased in response to haemorrhagic and endotoxic shock and cardiopulmonary bypass (Fletcher & Ramwell 1977, Cedro & Herbaczyńska-Cedro 1978). In addition, lung damage and pulmonary oedema may result in the production of vasoactive substances, while exposure to 100% oxygen (Said 1979) and hypoxia (Stalcup et al 1980) can inhibit their clearance.

The effects of the release of these hormones on whole-body metabolism is not clear, but there seems to be considerable potential for a vicious cycle of substrate deprivation, lung damage, hormone release and further substrate deprivation. These comments may also apply to other situations where the lung is damaged, such as pulmonary emboli and infarction.

The use of metabolic therapy under these circumstances awaits investigation. Corticosteroids have been used with variable success, as has glucose given by aerosol (Pennock et al 1977, Hewson et al 1976). A major difficulty has been the absence of a good guide to therapeutic response; it is here that the measurement of the metabolic indicators of lung function may prove to be of value.

CONCLUDING COMMENTS

The lung has long gone unrecognized as an organ of metabolism. It is hoped that the lung will now be recognized as having a dual respiratory and metabolic role. Perhaps we can anticipate the application of this knowledge to the treatment of pulmonary disorders and can instigate a search for clinical conditions characterized by abnormalities in the exogenous metabolic functions of the lung.

'Anon to sudden silence won,
In fancy they pursue,
The dream-child moving through a land
Of wonders wild and new
In friendly chat with bird or beast—
And half believe it true'.

Lewis Carroll: Alice's Adventures in Wonderland.

ACKNOWLEDGEMENTS

This paper owes much to the work and cooperation of numerous colleagues. I particularly wish to thank Professor C.J. Dickinson, Dr I. Morgan, Dr D. Kelly, Dr F. Walters, and the cardiothoracic and anaesthetic departments of St. Bartholomew's Hospital, London. This work was supported by the British Diabetic Association and the Edith Walsh Award of the British Medical Association. W.A.S. was in receipt of an MRC research fellowship.

References

Abe M, Tierney DF 1977 Lung lipid metabolism after seven days of hydrocortisone administration to adult rats. J Appl Physiol 42:202-205

Ballard PH 1980 Hormonal influences during fetal lung development. This volume, p 251-267

Barnett DB, Chesrown SE, Zbinden AF, Nisam M, Reed BR, Bourne HR, Melmon KR, Gold WM 1978 Cyclic AMP and cyclic GMP in canine peripheral lung: regulation *in vivo*. Am Rev Respir Dis 118:723-733

Bassett DJP, Fisher AB, Rabinowitz JL 1974 Effect of hypoxia on incorporation of glucose carbon into lipids by isolated rat lung. Am J Physiol 227:1103-1108

Bedwani JF, Marley PB 1975 Enhanced activation of prostaglandin E_2 by the rabbit lung during pregnancy or progesterone treatment. Br J Pharmacol 53:547-554

Berti F, Folco GC, Nicosia S, Omini C, Pasargiklian R 1979 The role of histamine H_1 and H_2 receptors in the generation of thromboxane A_2 in perfused guinea-pig lungs. Br J Pharmacol 65:629-633

Beyer A 1979 Shock lung. Br J Hosp Med 21:248-258

Boura ALA, Murphy RD 1978 Thromboxane B_2 inhibits prostaglandin E_2 inactivation by the rat isolated perfused lung. Clin Exp Pharmacol Physiol 5:387-392

Buchanan KD 1979 Gastrointestinal hormones: general concepts. Clin Endocrinol Metab 8:249-263

Cedro A, Herbaczyńska-Cedro K 1978 Increased blood level of prostaglandin-like substances during cardiopulmonary bypass in the dog. Cardiovasc Res 12:516-522

Chaisson CF, Massaro D 1978 2-Deoxy-D-glucose uptake by lung slices from fed and fasted rats. J Appl Physiol 44:380-383

Chochinov RH, Perlman K, Moorhouse JA 1978 Circulating alanine production and disposal in healthy subjects. Diabetes 27:287-295

Clark JM, Lambertson CJ 1971 Pulmonary oxygen toxicity: a review. Pharmacol Rev 23:37-133

Comroe JH 1952-1953 The function of the lung. Harvey Lect 48:110-144

d'A Semple P, Beastall GH, Watson WS, Hume R 1980 Serum testosterone depression associated with hypoxia in respiratory failure. Clin Sci 58:105-106

Datta H, Stubbs WA, Alberti KGMM 1980 Substrate utilization by the lung. This volume, p 85-99

Editorial 1974 Filtering aspects of lung function. Br Med J 2:681

Felts JM 1964 Biochemistry of the lung. Health Phys 10:973-979

Fisher AB 1978 Energy status of the rat lung after exposure to elevated pO_2. J Appl Physiol 45:56-59

Fisher AB, Steinberg H, Dodia C 1979 Reversal of 2-deoxyglucose inhibition of serotonin uptake in isolated guinea pig lung. J Appl Physiol 46:447-450

Fletcher JR, Ramwell PW 1977 Altered lung metabolism of prostaglandins during hemorrhagic and endotoxin shock. Surg Forum 28:184-189

Gacad G, Dickie K, Massaro D 1972 Protein synthesis in lung; influence of starvation on amino acid incorporation into protein. J Appl Physiol 33:281-284

Gluck L 1978 Evaluating functional fetal maturation. Clin Obstet Gynecol 21:547-559

Goodale RL, Goetzman B, Visscher MB 1970 Hypoxia and iodoacetic acid and alveolo-capillary barrier permeability to albumin. Am J Physiol 219:1226-1230

Gregorio CA, Gail DB, Massaro D 1976 Influence of fasting on lung oxygen consumption and respiratory quotient. Am J Physiol 230:291-294

Gross I 1977 Nutritional and hormonal influences on lung phospholipid metabolism. Fed Proc 36:2665-2669

Gryglewski RJ 1975 Corticosterone inhibits prostaglandin release from perfused mesenteric vessels of rabbit and from perfused lungs of sensitised guinea pig. Prostaglandins 10:343-355

Gryglewski RJ 1980 The lung as a generator of prostacyclin. This volume, p 147-156

Hewson JR, Holland DJC, McArdle AH 1976 Transalveolar metabolic protection to the lung. Arch Surg 111:812-815

Hitchcock KR 1979 Hormones and the lung. I. Thyroid hormones and glucocorticoids in lung development. Anat Rec 194:15-40

Holgate S, Stubbs WA, Wood P, McCaughey E, Alberti KGMM, Tattersfield A 1980 Airway and metabolic resistance to intravenous salbutamol: a study in normal man. Clin Sci, in press

Johnston DG, Alberti KGMM 1976 Carbohydrate metabolism in liver disease. Clin Endocrinol 5:675-702

Junod AF 1975 Metabolism, production and release of hormones and mediators in the lung. Am Rev Respir Dis 112:93-108

Krebs HA, Woods HF, Alberti KGMM 1975 Hyperlactataemia and lactic acidosis. Essays Biochem 1:81-103
Longmore WJ, Mourning JT 1977 Effect of CO_2 concentration on phosphatidylglycerol metabolism in surfactant and residual lung function. J Lipid Res 18:309-313
Mackay EM, Pecka EF 1950 Experimental pulmonary oedema. III. Hypoglycaemia. A cause of pulmonary oedema. Proc Soc Exp Biol Med 73:568-569
Moore PK, Hoult JRS 1978 Experimental hyperthyroidism in rats suppresses *in vitro* prostaglandin metabolism in lung and kidney. Prostaglandins 16:335-349
Morishige WK 1980 Endocrine influences on aspects of lung biochemistry. This volume, p 239-247
Moxley MA, Longmore WJ 1977 Effect of experimental diabetes and insulin on lipid metabolism in the isolated perfused rat lung. Biochim Biophys Acta 488:218-224
Nielsen JM, Ingham SD, Von Hagen DO 1938 Pulmonary oedema and embolism as complication of insulin shock in treatment of schizophrenia. J Am Med Assoc 3:2455-2458
Nuutinen LS, Mononen P, Kairaluoma M, Tuononen S 1977 Effects of open heart surgery on carbohydrate and lipid metabolism. J Thorac Cardiovasc Surg 73:680-683
Pennock JL, Pierce WS, Waldhausen JA 1977 The management of the lungs during cardiopulmonary bypass. Surg Gynecol Obstet 45:917-927
Pérez-Díaz J, Martin-Requero A, Ayuso-Parrilla MS, Parrilla R 1977a Metabolic features of isolated lung cells. Am J Physiol 232:394-400
Pérez-Díaz J, Martin-Requero A, Ayuso-Parrilla MS, Parrilla R 1977b Factors controlling the metabolic response to glucose in isolated rat lung cells. Life Sci 20:1599-1606
Picken J, Lurie M, Kleinerman J 1974 Mechanical and morphological effects of long-term corticosteroid administration on the rat lung. Am Rev Respir Dis 110:746-753
Piper PJ, Vane JR 1971 The release of prostaglandins from lung and other tissues. Ann NY Acad Sci 180:363-385
Rhoades RA 1974 Net uptake of glucose, glycerol and fatty acids by the isolated perfused rat lung. Am J Physiol 226:144-149
Rhoades RA 1975 Influence of altered O_2 tension on substrate metabolism in perfused rat lung. Am J Physiol 229:1476-1496
Robin ED, Cross CE, Zelis R 1973 Pulmonary edema. N Engl J Med 288:239-246
Rochester DF, Wichern WA, Fritts HW, Caldwell PRB, Lewis ML, Guintini G, Garfield JW 1973 Arteriovenous differences of lactate and pyruvate across healthy and diseased human lung. Am Rev Respir Dis 107:442-448
Roth RA, Gillis CN 1977 Effect of ventilation on removal of [^{14}C]mescaline by perfused rabbit lung. Biochem Pharmacol 26:1446-1447
Rubenstein AH, Zwi S, Miller K 1968 Insulin and the lung. Diabetologia 4:236-238
Sahebjami H, Vassallo CL, Wirman JA 1978 Lung mechanics and ultrastructure in prolonged starvation. Am Rev Respir Dis 177:77-83
Said SI 1979 Environmental injury of the lung: role of humoral mediators. Fed Proc 37:2504-2507
Said SI, Mutt V, Erdös EG 1980 The lung in relation to vasoactive polypeptides. This volume, p 217-232
Samuelsson B, Granström E, Green K, Hamberg M, Hammarström S 1975 Prostaglandins. Annu Rev Biochem 44:669-695
Schuyler MR, Niewoehn DE, Inkley SR, Kohn R 1976 Abnormal lung elasticity in juvenile diabetes mellitus. Am Rev Respir Dis 113:37-41
Searle GL 1976 The use of isotope turnover techniques in the study of carbohydrate metabolism in man. Clin Endocrinol Metab 5:783-804
Shaw MF, Rhoades RA 1977 Substrate metabolism in the perfused lung: response to changes in circulating glucose and palmitate levels. Lipids 12:930-935
Sole MJ, Drobac M, Schwartz L, Hussain MN, Vaughan-Neil EF 1979 The extraction of circulating catecholamines by the lungs in normal man and in patients with pulmonary hypertension. Circulation 60:160-163

Stalcup SA, Lipset JS, Mellins RB 1980 Modulation of converting enzyme activity by hypoxia and its physiological effects. This volume, p 293-307
Stubbs SM, Brudenell JM, Campbell J, Pyke DA, Watkins PJ, Burrin J 1978 Metabolism and fetal breathing in the pregnant diabetic. Diabetologia 15:273
Stubbs WA 1979 Metabolic studies of the lung. PhD thesis, University of Southampton
Stubbs WA, Morgan I, Lloyd B, Alberti KGMM 1977 The effect of insulin on lung metabolism in the rat. Clin Endocrinol (Oxf) 7:181-184
Stubbs WA, Stubbs SM 1978 Hyperinsulinism, diabetes mellitus, and respiratory distress of the newborn: a common link? Lancet 1:308-309
Tierney DF 1974 Lung metabolism and biochemistry. Annu Rev Physiol 26:209-231
Tierney DF, Young SL, O'Neil JJ, Abe M 1977 Isolated perfused lung – substrate utilization. Fed Proc 36:161-165
Thet NF, Delaney MD, Gregorio CA, Massaro D 1977 Protein metabolism by rat lung: influence of fasting, glucose and insulin. J Appl Physiol 43:463-467
Thomas DJB, Gill B, Brown P, Stubbs WA 1977 Salbutamol-induced diabetic ketoacidosis. Br Med J 2:438
Ueda E 1975 Metabolism of vasoactive substances and its significance in rabbits with experimental pneumonitis. Jpn Circ J 39:559-563
Wharton J, Polak JM, Bloom SR, Ghatei MA, Solcia E, Brown MR, Pearse AGE 1978 Bombesin-like immunoreactivity in the lung. Nature (Lond) 273:769-770
Wolfe RR, Hochachka PW, Trelstad RL, Burke JF 1979 Lactate oxidation in perfused rat lung. Am J Physiol 236:E276-282
Young SL, Tierney DF 1972 Dipalmitoyl lecithin secretion and metabolism by the rat lung. Am J Physiol 222:1539-1544

Discussion

Junod: You mentioned the work of Michael Sole, who showed that catecholamine uptake by lung was reduced in patients with primary pulmonary hypertension (Sole et al 1979). In fact, the basal levels of catecholamines in the systemic circulation did not differ in patients with primary pulmonary hypertension and in controls. This raises the question of the importance of this function in the body. You suggested that in patients with chronic obstructive pulmonary disease some of the metabolic abnormalities could be due to an increased plasma concentration of catecholamines, resulting from reduced clearance by the lung. It shouldn't be difficult to measure catecholamine concentrations in the blood of your patients, to find out whether this function of the lung is really essential.

Stubbs: Yes. We would have taken blood for catecholamine estimations had we known the metabolic abnormalities before starting the study!

Reid: Did you see any difference in patients with chronic obstructive lung disease according to whether they were severely ill, whether or not widespread severe emphysema was associated with airway obstruction, or whether right ventricular hypertrophy was present?

TABLE 1 (Stubbs)

Mean (± SEM) age, forced expiratory volume (FEV), forced vital capacity (FVC) and body weight in patients with lung disease and in controls (number of subjects in parentheses)

		Chronic lung disease		
	Controls	*No treatment*	*Steroids*	*Steroids + salbutamol*
	(12)	*(9)*	*(6)*	*(6)*
Age (years)	61 ± 3	67 ± 3	67 ± 4	66 ± 3
Body wt. (% ideal)	99 ± 1	97 ± 1	94 ± 3	97 ± 1
FEV (% normal)	72 ± 6	30 ± 4	14 ± 1	40 ± 8
FVC (% normal)	87 ± 5	48 ± 7	21 ± 2	54 ± 7

Stubbs: There were no obvious differences, but none of the patients was severely ill at the time of the study (see Table 1).

Alberti: In the group with severe lung disease there are nutritional changes, because the patients don't eat well; so this is another uncontrollable factor. This is why we studied the less severely ill group.

Ballard: I was interested in your observation that acute exposure to i.v. salbutamol increases lactate production, but after chronic exposure to the aerosol it does not. This seems like the effects of β-adrenergic drugs on bronchodilation. Does this reflect down-regulation of the adrenergic receptor, due to chronic exposure to agonist, with loss of receptor sites and sensitivity?

Stubbs: That is very possible. We have no direct evidence for this, although others have (see Holgate et al 1980). Airways resistance also becomes less sensitive to the effects of intravenously given salbutamol when normal subjects are treated for two weeks with salbutamol by aerosol (Holgate et al 1980). This could also be relevant to the use of salbutamol in the prevention of premature labour, if the uterine muscle were similarly affected.

Stalcup: We studied bradykinin levels in 11 infants undergoing hypothermic cardiopulmonary bypass (Pang et al 1979). With the onset of hypothermia, before bypass was instituted, there was a doubling or trebling of circulating bradykinin levels. When the infant was placed on bypass an abrupt further increase occurred, up to between 9 and 19 ng/ml. Then there was circulatory arrest. When the circulation was re-started we observed a large washout of kinin from the tissues, of 25–30 ng/ml. With restoration of the lung in the circuit these levels declined.

Vane: Did you also see increased levels of renin?

Stalcup: We haven't examined that. We and others have shown a catecholamine surge at the onset of cooling, especially with machine cooling – less so with surface cooling. Favre et al (1974) looked at the renin–angiotensin system and measured circulating angiotensin II in non-hypothermic pulmonary bypass. They found that shortly after going on to the bypass the patients showed an abrupt fall in AII. As bypass continued the levels over the next 20–60 minutes returned slowly to the original values. This was associated with stimulation of the renin–angiotensin system, meaning that there had to be more renin for the same amount of angiotensin II that was presumably being made in the tissues.

Moncada: Do kinin levels increase in the absence of an extracorporeal circuit during an operation?

Stalcup: There is a rise with hypothermia, but not without it. Bradykinin levels are raised in, for example, venous blood draining a wound, but in mixed venous blood (pulmonary artery blood) we can't detect an increase.

Woods: Has anyone measured bradykinin concentrations in accidental hypothermia?

Stalcup: Many people have tried to relate the reactive hyperaemia of chilblains to activation of kallikrein. If a hand is plunged in ice water, with the onset of hyperaemia there is a fall in kininogen concentration across the cold tissue. The difficulty in interpreting such experiments is that blood flow changes at the same time; flow has never been taken into account. We did the experiment in the intact child being chilled because it avoided the flow problems. My feeling is that the redness and pounding associated with hyperaemia after a cold injury probably has kallikrein activation as one of its components.

Alberti: You see notable changes in bradykinin in your hypothermic patients on bypass. We have measured 15 or 20 different hormones and metabolic parameters in similar patients who are on bypass, with or without hypothermia, and not one of the metabolic variables is normal. It would be useful to combine our data to see what is causing what.

Stalcup: Yes. I suspect that such changes are interrelated. Incidentally, a close correlation between temperature change and kinin formation has been shown for the umbilical cord. As little as 1°C change stimulates kallikrein (Melmon et al 1968).

Alberti: Are there any known effects of the kinins formed on metabolic parameters?

Stalcup: No; this is what is begging to be done!

Vane: Bradykinin levels in blood are vanishingly small (p 142); you have shown conditions where they can be increased. Is your hypoxic dog, where converting enzyme and bradykininase activity are reduced to very low levels, equivalent to the situation of cardiopulmonary bypass, where the lungs are out of the circulation?

Stalcup: We hope to answer that. We are now assaying AII and bradykinin in rats exposed to chronic hypoxia, and we find a chronic depression in AII relative to the amount of circulating renin. We suspect that part of the fall in blood pressure seen in chronically hypoxic patients will be due to increased bradykinin levels. The levels are very low normally, from 0.1 ng to 40 pg per ml plasma, depending on how you draw the blood.

Vane: A question that I posed at the beginning was related to the mode of action of captopril: does it act solely by inhibiting angiotensin conversion, or also through an increase in bradykinin?

Stalcup: I don't think bradykinin has been measured properly in patients on captopril. McCaa et al (1978) find that in sodium-depleted dogs receiving captopril, kinin levels rise on the second day, but this was not seen in sodium-replete dogs. McCaa et al correlated some of the fall in vascular resistance in the sodium-depleted dogs with the rise in kinin; the rest was attributed to reduced AII.

Bakhle: Johnston et al (1979) have measured kinin levels in the blood of patients receiving captopril and found no change.

Mellins: The result might depend on how much kinin was already being generated, if any? In the absence of kinin production, inhibition of bradykininase activity by captopril would not reveal any change.

Vane: Bradykinin can stimulate release of prostacyclin from the kidney (Moncada et al 1979). A local production of bradykinin in the kidney, which would be exaggerated by captopril, might cause prostacyclin to be secreted into the circulation. This would be a suitable system in which to look for an effect on kinin levels. Absence of kinin from the systemic blood does not mean that it is not contributing to vasodilatation by a local activity.

Soffer: The question of whether the effects of captopril are due to inhibition of AII production or the potentiation of bradykinin is difficult to answer conclusively. To look at this one has to take an experimental situation in which captopril has an effect, and in this situation use another specific pharmacological agent to interrupt the renin–angiotensin system at a different site. If the pharmacological effects of captopril and the other agent are similar, then it is likely that the effect of captopril in this experimental situation is due to interruption of the renin–angiotensin system rather than to potentiation of bradykinin.

One problem with this approach is that peptide angiotensin antagonists are also usually good converting enzyme inhibitors (Chiu et al 1976) and therefore unsatisfactory for use in this context. However, Dzau et al (1980) have examined the effect of anti-renin antibodies on renovascular hypertension in the dog. They had previously examined the effect of SQ 20 881 as a converting enzyme inhibitor in the same animal model (Miller et al 1972). In each case they observed a similar vasodepressor response, so that the effect of a converting enzyme inhibitor in this experimental situation seems to be mediated by interruption of the renin–angiotensin system rather than by bradykinin potentiation.

Vane: Tree & Morton (1980) measured blood concentrations of angiotensin II in dogs. They then gave captopril, which produced a fall in blood pressure, and infused enough angiotensin II to raise the blood concentration back to where it was before. The dose–response curve did not return to the original level, suggesting that reduction of plasma angiotensin II concentration was not the whole explanation for the fall in blood pressure. This was an acute experiment, over several hours.

Aiken: I would not expect blood pressure to come back to the previous level until a few days after infusing angiotensin II; you need to wait for an effect of angiotensin II on sodium and water excretion.

References

Chiu AT, Ryan JW, Stewart JM, Dorer FE 1976 Formation of angiotensin III by angiotensin-converting enzyme. Biochem J 155:189-192

Dzau VJ, Kopelman RI, Barger AC, Haber E 1980 Renin specific antibody for study of cardiovascular homeostasis. Science (Wash DC) 207:1091-1093

Favre L, Vallston MB, Muller AF 1974 Relationship between plasma concentration of angiotensin I, angiotensin II and plasma renin activity during cardio-pulmonary by-pass in man. Eur J Clin Invest 4:135-140

Holgate S, Stubbs WA, Wood P, McCaughey E, Alberti KGMM, Tattersfield A 1980 Airway and metabolic resistance to intravenous salbutamol: a study in normal man. Clin Sci, in press

Johnston CI, McGrath BP, Millar JA, Matthews PG 1979 Long term effects of captopril (SQ 14225) on blood pressure and hormone levels in essential hypertension. Lancet 2:493-495

McCaa RE, Hall JE, McCaa CS 1978 The effects of angiotensin I converting enzyme inhibitors on arterial blood pressure and urinary sodium excretion; role of the renal renin–angiotensin and kallikrein–kinin systems. Circ Res 43:32-39

Melmon KL, Cline MJ, Hughes T, Nies AS 1968 Kinins: possible mediators of neonatal circulatory changes in man. J Clin Invest 47:1295-1302

Miller ED, Samuels AL, Haber E, Barger AC 1972 Inhibition of angiotensin conversion in experimental renovascular hypertension. Science (Wash DC) 177:1108-1109

Moncada S, Mullane KM, Vane JR 1979 Prostacyclin-release by bradykinin *in vivo.* Br J Pharmacol 66:96P

Pang LM, Stalcup SA, Lipset JS, Hayes CJ, Bowman FO, Mellins RB 1979 Increased circulating bradykinin during hypothermia and cardiopulmonary bypass in children. Circulation 60:1503-1507

Sole MJ, Drobac M, Schwartz L, Hussain MN, Vaughan-Neil EF 1979 The extraction of circulating catecholamines by the lungs in normal man and in patients with pulmonary hypertension. Circulation 60:160-163

Tree M, Morton JJ 1980 Captopril lowers blood pressure by an additional mechanism independent of angiotensin II. (Proceedings of Medical Research Society) Clin Sci 58:2P (abstr)

General discussion

SURFACE CHARGE AND PULMONARY ENDOTHELIAL TRANSPORT

Vane: In this final discussion, may we take up some unresolved problems? Dr Simionescu mentioned the question of the negative surface charge of pulmonary endothelial cells. Are there situations in which this alters? The negativity will obviously repel other cells, but how important is this?

Simionescu: In experiments designed to investigate the capacity of isolated endothelial cells to take up macromolecules we found that anionic molecules are taken up by vesicles more readily than cationic probes. We then examined the charge distribution along the endothelial cell luminal surface. We used polycationic ferritin (pI 8.4) and examined capillaries of the pancreas, the endothelium of which is provided with all the features potentially involved in permeability: vesicles, transendothelial channels and fenestrae with diaphragms. Cationic ferritin was introduced by perfusion. To our surprise we found that binding of cationic ferritin is highly selective: it attaches to the cell membrane and to ~90% of the fenestral diaphragms and coated pits, but does not bind to the vesicles, channels or their diaphragms. After four hours ferritin is being accumulated in multivesicular bodies and is still present on fenestral diaphragms.

Perfusion of different enzymes before the cationic ferritin suggests that sulphated glycosaminoglycans and in particular heparan sulphate are the major components and bearers of anionic sites on the fenestral diaphragms. These results with cationic ferritin indicate the existence of even more refined differentiations along the cell surface of the same endothelial cell (M. Simionescu 1979).

Vane: A platelet, being approximately 2 μm across, is presumably not going to be affected by the variation in charge along the endothelial cell, but just by the general charge along the endothelial surface. Will the static charge difference across the endothelial cell membrane be likely to affect transport?

Soffer: Are protein–membrane interactions not more likely to be mediated by specific interactions of the lectin–sugar type? You could have heterogeneity along the membrane with respect to biologically cognitive molecules (see p 289). Why do you think that charge is important?

Simionescu: Most plasma proteins are negatively charged. They are transported across the endothelial cell via vesicles or channels and fenestrae. According to our experiments with cationized ferritin, vesicle and channel diaphragms either are positive or have no charge, so it looks as if vesicles and channels are a system devised to favour the transport of anionic molecules (such as plasma proteins).

Soffer: So these vesicles are tunnels bounded by membranes and the transported proteins do not actually enter the cytoplasm?

Simionescu: That is right. The vesicles shuttle from one side to the other of the cell. This is a short-cut between endocytosis and exocytosis for which the term 'transcytosis' has been proposed (N. Simionescu 1978).

Said: In pulmonary lymph, which represents interstitial fluid from the lung, the protein concentrations are normally about 60% of those in plasma (Warren & Drinker 1942, Staub 1971), which shows that plasma proteins are transported across the pulmonary endothelium.

Stalcup: We examined the concentration of protein in lymph in hypoxic sheep in which kinin was infused or was endogenously generated by acidosis. In the lung at normal P_{O_2} kinin does not produce any increase in lymph flow, which would reflect increased fluid movement, or any increased protein transfer. With the onset of hypoxia we see an increase in lymph flow and in the concentration of protein in lymph, suggesting that permeability to proteins has been increased. We also see a *selective* increase in permeability to larger protein molecules.

Soffer: The transport mechanism of shuttling vesicles that Dr Simionescu describes sounds like a rather non-specific process for protein transport out of the blood.

Reid: Under basal conditions it is probably highly selective, probably on the basis of size and charge of the different protein molecules.

Soffer: What is so selective about size and charge?

Bakhle: We are getting into a semantic problem! Dr Soffer considers specificity in terms of chemical or biochemical properties which may not be reflected in the size or charge of a protein molecule, whereas physiologists looking at protein permeability find size and charge to be major factors determining protein movement out of blood.

Stalcup: We are talking about different questions. One function of the capillary endothelium in the lung is to *prevent* the passage of water and proteins out of the blood. Many people are studying the extent to which the pulmonary capillary bed excludes water and protein and so prevents pulmonary oedema, and whether one can influence the extent of fluid and protein exchange across the lung capillary membrane. We induced either acidosis alone or hypoxia and acidosis in chronically catheterized sheep. Acidosis alone causes an abrupt 400% increase in lymph flow which declines. With superimposed hypoxia, lymph flow rises but stays up. The selectivity that I was speaking of is not the specific transfer of particular proteins but rather the *exclusion* of certain proteins. Normally, more albumin moves across the membrane, being a small protein, than IgM, a large protein. When bradykinin appears in blood as a result of acidosis, the proportions are reversed, with a relative increase in the flux of large proteins, which means that permeability, or vesicle transport, is increased. This reversal of the ratio of large to small proteins with bradykinin may specifically mean that vesicular transport increases in this condition.

Bakhle: Or it may mean that gaps between cells have opened up?

Simionescu: Yes; it is also possible that the junctions between endothelial cells of postcapillary (pericytic) venules – which are known to be sensitive to local mediators and to have a loose organization – open up.

Bakhle: Normally, how much protein goes through the cell, in vesicles or channels, and how much goes between endothelial cells?

Simionescu: Unfortunately, quantitative studies cannot be made with electron microscopy. From experiments with various probe molecules of different size (from ~ 2 to 30 nm diameter) we have observed that vesicles and channels transport these proteins across the endothelium in capillaries. In postcapillary venules, in addition to vesicles and channels, a small number of intercellular junctions are permeable to tracers up to 6 nm, which represents an additional pathway for small molecules of up to 6 nm diameter. The amount of protein passing through these intercellular spaces could not be determined but this may make a minor contribution to the overall transendothelial passage.

Vane: The size of the vesicle is large compared to that of any protein molecule, so how does the vesicle detect that it has only albumin inside it and not IgM?

Stalcup: Some people think that the diaphragm over these vesicles can be selective in the admission of proteins, on the basis of charge; but I hold to the opposite idea that in normal conditions fluid and proteins move through intercellular junctions, not by vesicles, but that in conditions of permeability change, vesicular transport increases.

Reid: Surely both processes operate? Different experiments are done in different organs and under different conditions. There are conditions in which with histamine you can show inflammation at the venular level with opening up of junctions, visible in electron micrographs (Majno & Palade 1961, Majno et al 1961). In endothelial cells of the aorta there are several different models of subintimal oedema; in one it is possible to identify opening of the intercellular junction; in another you cannot (Hüttner et al 1979).

Mellins: I would stress that in our experiment with high levels of bradykinin we see a change in the relationship of transport between two molecules of different size. This is already known to occur in the systemic circulation but it has been argued whether it happens in lung. This is the first time that a change in protein *permeability,* however one defines it, has been shown; it cannot be simply on a hydrostatic basis. How the molecules get across and the structural basis for that permeability is still unresolved.

Bakhle: And it would be very reasonable if bradykinin now (with hypoxia-induced loss of bradykininase), and only now, is able to survive and enter the venous side of the pulmonary vascular bed. Once there it could be exerting its effect, opening up cell junctions and increasing permeability to proteins.

Alberti: It would be interesting to know what insulin does to protein permeability. With insulin injection or secretion there is known to be a big increase in the number of vesicles passing across capillary endothelium (Østerby et al 1977) and a shift of albumin and fluid from the vascular to the extravascular space (Gundersen & Christensen 1977). The effect of insulin on such movements could be studied in your system.

Collier: Is there not a chemical selectivity in uptake as well as one based on size and charge?

Alberti: In liver there is chemical selectivity, in that similarly sized and (presumably) related molecules that are structurally somewhat different are taken up to different extents.

Soffer: The liver provides a good example of what I meant about specific protein removal from blood. The liver regulates the carbohydrate composition of circulating glycoproteins. There is a lectin on liver cell surfaces which specifically extracts from the blood those circulating glycoprotein molecules that contain an exposed terminal non-reducing galactosyl residue (Ashwell & Morell 1974). Presumably there are other such lectins, perhaps in other organs. I would expect cell–protein interactions to be mediated by that kind of specificity rather than by physical characteristics.

METABOLIC STUDIES AND CLINICAL APPLICATIONS

Said: I am often asked about the value of studies of the metabolic activities of the lung in the diagnosis and treatment of lung disease. It is therefore important to show the medical community as a whole and the general public that these studies do have clinical applications. One area where metabolic studies may be able to contribute is the early diagnosis of lung tumours. People have looked for hormones secreted by tumours as markers of malignant change; Dr Rosalyn Yalow has recently written (1979) about ACTH production by lung tumours and how this could be the first sign of a tumour. We all know how difficult the early diagnosis of lung cancer is. The promise of a specific marker has not yet been fulfilled, for ACTH or for any other hormonal secretion from lung. The discovery of such a marker would be immensely valuable, and would help convince others of the usefulness of our research.

Another example is the condition of pulmonary embolism. Numerous diagnostic tests have been proposed but no single, uniformly successful test has been devised which would diagnose all cases of pulmonary embolism without any false negatives either. If we could identify a vasoactive hormone that is secreted in excess, or is grossly deficient, in patients with pulmonary embolism, that would be an important advance.

Again, we talk about the lung inactivating a variety of hormones and activating others, but even in patients with severe emphysema or diffuse sarcoidosis, where the pulmonary vascular bed is grossly reduced, we have not yet identified major alterations in metabolic function that cause the serious difficulties in these patients. These are the types of problems where further basic research would pay off.

Woods: We have not given much consideration to drugs that are commonly used in everyday practice. Several lines of evidence have prompted people to think again about the lung as a site of drug metabolism and storage. There is plenty of evidence that the lung contains the necessary enzymic machinery to metabolize drugs; there is also evidence that this machinery can be induced by certain chemicals and in some cases by environmental factors such as cigarette smoking. Not only can the lung metabolize drugs but it also accumulates drugs and stores them to a concentration that in some experimental conditions may be quite large (Roth & Wiersma 1979, Junod 1976). Is this relevant to the treatment of patients? So far the evidence has been gathered by studying groups of patients with various pulmonary diseases and also the production of acute changes in man.

The evidence doesn't so far support strongly the idea that the lung has a major direct role in the overall pharmacokinetics of drugs. In many of the studies the observed changes may have come about through indirect effects. For example, the absorption of certain drugs from the gastrointestinal tract is decreased in chronic lung diseases (Cohen et al 1975). Others have reported that the half-life of many drugs has increased (Cumming 1976, Sotaniemi et al 1971) but, unfortunately, few studies have considered clearance as well. These effects may not reflect changes in drug accumulation or metabolizing systems solely in the lung; they may represent in part changes in other organs. If you acutely alter the acid–base balance by various respiratory manoeuvres you may also alter the blood supply to organs such as the liver and kidney, both of which play a role in the clearance of drugs. Other effects may also be indirect; there is evidence that the free fraction of drugs circulating in plasma may be altered by acute acid–base changes (see du Souich et al 1978 for review).

However, it is still attractive to propose a 'modulating' role for the lung and more investigation is needed in man and in animals, because there is no doubt that because of the huge blood flow through the lung even a small capacity to metabolize a drug can make a big difference to the economy of the body in the handling of that drug, and therefore potentially alter the response of a patient being treated with that drug.

The last piece of evidence is again indirect. Some studies suggest that for certain drugs, such as digoxin, the incidence of toxicity in long-term therapy is much increased in patients with chronic pulmonary disease (Hargreave 1965).

Soffer: One way of trying to understand what the lung does, from the perspective of clinical relevance, is to elaborate the biochemical features that seem somewhat specific to it, for example its relatively high content of guanylate cyclase activity. The identification of enzymes and reaction products which are selectively localized in the lung might suggest unexpected pulmonary functions. Furthermore, the presence of such molecules in the circulation might provide a useful criterion of pulmonary injury.

Vane: Is there any technique which detects cyclic GMP outside the cell, in the blood, or does it accumulate only inside the cell?

Stubbs: Dr P. Wood is measuring plasma levels of cyclic GMP by radioimmunoassay for us (Wood & Marks 1978) in blood taken from the pulmonary artery and aorta of patients undergoing open-heart surgery, but we still await the results.

Vane: This technique must produce a number of artifacts, however, so it isn't a good model of the normal lung?

Stubbs: We use this model at two levels: before the patients go onto cardiopulmonary bypass as a 'normal' lung (although it isn't), and then after cardiopulmonary bypass, when the lung has been exposed to various insults, as a 'shocked' lung.

Stalcup: I am not sure it is useful to think in terms of unique lung functions. It is central to this concept that part of the uniqueness of these functions is because they take place at the centre of the circulation, between the venous and arterial sides. They might not be so interesting if the lung was in the foot! It happens to lie between the venous and the arterial circulations and, because of that, its large endothelial surface can adjust the concentrations of substances before they reach arterial receptors. The argument as to whether this is a function unique to the lung or a generalized endothelial function should be seen from this point of view. We should really focus on the modulation of or interference with function, and how these things hook up together with downstream receptors.

Soffer: I don't mean to imply that this is the way to understand the lung's global role in physiology; obviously we can only look at physiology in terms of an integrated system. But if it were very simple to measure some circulating enzyme which derives specifically from the lung, it might be possible to find a human mutant lacking this enzyme and by correlating symptoms with the biochemical defect on a rational basis one could perhaps identify the normal physiological role of such an enzyme in the lung.

Morishige: I agree. In addition, there is a potentially valuable tool in the finding by King & Clements (1972) of a specific apoprotein associated with surfactant. There is a possibility that this protein might enter the circulation. With a specific radioimmunoassay to detect this apoprotein one could determine whether a relationship exists between surfactant secretion and circulating apoprotein levels; if such a relationship exists, this could prove to be a powerful diagnostic tool.

Alberti: We mustn't confuse physiological and diagnostic importance, however. They are very different things.

Moncada: We have suggested that the lungs play an important role in controlling platelet aggregability. My question to the lung specialists and clinicians is whether there is any pathological condition affecting the lung in which haemostatic changes are found. What is known about chronic lung pathology and atherosclerosis or thrombosis?

Said: One example is acute pulmonary embolism, where platelets are sequestered in the lung. Another is the group of conditions that lead to the adult respiratory distress syndrome, a disease similar to 'hyaline membrane disease' (respiratory distress syndrome) of the newborn. In this disorder we often see disturbances of clotting and of fibrinolysis, a syndrome called disseminated intravascular coagulation (Hopewell & Murray 1976, Colman et al 1979). We don't know which comes first, the coagulopathy or the lung lesion. They seem to happen at about the same time.

Stalcup: There are also early pathological changes in hyperoxic lung damage. Very soon (36–40 hours) after exposure to high oxygen tensions platelets are trapped in the lung and thereafter, with exposure of collagen, there is activation of coagulation proteases. Altered noradrenaline uptake is found in these lungs as early as 12 hours.

Said: Within 24 hours in that sort of experiment there is evidence of pulmonary oedema, so that we don't know which comes first, the aggregation of platelets or the injury to pulmonary endothelium.

Reid: In adult respiratory failure (also called the 'shock lung') there is probably even earlier damage. In the animal models there is probably platelet change within the first half hour, so this is likely to be important. Some of those patients who survive go on to develop pulmonary hypertension. Factor VIII is increased in many of these patients and its complexes show an abnormal pattern of migration in cross-immunoelectrophoresis (A.C.A. Carvalho et al, unpublished observations).

Herbaczyńska-Cedro: A platelet abnormality known to occur in lung pathology is shortened survival time, observed in hypoxaemic patients with chronic obstructive airway disease (Steele et al 1977). Platelet survival time increases when oxygen is given to such patients (Johnson et al 1978). Although the cause of this platelet abnormality is not clear, changes in platelet reactivity and/or endothelial injury produced by hypoxaemia were suggested as a possible explanation.

Reid: Professor Said rightly pointed out that it would be valuable to develop diagnostic tests for various lung diseases. One reason why our tests seem so insensitive is the enormous 'reserve' of the lung. In animal models of severe acute oedema our colleagues have followed the rate of destruction of $PGF_{2\alpha}$ as a test of lung function. They found no impairment (Kong et al 1980). In certain cases of chronic pulmonary hypertension, however, there is such severe loss of the lung's peripheral vascular bed that there is probably an order of magnitude difference in the damage to the lung's microcirculation. In some of these, carbon monoxide diffusion is greatly reduced (Meyrick et al 1974).

Junod: Is there really any one biochemical marker of lung function? I suspect there is not: there are 40 different cell types in the lung and it is not surprising that it is so difficult to relate lung function to one parameter, whether cyclic AMP, cyclic GMP, or anything else.

Secondly, I don't believe that one has to justify research on a particular biological phenomenon because it might turn out to be clinically important. I am not sure that some of the phenomena studied in the past and discussed here have any clinical relevance. If you take 5-HT uptake by the lung, for example, there is no evidence that this is a physiologically important process. But the fact that 5-HT is taken up by the lung, and by endothelial cells in particular, has been used by other investigators to study the functional state of the pulmonary endothelium in animals (Block & Fisher 1977). It may well be that in a few years clinicians will be able to use this property to assess the functional integrity of human lung endothelium when it is exposed to hyperoxia, to drugs and to various pathological conditions. An application of the research being done now may be found only years later.

Vane: I am a strong advocate of relatively unstructured basic research. After all, if we hadn't been studying the prostaglandins in general we should not have discovered prostacyclin.

Bakhle: I would point out that some attempts *have* been made to extend basic research results on lung metabolism to specific clinical uses. One of the difficulties is the lack of animal models for human lung disorders. There is no good animal model of asthma to study, for example. Two groups have looked at oxygen toxicity in rats and shown that 5-HT metabolism is decreased. This has been suggested as an 'early warning' of oxygen toxicity (Block & Fisher 1977). However, we found that prostaglandin E_2 metabolism was affected earlier, after a shorter exposure to oxygen, than 5-HT metabolism (Toivonen et al 1980). I offered this biochemical change as a marker of early oxygen toxicity at a meeting of respiratory clinicians but they said they didn't need it because they already knew by experience when to stop the oxygen treatment! It is also known that gaseous anaesthetics can change the metabolism of amines (Naito & Gillis 1973, Bakhle & Block 1976); exposing rats to tobacco smoke also changes the metabolism of angiotensin I and prostaglandin E_2 (Bakhle et al 1979). It is important to realize that attempts are being made to relate basic physiological research to pathological conditions and to discover a biochemical marker to alert the clinician *before* physical variables such as gas exchange or compliance are disturbed.

Vane: It would be very useful to have assay kits for measuring prostacyclin levels; they could well be diagnostic of cardiovascular diseases.

Stubbs: One problem in studying the hormonal function of the lung is that unlike the pancreas you can't remove it and see what happens to the hormones!

Professor Reid said earlier (p 50) that the response to a disease may become the disease itself. This could be an important concept for lung disease. I would like to know whether the metabolic abnormalities in my patients with chronic lung disease are further damaging the lung. I would also like to know whether in shock lung a vicious cycle develops, with the release of pulmonary peptides and amines producing further lung damage through vascular or metabolic effects. This concept is important because we may be able to break into the cycle at some point and treat the patient.

Stalcup: Along the line of the clinical applicability of non-respiratory functions of the lung, we started our emphysema experiments looking for a marker for decreased vascular surface area. We thought that angiotensin conversion might be a way of assessing vascular surface. We found that decreased angiotensin conversion was a good reflection of inhomogeneities of ventilation. It then occurred to us that if decreased angiotensin conversion reflected lung disease, to the extent that it produced regional hypoxia, there should be abnormalities in blood pressure. It was only at that point that we searched the literature and found that about every 10 years since the 1930s someone discovers that patients with lung disease have lower blood pressures than age-matched controls and that this is correlated to the extent of their disease. Patients with chronic obstructive pulmonary disease also have reduced blood pressures, also correlating with the extent of the disease and (in some hands) with the degree of inhomogeneity of ventilation. Heistad et al (1971) have shown that the reflex circulatory responses to hypotension are impaired in chronically hypoxic men because of obstructive pulmonary disease. There is in fact a large literature suggesting that the lung has a major role in regulating blood pressure and that loss of vascular surface, or inhomogeneities of ventilation, or both, have a direct clinical correlation in the regulation of blood pressure in people with chronic lung disease. So we can say that in this instance very basic physiological studies have led to advances in our understanding of pulmonary disease.

SUMMING-UP

Alberti: We have reached the end of a remarkable three days. On Tuesday morning several diverse groups of individuals sat down to discuss the metabolic functions of the lung. It was immediately obvious that the simple phrase 'metabolic activities' meant very different things to different people. To me it meant intermediary metabolism and energy production; to others it meant arachidonic acid, prostaglandins and prostacyclin, or alternatively the metabolism of peptides such as angiotensin and bradykinin. One group considered it to mean phospholipid metabolism and surfactant production, while Frank Woods, for instance, looks on the lung as an alternative site for drug metabolism.

If nothing else has been achieved, I hope that all of us in our various corners now realize that the title of the symposium encompasses *all* these aspects – that all are relevant, that all are exciting and, most important, that all are interrelated. In my own sphere we have already started to examine the effects of VIP, with the help of Dr Said, on glucose metabolism – and effects are there.

We shall now do the same for the prostaglandin family. I hope that others of you will now examine the effects of change in energy status, such as the fed state and the fasting state, on, for example, prostacyclin production or converting enzyme activity.

We have certainly all learned a great deal, but what specific conclusions can we draw and what are the important areas where we still need answers? It might be easiest to assess this if we return to the substance of the programme together with the questions that John Vane posed at the beginning of the symposium. I shall not attempt to cover all areas, but will concentrate on certain highlights.

We began with a crystal-clear exposition on the morphology of the lung, which immediately stressed one of our major problems. We are dealing with about 40 cell types and are faced with Dr Vane's first question: is the metabolic function of the lung related purely to the endothelial cell? I do not feel that we yet have a clear answer to this question. We have a reasonable idea of the site of production of surfactant, of the distribution of converting enzyme and of the disposition, as shown by Dr Said, of VIP. But I am still unclear about the precise localization of arachidonic acid metabolism; does it occur in the non-endothelial cells? And where are the insulin and other endocrine receptors, so well described by Dr Morishige and Dr Ballard, located and which of all these cells are the main sites of regulation of energy metabolism?

Again, we have had elegant presentations on hypoxia and its morphological and biochemical sequelae. Having established the effects we now need to establish the underlying mechanisms.

Another major and practical paper came on the methods used to study lung. What emerged from this and the discussion is that we have two sets of models: bad ones and worse ones! The perfused lung, appropriately cannulated whole animals, and isolated cells came through as the better of the available models, but it must be obvious that having a hyperoxic lung suspended in air gently dripping may not be a true reflection of physiology. For the time being I feel that we should be cross-checking our results in alternative models, and attempting to confirm our results in the whole animal, or man, before drawing final conclusions. This point was brought out well by Dr Bakhle in his studies of amine metabolism in homogenates and in whole cells, where he showed that uptake and not metabolism was the rate-limiting step.

From methodology we moved into the area of energy metabolism. Several important questions emerged to which answers are lacking. First, how much of the energy needs of the cell are met by glycolysis? Estimates vary from 30 to 100%, depending on the preparation and conditions. What role do alternative substrates have? I would also like to know the precise energy requirements for surfactant production, arachidonic acid metabolism and synthetic processes such as mucus production, the latter being a topic that has not been discussed here. The final major unanswered question on intermediary metabolism is what role the lung has in whole-body metabolism. We have heard plenty of speculative comments, but no facts.

Dr Vane's second question was: is there only one converting enzyme for bradykinin? A clear answer of 'no' has come through, primarily from Dr Bakhle. At the same time we have had a useful review of peptides and amines which are and are not metabolized by the lung. The physiological relevance of these observations now needs to be sorted out.

This leads into Dr Vane's next and, for me, most important question. Is the liberation of substances by the lung 'overspill', or 'purposeful', or 'stress related'? In other words, is the lung a real endocrine gland – or an accidental one? Dr Vane summarized the early work in this area, mostly done in his laboratory or at his prompting, which showed that in certain states many substances, such as histamine, bradykinin, prostaglandins, prostacyclin, and SRS-A can be released into the pulmonary circulation. I do not think, however, that we have a clear clean answer to his question, apart from angiotensin, and we need one.

Ryszard Gryglewski showed us beautiful data on the release of prostacyclin by the lung and how it may be increased, but is lung-derived prostacyclin important in preventing platelet aggregation in small distal blood vessels of the body? I remain sceptical, not about prostacyclin itself but about lung-derived prostacyclin. In contrast, as Dr Collier suggested, I am sure that the answer is positive to the question of whether prostacyclin is important in breaking up platelet clumps within the lung itself.

One important outcome of the symposium has been a clarification for many of us of the normal pathway of arachidonic acid metabolism, although again I feel we are short of information on the quantitative aspects of the pathway in health and disease. We heard impressive data from Dr Piper on the nature of at least one form of SRS; and a highlight for the novice in the field was Rod Flower's description of his steroid-induced protein inhibitor of phospholipase A_2, which prevents the provision of phospholipid-derived arachidonic acid for the prostaglandin biosynthetic pathway. The importance of this in understanding the mechanism whereby steroids reverse or prevent asthma is obvious. We have also had clearly expressed the manifold actions of different prostanoids on different aspects of lung function, with hints on mechanisms beginning to emerge.

Another major theme has been the role of the lung as a source of converting enzyme. The overriding importance of the lung has been established, but the presence of this enzyme in other sites is also well known. The logical construction of an inhibitor which is now in clinical use should be a strong pointer to other possible innovations in this whole area.

Finally, we moved to the fetus and newborn with encyclopaedic documentation of changes in the important peptides, and interesting data on the effects of hypoxia, particularly on converting enzyme. The possible interplay with prostacyclins and with the marked changes in fuel homeostasis that occur here will be of interest in the future. The role of prostaglandins and prostacyclins in the maturation of the fetal lung is also ripe for further attack. We have heard about the interrelations of steroids and triiodothyronine in surfactant production but, as Dr Ballard showed, there are myriad possible substances affecting surfactant biosynthesis, and much hard work and knowledge is still needed in this area.

In summary, I feel that much has been gained in the past three days by the fusing of disciplines and the blurring of boundaries. Perhaps we should not forget some of the other functions of the lung; it *is* a pair of bellows; it *is* a critical regulator of acid-base homeostasis; it *is* a massive synthesizer of glycoprotein. Eventually, perhaps, we shall develop an integrated picture of the field and be able to apply our knowledge to clinical situations.

Finally, we should thank John Vane, not only for spawning many of the participants and for fathering (theoretically at least) a large part of the field, but also for his magnificent chairmanship. He has guided the meeting gently but firmly, so that a coherent whole has emerged. To him, and to Ruth Porter, we are deeply indebted.

References

Ashwell G, Morell AG 1974 The role of surface carbohydrates in the hepatic recognition and transport of circulating glycoproteins. Adv Enzymol Relat Areas Mol Biol 41:91-128

Bakhle YS, Block AJ 1976 Effects of halothane on pulmonary inactivation of noradrenaline and prostaglandin E_2 in anaesthetized dogs. Clin Sci Mol Med 50:87-90

Bakhle YS, Hartiala J, Toivonen H, Uotila P 1979 Effects of cigarette smoke on the metabolism of vasoactive hormones in rat isolated lungs. Br J Pharmacol 65:495-500

Block ER, Fisher AB 1977 Depression of serotonin clearance by rat lungs during oxygen exposure. J Appl Physiol 42:33-38

Cohen MD, Raeburn JA, Devine J, Kirkwood J, Elliott B, Cockburn F, Forfar JO 1975 Pharmacology of some oral penicillins in the newborn infant. Arch Dis Child 50:230-234

Colman RW, Robboy SJ, Minna JD 1979 Disseminated intravascular coagulation: a reappraisal. Annu Rev Med 30:359-374

Cumming JF 1976 The effect of arterial oxygen tension on antipyrine half-time in plasma. Clin Pharmacol Ther 19:468-471

du Souich P, McLean AJ, Lalka D, Erill S, Gibaldi M 1978 Pulmonary disease and drug kinetics. Clin Pharmacokinet 3:257-266

Gundersen HJG, Christensen NJ 1977 Intravenous insulin causing loss of intravascular water and albumin and increased adrenergic nervous activity in diabetics. Diabetes 26:551-557
Hargreave FE 1965 Digitalis and cor pulmonale. Br Med J 2:943
Heistad DD, Abboud FM, Mark AL, Schmid PG 1971 Impaired reflex vasoconstriction in chronically hypoxemic patients. J Clin Invest 51:331-337
Hopewell PC, Murray JF 1976 The adult respiratory distress syndrome. Annu Rev Med 27:343-356
Hüttner I, Badonnel M-C, Elemer G, Gabbiani G 1979 Aortic intima of the rat in various phases of hypertension. Exp Mol Pathol 31:191-200
Johnson TS, Ellis JH, Steele P 1978 Improvement of platelet survival time with oxygen in patients with chronic obstructive airway disease. Am Rev Respir Dis 117:255-257
Junod AF 1976 Uptake, release and metabolism of drugs in the lungs. Pharmacol Ther B 2:511-521
King RJ, Clements JA 1972 Surface active materials from dog lung. I. Method of isolation. Am J Physiol 223:707-714
Kong DL, Watkins WD, Zapol WM, Peterson MB 1980 Effects of hypoxemia and acute lung injury on transpulmonary metabolism of prostaglandin $F_{2\alpha}$ in anesthetized sheep. Fed Proc 39:765 (abstr 2625)
Majno G, Palade GE 1961 Studies on inflammation. 1. The effect of histamine and serotonin on vascular permeability: an electron microscopic study. J Biophys Biochem Cytol 11:571-606
Majno G, Palade GE, Schoefl GI 1961 Studies on inflammation. 2. The site of action of histamine and serotonin along the vascular tree: a topographical study. J Biophys Biochem Cytol 11:607-626
Meyrick B, Clarke SW, Symons C, Woodgate DJ, Reid L 1974 Primary pulmonary hypertension. A case report including electron microscopic study. Br J Dis Chest 68:11-20
Naito H, Gillis CN 1973 Effects of halothane and nitrous oxide on removal of noradrenaline from the pulmonary circulation. Anesthesiology 39:575-580
Østerby R, Gundersen HJG, Christensen NJ 1977 The acute effect of insulin on function and morphology of capillaries in diabetics and in rats with experimental diabetes. Diabetologia 13:423
Roth RA, Wiersma DA 1979 Role of the lung in total body clearance of circulating drugs. Clin Pharmacokinet 4:355-367
Simionescu M 1979 Structural and functional differentiation of microvascular endothelium. In: Blood cells and vessel walls: functional interactions. Excerpta Medica, Amsterdam (Ciba Found Symp 71), p 39-50
Simionescu N 1978 The microvascular endothelium: segmental differentiations; transcytosis; selective distribution of anionic sites. In: Weissmann G (ed) Advances in inflammation research. Raven Press, New York, vol 1:61-70
Sotaniemi E, Arvela P, Huhti E, Koivisto O 1971 Half-life of tolbutamide in patients with chronic respiratory failure. Eur J Clin Pharmacol 4:29-31
Staub NC 1971 Steady state pulmonary transvascular water filtration in unanesthetized sheep. Circ Res 28:suppl 1:35-39
Steele P, Ellis JH Jr, Weily HS, Genton E 1977 Platelet survival time in patients with hypoxemia and pulmonary hypertension. Circulation 55:660-662
Toivonen H, Hartiala J, Bakhle YS 1980 Effects of high oxygen tension on the metabolism of vasoactive hormones in isolated perfused rat lung. Acta Physiol Scand, in press
Warren MF, Drinker CK 1942 The flow of lymph from the lungs of the dog. Am J Physiol 136:207-221
Wood PJ, Marks V 1978 Direct measurement of cGMP in blood plasma and urine by radioimmunoassay. Ann Clin Biochem 15:25-30
Yalow RS 1979 Big ACTH and bronchogenic carcinoma. Annu Rev Med 30:241-248

Index of contributors

Entries in **bold** *type indicate papers; other entries refer to discussion contributions*

Indexes compiled by William Hill

Subject index